Clinical Assessment and Treatment of Fractures

Clinical Assessment and Treatment of Fractures

Editor: Brandon Gomez

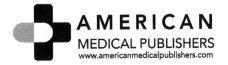

AMERICAN
MEDICAL PUBLISHERS
www.americanmedicalpublishers.com

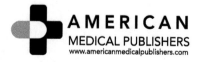

Cataloging-in-Publication Data

Clinical assessment and treatment of fractures / edited by Brandon Gomez.
    p. cm.
Includes bibliographical references and index.
ISBN 978-1-63927-990-6
    1. Fractures. 2. Fractures--Diagnosis. 3. Fractures--Treatment. 4. Bones--Wounds and injuries. I. Gomez, Brandon.
RD101 .C55 2023
617.15--dc23

American Medical Publishers,
41 Flatbush Avenue,
1st Floor, New York,
NY 11217, USA

ISBN 978-1-63927-990-6 (Hardback)

Contents

Preface

A fracture refers to a break in a bone, which can happen due to injuries, falls or car accidents. The common symptoms of a fracture are intense pain, deformity, swelling, bruising, or tenderness around the injury, difficulty in moving a limb, inability to move the affected part, and numbness. There are various types of fractures including avulsion fracture, comminuted fracture, fracture dislocation, hairline fracture, oblique fracture, and pathological fracture. The diagnosis involves physical examination and diagnostic tests like bone scan, X-ray, MRI and CT scan. The treatment of fractures involves covering the fractures with a hard protection such as a cast or splint. In some cases, the method of traction is used for aligning the bone that promotes the healing process. This method involves the use of pulleys and weights to stretch the muscles and tendons around the broken bone. Surgery is also a treatment option for severe cases of fractures. This book outlines the clinical assessment and treatment of fractures in detail. It presents researches and studies performed by experts across the globe. Researchers and students in this field will be assisted by this book.

Various studies have approached the subject by analyzing it with a single perspective, but the present book provides diverse methodologies and techniques to address this field. This book contains theories and applications needed for understanding the subject from different perspectives. The aim is to keep the readers informed about the progresses in the field; therefore, the contributions were carefully examined to compile novel researches by specialists from across the globe.

Indeed, the job of the editor is the most crucial and challenging in compiling all chapters into a single book. In the end, I would extend my sincere thanks to the chapter authors for their profound work. I am also thankful for the support provided by my family and colleagues during the compilation of this book.

Editor

Total Hip Arthroplasty for Bilateral Femoral Neck Stress Fracture

Kevin Moerenhout ⊚,[1,2] Georgios Gkagkalis,[1] G.-Yves Laflamme,[1] Dominique M. Rouleau,[1] Stéphane Leduc,[1] and Benoit Benoit[1]

[1]*Orthopedic Surgery, Department of Surgery, Hôpital Sacré-Cœur de Montréal, 5400 Boul. Gouin O., Montréal, Québec H4J 1C5, Canada*
[2]*Department of Orthopaedics and Traumatology, Lausanne University Hospital, Rue du Bugnon 46, CH-1011 Lausanne, Switzerland*

Correspondence should be addressed to Kevin Moerenhout; kevin.moerenhout@chuv.ch

Academic Editor: Benjamin Blondel

Femoral neck stress fractures (FNSFs) can be treated conservatively or surgically, depending on initial displacement and patient condition. Surgical treatment options include internal fixation, with or without valgus osteotomy or hip arthroplasty, either hemi or total. The latter is mainly considered when initial treatment fails. A review of the literature shows that total hip arthroplasty (THA) is only considered as primary treatment in displaced fractures (type 3) in low-demand patients. We present a case of successive bilateral FNSF in a young active patient, where a THA was performed on one side, after failed internal fixation, and where it was chosen as primary treatment on the other side after failed conservative treatment.

1. Introduction

Stress fractures are infrequent lesions due to overloading and/or repetitive overuse and can occur at several sites, with the more common being the metatarsals, femoral/tibial shaft, and femoral neck. They can be subcategorized into insufficiency fractures when an abnormal bone fractures under normal stresses and into fatigue fractures when a normal bone fractures under abnormal stresses [1]. The physiopathologic substrate is the combination of an imbalance between bone remodeling capacity and repetitive stress. Endocrine, metabolic, and pharmacologic causes have been described.

Femoral neck stress fractures (FNSFs) represent 5% of all stress fractures in the general population and are encountered more often, up to 15%, in athletes [1]. More specifically, it is seen in long-distance runners and can be associated with the "female athlete triad" [2, 3]. In nondisplaced incomplete femoral stress fractures, treatment is nonoperative with non-weight-bearing and activity cessation. In complete fractures, or when conservative treatment fails, internal fixation by percutaneous screw fixation or dynamic hip screw (DHS) is applied. Other treatment possibilities are intertrochanteric osteotomy or hip arthroplasty, either hemi or total (THA). The latter is mainly reserved as a salvage option in cases where previous surgical treatment has failed. We present the case of a young patient who presented with femoral neck stress fractures on both sides within a two-year span. THA has been chosen as a salvage procedure after nonunion following internal fixation on one side and as the primary surgical treatment on the other side.

2. Case Report

A 46-year-old female patient, who used to run three times a week (20 km/week), presented to our outpatient clinic in 2016 with right groin pain, which had begun a few days before without trauma. She was under treatment for multiple sclerosis since 2002, taking teriflunomide daily. Initial X-rays

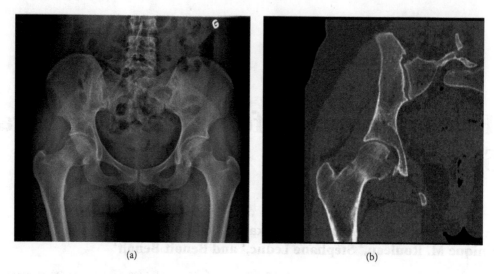

FIGURE 1: (a) AP pelvic X-ray showing a stress fracture of the right femoral neck. (b) Frontal view on CT scan of the right hip confirming the femoral neck fracture.

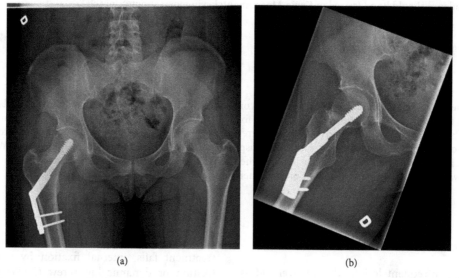

FIGURE 2: (a) AP pelvic X-ray and (b) lateral view of the right hip after dynamic hip screw (DHS), 6 weeks after surgery. The implant is in good position.

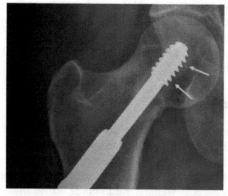

FIGURE 3: Right hip X-ray showing mobility around the DHS (arrows) and a fracture line on the compression side.

showed a dense line in the femoral neck, with lateral cortex disruption on the tension side. A stress fracture was suspected and confirmed on CT scan (Figures 1(a) and 1(b)). The patient underwent internal fixation by DHS with a good radiographic result (Figure 2). However, groin pain was still present after 1 year, disabling all sports activity. X-rays were taken, showing radiolucency around the cervicocephalic screw, probably due to interfragmentary mobility, and signs of nonunion, mainly on the compression side (Figure 3). A THA using a cementless stem and a press-fit cup (AMIS/Versafit, Medacta®, Switzerland) with ceramic on ceramic bearing was performed (Figure 4), without complications. Pathological exam of the retrieved femoral head showed avascular necrosis.

Two years later, aged 48 years, the patient returned because of pain in her left groin, with no traumatic event

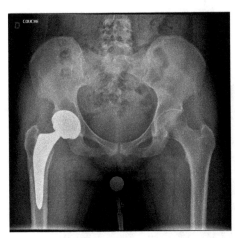

FIGURE 4: AP pelvic X-ray 6 weeks after right noncemented THA.

present in the previous days. Initial X-rays and CT scan were normal. Due to the history of the patient, non-weight-bearing was applied and an MRI was taken. This MRI showed bone marrow edema of the left hip on the compression side. Follow-up X-rays showed a minimally displaced femoral neck fracture of the left hip (Figure 5).

Blood samples and metabolic analysis (vitamin D, Ca, P, TSH, PTH, and VIH) were normal. Body mass index was normal, and "female athlete triad" syndrome was excluded as there were no menstrual abnormalities. Osteoporosis was excluded by DEXA scan. Four months of nonoperative treatment with non-weight-bearing protocol found the patient still in pain. X-rays confirmed a nondisplaced complete fracture of the femoral neck. After discussion with the patient, we opted for primary THA (Figure 6). The same combination of implants as the contralateral side was used. The patient was discharged from hospital one day after surgery with no adverse events, with a Harris Hip Score (HHS) of 94 and a Hip disability and Osteoarthritis Outcome Score (HOOS) of 85.6 for her left hip at 5 months postoperatively. HHS and HOOS were, respectively, 99.9 and 94.6 for her right hip at two years after surgery. The patient regained walking activity without support four weeks after surgery but has yet to regain all previous sports activity.

3. Review of the Literature

A medical literature search was performed in MEDLINE (PubMed) database. The keywords used were bilateral, femoral, neck, stress, fatigue, and fractures. Only papers published in English were considered. Radiology papers as well as papers with fractures due to trauma or located elsewhere than the femoral neck were rejected. Three case series and 36 case reports matched the search criteria and were retained for review.

Bilateral FNSFs are only described in case reports or minor case series, with various management and failure rates (Table 1). Miller has reported the first documented case of bilateral FNSF in the literature in 1950 [4]. Cases of bilateral femoral neck fractures, even simultaneous, have been reported in healthy military recruits [5–9] as well as in healthy

nonathletes [10, 11]. Insufficiency or fatigue bilateral fractures of the femoral neck have been described in various conditions such as pregnancy [12]; bone metabolic diseases, caused by osteomalacia associated with coxa vara [13] or by celiac disease [14]; vitamin D deficiency [15]; and rare genetic syndromes like Marfan [16] and autosomal dominant osteopetrosis [17]. Other more common risk factors, such as steroid treatment [18, 19] and anorexia nervosa [20], have also been involved in cases of bilateral insufficiency femoral neck fractures. Bilateral FNSF has also been described as a very rare complication following simultaneous bilateral total knee arthroplasty [21].

Among the 46 patients with bilateral FNSF found in the literature, 23 were male and 23 were female, with a mean age of 35 years. Fifty-six percent were on compression, 18% were on the tensile side, and 26% were displaced. Twenty-three percent were treated conservatively; 56% were treated by internal fixation; 12% had an osteotomy; and eight (9%) out of 92 patients had a prosthetic implant, among them only two had a total hip replacement. Failure rate for internal fixation was 11.5%. Internal fixation methods used in those cases were screws in four patients and gamma nails in one patient, bilaterally. Two (10%) of the 21 patients with conservative treatment were eventually operated, with screws in one case and hemiarthroplasty in the other. One patient went on being treated conservatively using bisphosphonates, although the femoral neck fracture on one side was still visible in the X-rays at 24 months of follow-up postinternal fixation [22]. Failure rate for conservative treatment was three (14%) out of 21 patients.

No complications were recorded with the osteotomy treatment in those series nor with the prosthetic implants. Follow-up was inconsistent, ranging from 2 weeks to 15 years. No quality of life questionnaire or other outcome measuring score was reported in any of the case reports.

4. Discussion

Different classifications exist regarding FNSF. Fullerton and Snowdy proposed a classification of FNSF in three types, based on biomechanics and degree of displacement: type 1 is a compression-sided fracture; type 2 is a tension-sided fracture; and type 3 is a displaced fracture [23]. If fracture lines are less than 50% of the neck, treatment of femoral neck stress fractures is nonoperative, consisting of non-weight-bearing and activity cessation. If compression or tension-sided fractures have fracture lines greater than 50% of the neck, percutaneous screw fixation must be strongly considered [23]. Type 2 stress fractures, as found in the right hip of our patient, often heal poorly and therefore require treatment that is more aggressive in order to avoid malunion, nonunion, or osteonecrosis, leading to hip osteoarthritis [24]. After nonunion following DHS on the right hip, we opted for THA. Other treatment options, such as valgus intertrochanteric osteotomy with DHS or blade plate fixation in order to compress and stabilize the stress fracture by converting shear forces to compressive ones, have been described with variable failure rates [25, 26]. Valgus intertrochanteric osteotomy permits a more horizontal

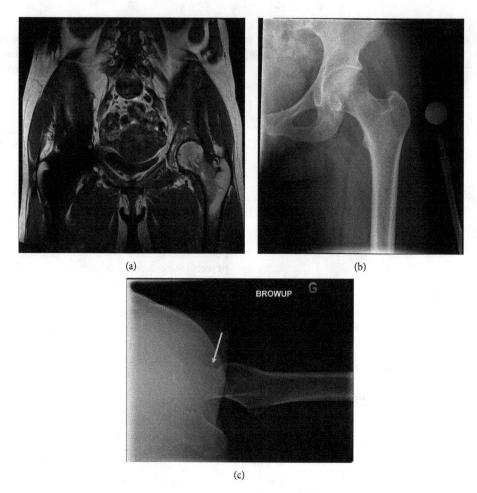

(a)

(b)

(c)

FIGURE 5: (a) Pelvic MRI showing bone marrow edema of the left hip on the compression side. (b) AP and (c) profile follow-up X-ray of the left hip showing a minimally displaced complete femoral neck fracture (arrow).

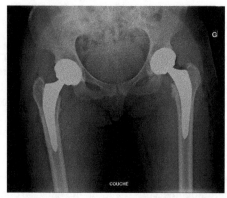

FIGURE 6: Postoperative pelvic X-ray after left total hip arthroplasty and three years after right total hip arthroplasty. Implants are in good position.

reorientation of the stress fracture line by subtracting a wedge on the lateral femur (Figure 7). THA has given good results and more predictable failure rates.

We opted for primary THA on the patient's left hip once conservative treatment failed. This treatment option can be disputed. As the second femoral neck stress fracture was on the compression side, it would have had more healing potential than the contralateral tension-sided stress fracture. These two fractures are therefore not comparable in outcome. Although valgus intertrochanteric osteotomy was a valid therapeutic option age wise, we believed it presented a potential failure risk, resulting from avascular necrosis of the femoral head, given that this was the pathological finding on the contralateral side. In such a case, we would have been confronted with a more complicated primary THA requiring the extraction of material and a hip with altered biomechanics from the valgus orientation of the proximal femur. This was explained to the patient, but she refused to go through the same process with the risk of a potential failed internal fixation and preferred the option of THA. Another reason for her decision is that, as an independent worker, she needed to get rapidly back to work. Taking a longer leave of absence from work was no longer an option for her.

This case highlights the potential of primary THA in femoral neck stress fractures. We found only one case of bilateral femoral neck stress fractures treated by THA in the literature, but this case reported on a debilitated cerebral palsy patient [27]. To the best of our knowledge, this case is the first to report on a young active patient treated by THA for bilateral femoral neck stress fractures. Although this

TABLE 1: Case series of bilateral femoral neck fractures with their treatment, failure rates, and follow-up duration.

Author	Tensile/ compressive	Treatment	Failure/ treatment	Follow-up	Patient age/sex
Naik et al.					
Case 1	L: n.a.; R: 1	L: OS screw; R: OT	L: HA	28 m	38 M
Case 2	L: 1; R: 3	L: OS screw; R: OT	No	12 m	38 F
Case 3	L: 3; R: 1	L: OT; R: OT	No	6 m	48 F
Case 4	L: 2; R: 3	L: OT; R: OT	No	7 y	40 F
Selek et al.					
Case 1	L: n.a.; R: n.a.	L: OS screws; R: OS screws	No	4 y	30 F
Case 2	L: n.a.; R: n.a.	L: OS screws; R: OS screws	No	28 m	35 F
Case 3	L: n.a.; R: n.a.	L: OS screws; R: OS screws	No	2 y	30 F
Moo et al.					
Case 1	L: 2; R: 1	L: OS screws; R: cons	No	28 m	19 M
Case 2	L: 1; R: 3	L: cons; R: OS screws	No	4 m	18 M
Case 3	L: n.a.; R: 2	L: OS screws; R: OS screws	No	24 m	20 M
Cakmak et al.	L: 2; R: 3	L: OS screws; R: HA	No	18 m	82 F
Nagao et al.	L: 2; R: 3	L: OS screws; R: cons	L: HA; R: HA	24 m	36 M
Hernigou et al.	L: 1; R: 1	L: OS DHS; R: OS DHS	No	2 w	38 F
Vaishya et al.	L: 1; R: 1	L: OS screws; R: OS screws	No data	No data	50 M
Santoso et al.	L: 1; R: 1	L: cons; R: cons	No	5 m	37 M
Oliveira et al.	L: 1; R: 1	L: OS; R: OS	No data	No data	43 M
Sariyilmaz et al.	L: 1; R: 1	L: VOT (blpl); R: VOT (blpl)	No	2 y	26 F
Baki et al.	L: 1; R: 1	L: OS screws; R: OS screws	No	6 m	22 F
Nemoto et al.	L: 1; R: 1	L: OS screws; R: OS screws	No	2 y	24 M
Webber et al.	L: 1; R: 1	L: OS screws; R: OS screws	No	No data	23 M
Wright et al.	L: 3; R: 3	L: OS screws; R: OS screws	No access to full article	No access	24 M
Bouchoucha et al.	L: 3; R: 2	L: VOT (blpl) R: OS (DHS)	No data	No data	15 F
Naranje et al.	L: 3; R: 2	L: OS screws; R: OS screws	No	12 m	34 M
Carpintero et al.	L: 2 ; R: 3	L: OS gamma; R: OS gamma	R: AVN L: AVN/THA	No data	32 M
Khadabadi et al.	L: n.a.; R: n.a.	L: OS DHS; R: OS DHS	No	12 m	25 M
Romero et al.	L: 2; R: 1	L: OS screws; R: OS screws	No	6 m	19 M
Chameseddine et al.	L: 3; R: 3	L: HA; R: HA	No	6 m	71 F
Pankaj et al.	L: 2; R: 3	R: HA; R: OS screws	No	±5 y	58 M
Haddad et al.	L: 3; R: n.a.	L: OS screws; R: OS screws	L: delayed union/conservative	4 m	56 F
Mariani et al.	L: 3; R: 3	L: THA; R: THA	No	24 m	24 M
Eberle et al.	L: 2; R: 1	L: cervical nail ("three-flanged nail"); R: cons	No	40 m	54 F
Zuckerman et al.	L: 1; R: 1	L: OS DHS; R: OS DHS	No	24 m	46 F
Voss et al.	L: 1; R: 1	L: cons; R: OS screws	R/L: nonunion	24 m	30 F
Bailie et al.	L: 1; R: 1	L: cons; R: cons	No	2 m	15 M
Annan et al.	L: n.a.; R: n.a.	L: DHS + VOT R: DHS + VOT	No	6 m	29 F
Ichikawa et al.	L: 2; R: 2	L: OS screws; R: OS screws			61 F
Chouhan et al.	L: 1; R: 1	L: cons; R: cons	No	6 m	32 M
Hootkani et al.	L: 3; R: 3	L: HA; R: HA	No	24 m	28 M
Scheerlinck et al.	L: 1; R: 1	L: cons; R: cons	L: displaced fracture after accidental fall/ OS by 2 screws	14 w	8 F
Kharazzi et al.	n.a.	L: OS pins; R: OS pins	No	15 y	22 M
Rengman	n.a.	L: cons; R: cons	No	No data	21 M
Vento et al.	n.a.	L: OS pins; R: OS pins & DHS	No data	No data	53 M
Miller	L: 1; R: 1	L: cons; R: cons	No	8 m	36 F
Slipman et al.	L: 1; R: 1	L: cons; R: cons	No data	No data	36 F
Kalaci et al.	L: 1; R: 1	L: OS screws; R: OS screws	No	6 w	18 F
Gurdezi et al.	L: 1; R: 1	L: cons; R: cons	No	12 m	61 F

TABLE 1: Continued.

Author	Tensile/ compressive	Treatment	Failure/ treatment	Follow-up	Patient age/sex
N total	Type 1: 41 (56%) Type 2: 13 (18%) Type 3: 19 (26%) Total known: 73 Total unknown: 21	% of prosthesis Cons: 21 (23%) OS: 52 (56%) OT: 11 (12%) Arthroplasty (6HA, 2THA): 8 (9%) Total known: 92 Total unknown: 2	% of failure 2 screws: HA 1 screw: delayed union 1 screw: nonunion 1 cons: nonunion 1 cons: HA 1 cons: OS 1 nail: AVN 1 nail: THA	Mean: 23, 4 m	Mean: 35 y Mean M: 30 y Mean F: 40 y

L: left hip; R: right hip; OS: osteosynthesis; HA: hemiarthroplasty; OT: osteotomy; cons: conservative treatment; DHS: dynamic hip screw; VOT: valgus osteotomy; blpl: blade plate; THA: total hip arthroplasty; NS: no score; AVN: avascular necrosis; Type 1: compression fracture; type 2: tension fracture; type 3: displaced fracture; n.a.: not available.

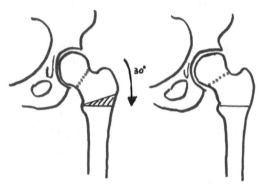

FIGURE 7: Valgus intertrochanteric osteotomy: by subtracting a 30° wedge on the lateral femur (black hatched), the vertical stress fracture (red hatched) on the left becomes 30° more horizontal on the right.

should not be the gold standard, it should be considered as a treatment option, especially in young high-demand patients who want to quickly regain unrestricted and painless mobility of their hips. Failure rate following internal fixation of femoral neck fractures in the nonelderly population has been reported as high as 59% [28]. Complications associated with treatment by internal fixation, such as avascular necrosis (12–86%), nonunion (10–59%), as well as early-onset hip osteoarthrosis, are avoided with the THA option [29]. Although all the risk factors associated with traumatic femoral neck fractures are well described in the literature, data about the incidence of these complications in femoral neck stress fractures are lacking. The incidence is dependent on the situation (tensile versus compression side), fracture line (complete versus partial), and initial displacement of the fracture. Potential complications associated with THA, such as infection or dislocation, must be considered and clearly explained to the patient. The incidence of infection and dislocation following THA for femoral neck fractures are probably the same as those in the general population, but we do not have the data to back this assumption. However, salvage THA after failed internal fixation of the neck fracture is associated with higher complication rates [30–32].

In cases of uni- or bilateral neck stress fractures, a metabolic and systemic assessment is mandatory in order to

rule out a metabolic cause favoring the stress fracture. Menstrual abnormalities and eating disorders must always be investigated when femoral neck stress fractures are present. In the present case, blood and metabolic workup were normal. The patient had no risk factor other than running three times a week, for a total of 20 km/week. Her treatment for multiple sclerosis is not known to be associated with bone metabolism and thus cannot be held responsible for playing a role in the pathogenesis of her stress fractures. Bazelier et al. found that multiple sclerosis itself is associated with an increased risk of osteoporotic fractures—especially hip fractures—mainly resulting from an increased risk of falls, particularly when taking glucocorticoids or antidepressants [33]. However, in our case, the patient sustained no fall, had a normal osteoporotic workup, and took no glucocorticoid or antidepressant medication.

5. Conclusion

Although internal fixation remains the gold standard in nondisplaced femoral neck stress fractures, femoral osteotomy and THA must be part of the treatment options. Total hip arthroplasty, especially with the advances in material technology, tribology, and surgical technique, has excellent clinical outcomes and high patient satisfaction rates, making it now a more interesting avenue for young and active patients. Thus, when it comes to femoral neck stress fractures, it should be considered in cases of failed internal fixation or in those cases not responding to conservative treatment.

Conflicts of Interest

Kevin Moerenhout was supported by the Edouard-Samson Scholarship Fund, Canada; the Fonds de bourse Swiss Orthopaedics, Switzerland; and Fonds de Perfectionnement du CHUV (Centre Hospitalier Universitaire Vaudois), Switzerland. Georgios Gkagkalis was supported by the Edouard-Samson Scholarship Fund, Canada; the Fond de bourses Swiss Orthopaedics, Switzerland; and the Fondation Profectus, Switzerland. G.-Yves Laflamme is a consultant for Stryker, and the institution (HSCM) has received funding for research and educational purposes from Arthrex, CONMED, Depuy, Linvatec, Medacta, Smith & Nephew, Stryker, Synthes, Tornier, Wright, and Zimmer Biomet. Dominique M. Rouleau is a consultant for Bioventus and Wright Medical. The institution (HSCM) has received funding for research and educational purposes from Arthrex, CONMED, Depuy, Linvatec, Medacta, Smith & Nephew, Stryker, Synthes, Tornier, Wright, and Zimmer Biomet. Stéphane Leduc is a consultant for Stryker, and the institution (HSCM) has received funding for research and educational purposes from Arthrex, CONMED, Depuy, Linvatec, Medacta, Smith & Nephew, Stryker, Synthes, Tornier, Wright, and Zimmer Biomet. Benoit Benoit is a consultant for Medacta, Stryker, and Bioventus. The institution (HSCM) has received funding for research and educational purposes from Arthrex, CONMED, Depuy, Linvatec, Medacta, Smith & Nephew, Stryker, Synthes, Tornier, Wright, and Zimmer Biomet.

Acknowledgments

The authors wish to thank Julie Fournier and Karine Tardif for research support as well as Kathleen Beaumont for manuscript review and preparation.

References

[1] D. S. Bailie and D. E. Lamprecht, "Bilateral femoral neck stress fractures in an adolescent male runner: a case report," *The American Journal of Sports Medicine*, vol. 29, no. 6, pp. 811–813, 2001.

[2] C. A. Moreira and J. P. Bilezikian, "Stress fractures: concepts and therapeutics," *The Journal of Clinical Endocrinology & Metabolism*, vol. 102, no. 2, pp. 525–534, 2017.

[3] G. Ducher, A. I. Turner, S. Kukuljan et al., "Obstacles in the optimization of bone health outcomes in the female athlete triad," *Sports Medicine*, vol. 41, no. 7, pp. 587–607, 2011.

[4] L. F. Miller, "Bilateral stress fracture of the neck of the femur; report of a case," *The Journal of Bone & Joint Surgery*, vol. 32, no. 3, pp. 695–697, 1950.

[5] B. J. Webber, W. E. Trueblood, J. N. Tchandja, S. P. Federinko, and T. L. Cropper, "Concurrent bilateral femoral neck stress fractures in a military recruit: a case report," *Military Medicine*, vol. 180, no. 1, pp. e134–e137, 2015.

[6] O. Nemoto, M. Kawaguchi, and T. Katou, "Simultaneous bilateral femoral neck stress fractures in a 24-year old male recruit: a case report," *West Indian Medical Journal*, vol. 62, no. 6, pp. 552–553, 2013.

[7] I. H. Moo, Y. H. Lee, K. K. Lim, and K. V. Mehta, "Bilateral femoral neck stress fractures in military recruits with unilateral hip pain," *Journal of the Royal Army Medical Corps*, vol. 162, no. 5, pp. 387–390, 2016.

[8] S. Naranje, N. Sezo, V. Trikha, R. Kancherla, L. Rijal, and R. Jha, "Simultaneous bilateral femoral neck stress fractures in a young military cadet: a rare case report," *European Journal of Orthopaedic Surgery & Traumatology*, vol. 22, no. 1, pp. 103–106, 2012.

[9] A. N. Romero and S. R. Kohart, "19-year-old male adolescent with bilateral femoral neck stress fractures: a case report," *Military Medicine*, vol. 173, no. 7, pp. 711–713, 2008.

[10] M. A. Naik, P. Sujir, S. K. Tripathy, S. Vijayan, S. Hameed, and S. K. Rao, "Bilateral stress fractures of femoral neck in non-

athletes: a report of four cases," *Chinese Journal of Traumatology*, vol. 16, no. 2, pp. 113–117, 2013.

[11] U. S. Oliveira, P. J. Labronici, A. João Neto, A. Y. Nishimi, R. E. Pires, and L. H. Silva, "Bilateral stress fracture of femoral neck in non-athlete-case report," *Revista Brasileira de Ortopedia*, vol. 51, no. 6, pp. 735–738, 2016.

[12] M. E. Baki, H. Uygun, B. Arı, and H. Aydın, "Bilateral femoral neck insufficiency fractures in pregnancy," *Joint Diseases and Related Surgery*, vol. 25, no. 1, pp. 60–62, 2014.

[13] K. Sariyilmaz, O. Ozkunt, M. Sungur, F. Dikici, and O. Yazicioglu, "Osteomalacia and coxa vara. An unusual coexistence for femoral neck stress fracture," *International Journal of Surgery Case Reports*, vol. 16, pp. 137–140, 2015.

[14] O. Selek, K. Memisoglu, and A. Selek, "Bilateral femoral neck fatigue fracture due to osteomalacia secondary to celiac disease: report of three cases," *Archives of Iranian Medicine*, vol. 18, no. 8, pp. 542–544, 2015.

[15] S. Nagao, K. Ito, and I. Nakamura, "Spontaneous bilateral femoral neck fractures associated with a low serum level of vitamin D in a young adult," *The Journal of Arthroplasty*, vol. 24, no. 2, pp. 322.e1–322.e4, 2009.

[16] F. D. Kharrazi, W. B. Rodgers, D. L. Coran, J. R. Kasser, and J. E. Hall, "Protrusio acetabuli and bilateral basicervical femoral neck fractures in a patient with Marfan syndrome," *The American Journal of Orthopedics*, vol. 26, no. 10, pp. 689–691, 1997.

[17] A. H. Krieg, B. M. Speth, H. Y. Won, and P. D. Brook, "Conservative management of bilateral femoral neck fractures in a child with autosomal dominant osteopetrosis," *Archives of Orthopaedic and Trauma Surgery*, vol. 127, no. 10, pp. 967–970, 2007.

[18] F. S. Haddad, P. N. Mohanna, and N. J. Goddard, "Bilateral femoral neck stress fractures following steroid treatment," *Injury*, vol. 28, no. 9-10, pp. 671–673, 1997.

[19] S. Gurdezi, R. K. Trehan, and M. Rickman, "Bilateral undisplaced insufficiency neck of femur fractures associated with short-term steroid use: a case report," *Journal of Medical Case Reports*, vol. 2, no. 1, p. 79, 2008.

[20] P. Carpintero, E. Lopez-Soroche, R. Carpintero, and R. Morales, "Bilateral insufficiency fracture of the femoral neck in a male patient with anorexia nervosa," *Acta Orthopaedica Belgica*, vol. 79, no. 1, pp. 111–113, 2013.

[21] S. Cakmak, M. Mahiroğulları, M. Kürklü, and C. Yıldız, "Bilateral femoral neck stress fracture following bilateral total knee arthroplasty: a case report," *Acta Orthopaedica et Traumatologica Turcica*, vol. 46, no. 4, pp. 312–315, 2012.

[22] L. Voss, M. DaSilva, and P. G. Trafton, "Bilateral femoral neck stress fractures in an amenorrheic athlete," *The American Journal of Orthopedics*, vol. 26, no. 11, pp. 789–792, 1997.

[23] L. R. Fullerton Jr., H. A. Snowdy, Femoral neck stress fractures," *The American Journal of Sports Medicine*, vol. 16, no. 4, pp. 365–377, 1988.

[24] A. Y. Shin and B. L. Gillingham, "Fatigue fractures of the femoral neck in athletes," *Journal of the American Academy of Orthopaedic Surgeons*, vol. 5, no. 6, pp. 293–302, 1997.

[25] J. Petrie, A. Sassoon, and G. J. Haidukewych, "When femoral fracture fixation fails: salvage options," *The Bone & Joint Journal*, vol. 95, no. 11, pp. 7–10, 2013.

[26] V. D. Varghese, A. Livingston, P. R. Boopalan, and T. S. Jepegnanam, "Valgus osteotomy for nonunion and neglected neck of femur fractures," *World Journal of Orthopedics*, vol. 7, no. 5, pp. 301–307, 2016.

[27] P. Mariani, M. Buttaro, F. Comba, E. Zanotti, P. Ali, and F. Piccaluga, "Bilateral simultaneous femoral neck fracture mimicking abdominal pain in a cerebral palsy patient," *Case

Reports in Orthopedics, vol. 2014, Article ID 925201, 4 pages, 2014.

[28] C. Rogmark, M. T. Kristensen, B. Viberg, S. S. Rönnquist, S. Overgaard, and H. Palm, "Hip fractures in the non-elderly-who, why and whither?," Injury, vol. 49, no. 8, pp. 1445–1450, 2018.

[29] S. Henari, M. Leonard, M. Hamadto, and D. Cogley, "Review of a single contemporary femoral neck fracture fixation method in young patients," Orthopedics, vol. 34, no. 3, p. 171, 2011.

[30] S. S. Mahmoud, E. O. Pearse, T. O. Smith, and C. B. Hing, "Outcomes of total hip arthroplasty, as a salvage procedure, following failed internal fixation of intracapsular fractures of the femoral neck: a systematic review and meta-analysis," The Bone & Joint Journal, vol. 98, no. 4, pp. 452–460, 2016.

[31] P. C. Krause, J. L. Braud, and J. M. Whatley, "Total hip arthroplasty after previous fracture surgery," Orthopedic Clinics of North America, vol. 46, no. 2, pp. 193–213, 2015.

[32] J. Jiang, C. H. Yang, Q. Lin, X. D. Yun, and Y. Y. Xia, "Does arthroplasty provide better outcomes than internal fixation at mid- and long-term followup? a meta-analysis," Clinical Orthopaedics and Related Research, vol. 473, no. 8, pp. 2672–2679, 2015.

[33] M. T. Bazelier, T. van Staa, B. M. Uitdehaag et al., "The risk of fracture in patients with multiple sclerosis: the UK general practice research database," Journal of Bone and Mineral Research, vol. 26, no. 9, pp. 2271–2279, 2011.

2

Prophylactic Topical Antibiotics in Fracture Repair and Spinal Fusion

Eric K. Kim ⓘ,[1] Claire A. Donnelley ⓘ,[2] Madeline Tiee,[1] Heather J. Roberts,[3] Ericka Von Kaeppler,[2] David Shearer,[3] and Saam Morshed ⓘ[3,4]

[1]University of California San Francisco, School of Medicine, San Francisco, California, USA
[2]Institute for Global Orthopaedics and Traumatology, Department of Orthopaedics, University of California, San Francisco, California, USA
[3]University of California San Francisco, Department of Orthopaedic Surgery, San Francisco, California, USA
[4]University of California San Francisco, Department of Epidemiology and Biostatistics, San Francisco, California, USA

Correspondence should be addressed to Saam Morshed; saam.morshed@ucsf.edu

Academic Editor: Benjamin Blondel

Introduction. The objective of this systematic review with meta-analysis is to determine whether prophylactic local antibiotics prevent surgical site infections (SSIs) in instrumented spinal fusions and traumatic fracture repair. A secondary objective is to investigate the effect of vancomycin, a common local antibiotic of choice, on the microbiology of SSIs. *Methods.* An electronic search of PubMed, EMBASE, and Web of Science databases and major orthopedic surgery conferences was conducted to identify studies that (1) were instrumented spinal fusions or fracture repair and (2) had a treatment group that received prophylactic local antibiotics. Both randomized controlled trials (RCTs) and comparative observational studies were included. Meta-analysis was performed separately for randomized and nonrandomized studies with subgroup analysis by study design and antibiotic. *Results.* Our review includes 44 articles (30 instrumented spinal fusions and 14 fracture repairs). Intrawound antibiotics significantly decreased the risk of developing SSIs in RCTs of fracture repair (RR 0.61, 95% CI: 0.40–0.93, $I^2 = 32.5\%$) but not RCTs of instrumented spinal fusion. Among observational studies, topical antibiotics significantly reduced the risk of SSIs in instrumented spinal fusions (OR 0.34, 95% CI: 0.27–0.43, $I^2 = 52.4\%$) and in fracture repair (OR 0.49, 95% CI: 0.37–0.65, $I^2 = 43.8\%$). Vancomycin powder decreased the risk of Gram-positive SSIs (OR 0.37, 95% CI: 0.27–0.51, $I^2 = 0.0\%$) and had no effect on Gram-negative SSIs (OR 0.95, 95% CI: 0.62–1.44, $I^2 = 0.0\%$). *Conclusions.* Prophylactic intrawound antibiotic administration decreases the risk of SSIs in fracture surgical fixation in randomized studies. Therapeutic efficacy in instrumented spinal fusion was seen in only nonrandomized studies. Vancomycin appears to be an effective agent against Gram-positive pathogens. There is no evidence that local vancomycin powder is associated with an increased risk for Gram-negative infection.

1. Introduction

Surgical site infections (SSIs) are a significant source of morbidity and cost for patients undergoing orthopedic procedures. SSIs are challenging to treat because of the potential formation of a bacterial biofilm, an extracellular matrix that can attach to implants and protect pathogens from host immunity and systemic antibiotics [1]. Both instrumented spinal procedures and fracture surgeries have in common the use of metallic hardware, and each suffer from a nontrivial rate of SSIs, ranging from 9.4% of noninstrumented spinal trauma cases [2] to over 30% in lower extremity fracture cases [3, 4]. SSIs lead to delayed healing, nonunion, irreversible loss of function, or amputation of the infected limb [3, 4].

The current standard of care for SSI prevention is systemic antibiotics [5, 6]. However, parenterally administered antibiotics have the disadvantages of delivering a reduced concentration of antibiotics to the targeted site, failing to reach poorly vascularized tissues, and potentially causing systemic toxicity. Alternatively, locally delivered antibiotics can achieve a high local concentration with low systemic levels, thereby avoiding dangerous side effects such as nephrotoxicity or ototoxicity [1].

Despite these strengths associated with local antibiotic therapy, there are also concerns. One is that a high concentration of antibiotics can potentially inhibit new bone formation [7]. Another concern is the development of antibiotic resistance [8] or the emergence of pathogens not covered under the narrow spectrum of commonly used antibiotics such as vancomycin [9–11]. Additionally, prophylaxis with local antibiotics is an off-label usage and may cause unforeseen adverse events.

Previous systematic reviews have examined the effect of intrawound antibiotics in either instrumented spinal procedures or open limb fractures [9, 12–16]. Because both fields share a high risk of infection and the objective of achieving bony union, which may be affected by local antibiotics, we believe there is value in reporting pooled outcomes of local antibiotics comprehensively from both specialties. The outcomes of local antibiotics in extremity fracture treatment may therefore be generalizable to spinal fusion surgery and vice versa.

Therefore, the aim of this systematic review is to assess the efficacy of locally administered antibiotics in preventing SSIs in instrumented spinal procedures and fracture surgeries and to investigate the effect of local vancomycin powder on SSIs caused by Gram-negative organisms.

2. Materials and Methods

2.1. Search Strategy.
We searched the PubMed, EMBASE, and Web of Science databases for our systematic review and meta-analysis. Keywords and phrases that guided our search strategy included "intrawound OR local" and "fracture OR fusion" and "prophylaxis OR prevent." The following MeSH terms were developed from key articles and used on PubMed: "anti-infective agents, local" and "antibiotic prophylaxis" (full search strategy in Appendix A). All relevant abstracts presented at major orthopedic conferences (Orthopaedic Trauma Association Conference, American Academy of Orthopaedic Surgeons Conference, North American Spine Society, Scoliosis Research Society) and available on the conference databases were included. Two additional articles were identified from the bibliographies of included articles and relevant review papers. Our initial search was performed in 2019; a secondary search was performed in 2021 to identify updated, relevant articles.

2.2. Eligibility Criteria.
Criteria for inclusion in this systemic review were studies that (1) included patients undergoing acute fracture repair or spinal fusion with instrumentation, (2) had a treatment group that received prophylactic local antibiotics, and (3) reported SSI as a primary outcome. We wanted to assess local antibiotic prophylaxis in instrumented procedures meant to achieve bone healing in adult studies.

We excluded studies of only pediatric patients. We included studies whose patient age range spanned children and adults because the age means with standard deviations of these articles indicated that the majority of the patients

were adults. Studies of craniofacial surgeries were excluded because of the unique bacterial flora and vasculature of this anatomic region [17]. We excluded case series and studies without a control group. Studies of spinal decompression procedures without fusion (e.g., laminectomy) were excluded. For articles that investigated both decompression and/or instrumented procedures, only the infection results of instrumented cases were included. Studies in which the treatment group received other experimental therapies (e.g., antiseptics) in addition to local antibiotics were also excluded. Furthermore, there were some groups that published multiple studies on the same patient cohort, either at different time points during one collection period or with different subsets of the same data. In such cases, only the article with the greatest sample size was included. Finally, any articles that did not report patient data were excluded, such as narrative reviews, pharmacokinetic studies, and articles on novel antibiotic delivery systems. Any conflicts were resolved through discussion and consensus.

2.3. Study Identification and Data Extraction.
Two authors (EK and MT) individually conducted a title and abstract screening with DistillerSR (Evidence Partners, Ottawa, Canada). The full text articles of selected studies were separately assessed by two authors (EK and CD). The data were extracted independently by two authors (EK and CD), including an assessment of patient population, local antibiotic of choice, sample size, method of controlling for bias, number of infections, and the culture results, if available. The Preferred Reporting Items for Systematic Reviews and Meta-Analyses (PRISMA) flow diagram details the number of articles retrieved and excluded at each stage of the review (Figure 1).

2.4. Meta-Analysis and Subgroup Analysis.
To study whether prophylactic local antibiotics reduce the risk of SSIs, separate meta-analyses were performed for the instrumented spinal procedure and fracture repair. Further, RCTs and observational studies were pooled separately, with subgroups of study design among nonrandomized studies (propensity-matched cohort study or nonpropensity-matched cohort study) (Figures 2–5). Risk ratios (RRs) and odds ratios (ORs) were calculated in the meta-analyses of RCTs and observational studies, respectively.

To evaluate the effect of vancomycin on Gram-positive and Gram-negative infections, data were pooled from articles that studied the use of vancomycin powder and reported SSI culture results. These data were grouped into meta-analyses of Gram-positive vs. Gram-negative organisms with subgroup analysis for spine and fracture studies (Figures 6 and 7). Negative or mixed polymicrobial results (both Gram-positive and Gram-negative pathogens cultured in the same infection) were omitted. When multiple organisms that were either all Gram-positive or all Gram-negative were cultured in one SSI, they were counted as one. Studies that provided bacterial data for only a portion of the SSIs were excluded from this subgroup analysis.

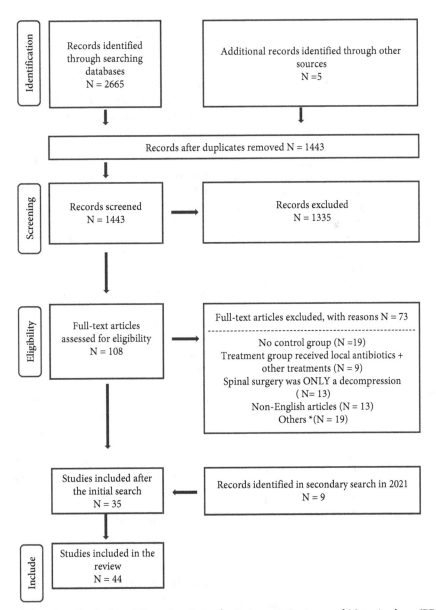

FIGURE 1: Literature search flowchart for Preferred Reporting Items for Systematic Reviews and Meta-Analyses (PRISMA). * Excluded for the following reasons: no patient data, pediatric study, no local antibiotic usage, repeat study, animal study, not accessible, and includes surgeries that are not instrumented spinal fusion or fracture surgeries.

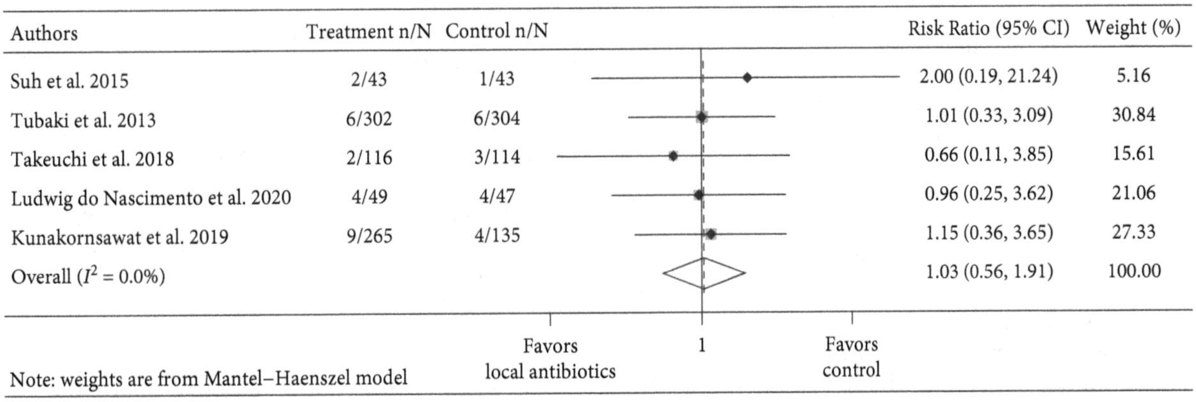

Authors	Treatment n/N	Control n/N		Risk Ratio (95% CI)	Weight (%)
Suh et al. 2015	2/43	1/43		2.00 (0.19, 21.24)	5.16
Tubaki et al. 2013	6/302	6/304		1.01 (0.33, 3.09)	30.84
Takeuchi et al. 2018	2/116	3/114		0.66 (0.11, 3.85)	15.61
Ludwig do Nascimento et al. 2020	4/49	4/47		0.96 (0.25, 3.62)	21.06
Kunakornsawat et al. 2019	9/265	4/135		1.15 (0.36, 3.65)	27.33
Overall ($I^2 = 0.0\%$)				1.03 (0.56, 1.91)	100.00

Favors local antibiotics — 1 — Favors control

Note: weights are from Mantel–Haenszel model

FIGURE 2: Forest plot of infection data of 5 instrumented spinal fusion randomized controlled trials. Treatment n/N: number of infections in the treatment group/total number of patients in the treatment group. Control n/N: number of infections in the control group/total number of patients in the control group.

2.5. Statistical Analysis. STATA 16 software (Statacorp, College Station, TX) was used to conduct random-effects meta-analyses using the admetan command, which is built on the Mantel and Haenszel model to develop RRs and ORs for binary and continuous data [18, 19]. The heterogeneity of the included studies was quantified with the I^2 statistic.

3. Results

3.1. Spinal Instrumentation. Thirty spinal instrumentation studies were included, with five RCTs, two prospective observational studies, and 23 retrospective studies (Table 1) [20–49]. A total of 17,756 patients were included. Among the nonrandomized studies, three studies were propensity-matched [23, 29, 35]. There was a wide variety in the type of instrumented procedure performed, reflecting a range of diagnoses across studies. Twenty-two of the 30 studies exclusively included fusion cases. The treatment group in 29 of 30 studies received vancomycin with varying dosages (0.5–2 g) and methods of application. The study that did not report the use of vancomycin did not specify either the antibiotic type or the dosage [23]. The primary outcome of included studies was SSI.

The pooled RR of infection in the treatment group compared to the control group across five spinal instrumentation RCT studies was 1.03 (95% CI: 0.56–1.91, $I^2 = 0.0\%$) (Figure 2). The pooled odds ratio (OR) of infection in the treatment group compared to the control group across all 25 spinal instrumentation observational studies was 0.34 (95% CI: 0.27–0.43, $I^2 = 52.4\%$ (Figure 3). Subgroup analyses by the study type (propensity-matched cohort or non-propensity-matched cohort) among observational studies were performed. The pooled OR of the three propensity-matched cohort studies was 0.77 (95% CI: 0.52–1.12, $I^2 = 0.0$). The remaining 22 studies had a pooled OR of 0.24 (95% CI: 0.17–0.32, $I^2 = 42.8\%$).

3.2. Fracture Repair. Fourteen fracture studies were included, with three RCTs, two prospective observational studies, and nine retrospective studies (Table 2) [50–63]. A total of 4,635 patients were included. Similar to the spine studies, the fracture studies reported SSI as the primary outcome. There was considerable clinical heterogeneity among the studies, such as fracture location, antibiotic type, and definition of SSI. Data from Bibbo and Patel [50] did not contribute to the meta-analysis because both the treatment and control groups had a 0% SSI incidence.

The pooled RR of infection in the treatment group in the three RCTs was 0.61 (95% CI: 0.40–0.93, $I^2 = 32.5\%$) (Figure 4). Subgroup analyses by the study type (propensity-matched cohort or non-propensity-matched cohort studies) among observational studies were also performed. Because there was only one propensity-matched cohort study, it was not pooled. The pooled odds ratio (OR) of infection in the treatment group compared to the control group across 10 observational fracture studies was 0.49 (95% CI: 0.37–0.65 $I^2 = 43.8\%$) (Figure 5). In the subgroup analysis

by study type, the pooled OR for nine non-propensity matched cohort studies was 0.51 (95% CI: 0.39–0.68, $I^2 = 44.9\%$).

Because the fracture studies used a variety of antibiotics, subgroup analysis by antibiotic type was conducted, which pooled studies of all designs together (Appendix B). For the five vancomycin studies, the pooled OR was 0.71 (95% CI: 0.51–0.98, $I^2 = 0.0\%$). The pooled OR for the three tobramycin studies was 0.31 (95% CI: 0.19–0.50, $I^2 = 27.4\%$). Two studies used both vancomycin and tobramycin and showed a pooled OR of 0.41 (95% CI: 0.18–0.94, $I^2 = 0.0\%$). The study by Bibbo and Patel [50] was not included because both the treatment and control groups had a 0% SSI incidence. Three remaining studies [52, 54, 55] each had a unique antibiotic regimen and were not pooled with other studies.

3.3. Microbiology in Instrumented Spinal Procedures and Fracture Surgeries That Used Vancomycin. To address the concern that the use of local vancomycin powder can affect the incidence of Gram-negative infection, two meta-analyses spanning 20 studies that studied local vancomycin and reported culture data were conducted. The pooled OR for an infection caused by Gram-positive bacteria in the vancomycin group compared to the control group was 0.37 (95% CI: 0.27–0.51, $I^2 = 0.0\%$) (Figure 6). Subgroup analysis by spine and fracture cases revealed an OR of 0.33 (95% CI: 0.22–0.50, $I^2 = 12.6\%$) in instrumented spinal procedures and OR of 0.46 (95% CI: 0.26–0.83, $I^2 = 0.0\%$) in fracture repairs. The pooled OR for Gram-negative infection in the vancomycin group was 0.95 (95% CI: 0.62–1.44, $I^2 = 0.0\%$) (Figure 7). The subgroup analysis showed that the OR was 0.83 (95% CI: 0.50–1.39, $I^2 = 0.0\%$) for spinal instrumentation and 1.23 (95% CI: 0.60–2.55, $I^2 = 0.0\%$) for fracture surgeries. Three studies were excluded in the meta-analysis of Gram-negative infections because both control and treatment groups had no Gram-negative SSIs. Subgroup analyses by study type showed a similar trend towards greater effect size among nonrandomized studies.

4. Discussion

We performed a meta-analysis of 44 studies evaluating the effect of locally administered antibiotics on rates of infection after instrumented spine and fracture surgeries. Notable findings include a significant reduction in the pooled incidence of infection in both patient populations, but this effect was weaker or absent with more rigorous study designs. The pooled effect of vancomycin was significant for the reduction in Gram-positive infection and did not show any association with Gram-negative infection compared to no local antibiotics.

4.1. Spinal Instrumentation. Previous systematic reviews have demonstrated the benefit of local antibiotics and antiseptic prophylaxis. Dodson et al. [9] pooled 21 studies (2 RCTs and 19 observational studies) and found that

TABLE 1: Summary of infection rates and methodology of studies of instrumented spinal procedure.

Authors/year	Study design/ method of controlling for bias	No. of pts	Age range of pts	Included spinal diagnoses/procedures	Intervention	Wound infection rates in treatment group	Wound infection rates in control group
Adhikari et al. 2020 [20][‡]	RC/NR	141	Adults	Deformity, degenerative, trauma, neoplastic/ posterior instrumented fusion	Vancomycin powder 1 g	3.53% (3/85)	1.79% (1/56)
Caroom et al. 2013 [21][*]	RC/NR	112	NR	Cervical spondylotic myelopathy/posterior instrumented fusion	Vancomycin powder 1 g	0% (0/40)	15.28% (11/ 72)
Dewan et al. 2013 [22][a,*]	RC/NR	455	NR	Degenerative/posterior spinal fusion	Vancomycin powder 1 g	0% (0/137)	5.66% (18/ 318)
Ehlers et al. 2016 [23][b]	PC/propensity score matching	6910	NR	Instrumented cervical or lumbar fusion	Intrawound antibiotics (type and dose NR)	0.93% (32/ 3455)	1.30% (45/ 3455)
Emohare et al. 2014 [24][c]	RC/multivariate analysis, pseudo-randomization by surgeon[d]	200	NR	Degenerative/posterior instrumented thoracic, thoracolumbar, lumbar fusion	Vancomycin powder 1 g	0% (0/78)	3.28% (4/122)
Gaviola et al. 2016 [25]	RC/multivariate analysis	326	40–71	Instrumented multilevel fusion	Vancomycin powder 2 g	5.17% (6/116)	11.0% (23/ 210)
Haimoto et al. 2018 [26][*]	RC/NR	515	18 and above	Posterior instrumented cervical, thoracic, lumbar fusion	Vancomycin powder 1 g	0% (0/247)	5.60% (15/ 268)
Heller et al. 2015 [27][‡]	RC/NR	683	NR	Degenerative, deformity, neoplastic, others/ posterior instrumented fusion	Vancomycin powder 0.5–2 g	2.63% (9/342)	5.28% (18/ 341)
Hey et al. 2017 [28][*]	RC/multivariate analysis, pseudo-randomization	389	11–85	Degenerative, trauma, neoplastic/open instrumentation	Vancomycin powder 1 g	0.85% (1/117, 1 deep)	6.25% (17/ 272, 10 deep, 7 superficial)
Horii et al. 2018 [29][b]	RC/propensity score matching	1014	15 and above	Degenerative, deformity, trauma, neoplastics/ posterior instrumentation	Vancomycin powder 1–2 g	1.58% (8/507)	1.78% (9/507)
Kim et al. 2013 [30][*]	RC/logistic regression, multivariate analysis, and cox regression	74	NR	Spinal instability/ posterior instrumented fusion	Vancomycin powder 1 g	0% (0/34)	12.5% (5/40, 3 deep, 2 superficial)
Kunakornsawat et al. 2019 [31][‡]	RCT/ randomizations	400	11–82	Trauma, degenerative, congenital, neoplastic, infectious/posterior instrumented thoracic or lumbosacral fusions	Vancomycin powder 1–2 g	3.40% (9/265)	2.96% (4/135)
Lemans et al. 2017 [32][*]	RC/NR	505	Adults	Open posterior instrumentation	Vancomycin powder 1–2 g	4.44% (8/180, 5 deep, 3 superficial)	13.85% (45/ 325, 31 deep, 14 superficial)
Liu et al. 2015 [33][‡]	RC/NR	334	53.5–74	Deformity, degenerative, neoplastic/posterior instrumentation	Vancomycin powder 0.5–2 g	2.78% (5/180)	7.14% (11/ 154)
Ludwig do nascimento et al. 2020 [34]	RCT/randomization, double blinding	96	17–74	Degenerative, trauma/ thoracolumbar spine arthrodesis	20 ml of saline with 2 g of diluted vancomycin	8.16% (4/49)	8.51% (4/47)
Martin et al. 2014 [35][b,‡]	RC/logistic regression, propensity score matching	306	18 and above	Deformity/posterior instrumented fusion	Vancomycin powder 2 g	5.12% (8/156)	5.33% (8/150)

TABLE 1: Continued.

Authors/year	Study design/ method of controlling for bias	No. of pts	Age range of pts	Included spinal diagnoses/procedures	Intervention	Wound infection rates in treatment group	Wound infection rates in control group
Ogihara et al. 2021 [36][‡]	RC/multivariable analysis	2913	18–93	Degenerative/posterior instrumented fusion in the thoracic/lumbar spines	Vancomycin powder	1.52% (7/460)	1.14% (28/ 2453)
Oktay et al. 2020 [37][*]	RC/NR	209	14–90	Degenerative, trauma, neoplastic, revision/ posterior instrumentation	Vancomycin powder 1 g	1.96% (2/102, 1 deep, 1 superficial)	6.54% (7/107, 4 deep, 3 superficial)
O'Neill et al. 2011 [38][*]	RC/pseudo-randomization	110	18 and above	Trauma/posterior instrumented fusion	Vancomycin powder 1 g	0% (0/56)	12.96% (7/54, 5 deep, 2 superficial)
Satake et al. 2015 [39][‡,*]	PC/NR	207	Not given	Open posterior instrumented thoracic, lumbar fusion	Vancomycin powder with fibrin glue (dosage NR)	0% (0/59)	6.08% (9/148)
Scheverin et al. 2015 [40][*]	RC/pseudo-randomization	513	18–78	Degenerative/posterior instrumented lumbar fusion	Vancomycin powder 1 g mixed with bone graft	1.29% (3/232)	4.98% (14/ 281)
Strom et al. 2013 [41][*]	RC/NR	171	Adult patients	Degenerative, infectious, neoplastic, trauma/ posterior cervical instrumented fusion	Vancomycin powder 1 g	2.53% (2/79)	10.87% (10/ 92)
Strom et al. 2013 [42][*]	RC/stratification	165	NRs	Degenerative, infectious, neoplastic, trauma/ lumbar laminectomy and posterior instrumented fusion	Vancomycin powder 1 g	0% (0/88)	11.69% (9/77)
Suh et al. 2015 [43]	RCT/NR	86	23–83	Degenerative/posterior instrumented lumbar fusion	Vancomycin powder 2 g	4.65% (2/43)	2.33% (1/43)
Sweet et al. 2011 [44][‡,*]	RC/NR	1732	12–86	Posterior instrumented thoracolumbar fusions	Vancomycin powder 2 g	0.22% (2/911)	2.56% (21/ 821)
Takeuchi et al. 2018 [45][d]	RCT/randomization, blinding	230	NR	Deformity, degenerative, trauma/thoracic, lumbar fusion	Vancomycin powder 1 g	1.72% (2/116, 1 deep, 1 superficial)	2.63% (3/114, 1 deep, 2 superficial)
Takeuchi et al. 2019 [46][*]	RC/NR	668	16–89	Degenerative, fracture/ posterior spinal instrumentation	Vancomycin powder 1 g	0.32% (1/314)	2.54% (9/354)
Theologis et al. 2014 [47][*]	RC/NR	215	18–88	Deformity/fusion greater than 3 levels	Vancomycin powder 2 g	2.65% (4/151)	10.93% (7/64)
Tofuku et al. 2012 [48][‡,*]	RC/NR	384	7–89	Degenerative, neoplastic, trauma, infectious/spinal instrumentation	0.5 g Vancomycin-impregnated fibrin sealant	0% (0/196)	5.85% (11/ 188)
Tubaki et al. 2013 [49][‡]	RCT/randomization	606	3–84	Listhesis, disc prolapse/ open instrumentation	Vancomycin powder 1 g	1.99% (6/302)	1.97% (6/304)

Abbreviations: No., number; pts, patients; RCT, randomized controlled trial; PC, prospective cohort; RC, retrospective cohort; NR, not reported. [a]We included only deep SSI that occurred in fusion cases. Superficial SSI were excluded because the paper reports that 5 occurred in both control and treatment groups, but the paper did not discern whether these occurred in instrumented or noninstrumented cases. [b]There is another paper by O'Neill et al. that looked at only the spine trauma cases, but Dewan et al. look at the same trauma cases plus degenerative spine disease cases. The numbers included pertain to only the degenerative spine disease cases. [c]Sample size reflects the propensity score matched cohorts. [g]Control group received ampicillin powder. [‡]Only deep infections were reported in this study. [*]Studies showed a significant difference between the control and treatment groups.

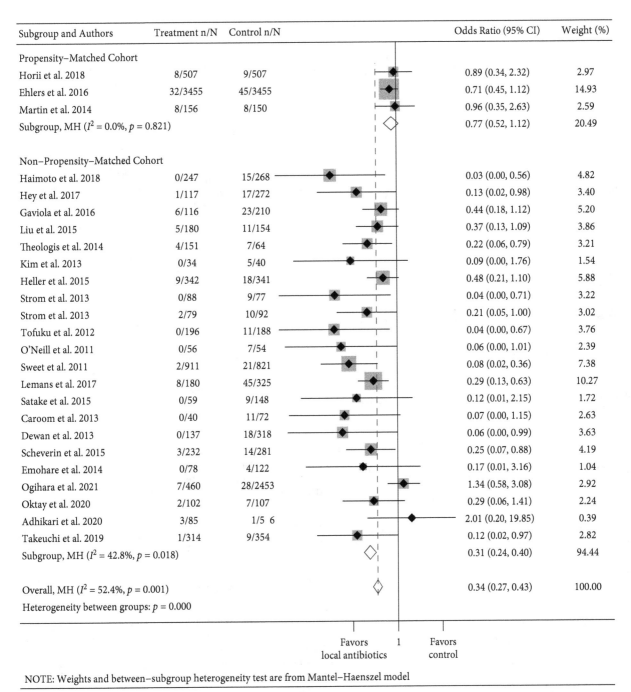

Subgroup and Authors	Treatment n/N	Control n/N	Odds Ratio (95% CI)	Weight (%)
Propensity–Matched Cohort				
Horii et al. 2018	8/507	9/507	0.89 (0.34, 2.32)	2.97
Ehlers et al. 2016	32/3455	45/3455	0.71 (0.45, 1.12)	14.93
Martin et al. 2014	8/156	8/150	0.96 (0.35, 2.63)	2.59
Subgroup, MH ($I^2 = 0.0\%$, $p = 0.821$)			0.77 (0.52, 1.12)	20.49
Non–Propensity–Matched Cohort				
Haimoto et al. 2018	0/247	15/268	0.03 (0.00, 0.56)	4.82
Hey et al. 2017	1/117	17/272	0.13 (0.02, 0.98)	3.40
Gaviola et al. 2016	6/116	23/210	0.44 (0.18, 1.12)	5.20
Liu et al. 2015	5/180	11/154	0.37 (0.13, 1.09)	3.86
Theologis et al. 2014	4/151	7/64	0.22 (0.06, 0.79)	3.21
Kim et al. 2013	0/34	5/40	0.09 (0.00, 1.76)	1.54
Heller et al. 2015	9/342	18/341	0.48 (0.21, 1.10)	5.88
Strom et al. 2013	0/88	9/77	0.04 (0.00, 0.71)	3.22
Strom et al. 2013	2/79	10/92	0.21 (0.05, 1.00)	3.02
Tofuku et al. 2012	0/196	11/188	0.04 (0.00, 0.67)	3.76
O'Neill et al. 2011	0/56	7/54	0.06 (0.00, 1.01)	2.39
Sweet et al. 2011	2/911	21/821	0.08 (0.02, 0.36)	7.38
Lemans et al. 2017	8/180	45/325	0.29 (0.13, 0.63)	10.27
Satake et al. 2015	0/59	9/148	0.12 (0.01, 2.15)	1.72
Caroom et al. 2013	0/40	11/72	0.07 (0.00, 1.15)	2.63
Dewan et al. 2013	0/137	18/318	0.06 (0.00, 0.99)	3.63
Scheverin et al. 2015	3/232	14/281	0.25 (0.07, 0.88)	4.19
Emohare et al. 2014	0/78	4/122	0.17 (0.01, 3.16)	1.04
Ogihara et al. 2021	7/460	28/2453	1.34 (0.58, 3.08)	2.92
Oktay et al. 2020	2/102	7/107	0.29 (0.06, 1.41)	2.24
Adhikari et al. 2020	3/85	1/5 6	2.01 (0.20, 19.85)	0.39
Takeuchi et al. 2019	1/314	9/354	0.12 (0.02, 0.97)	2.82
Subgroup, MH ($I^2 = 42.8\%$, $p = 0.018$)			0.31 (0.24, 0.40)	94.44
Overall, MH ($I^2 = 52.4\%$, $p = 0.001$)			0.34 (0.27, 0.43)	100.00
Heterogeneity between groups: $p = 0.000$				

Favors local antibiotics | 1 | Favors control

NOTE: Weights and between–subgroup heterogeneity test are from Mantel–Haenszel model

FIGURE 3: Forest plot of observational instrumented spinal fusion studies. Treatment n/N: number of infections in the treatment group/total number of patients in the treatment group. Control n/N: number of infections in the control group/total number of patients in the control group.

prophylactic vancomycin powder significantly reduced the risk of developing SSIs in spinal surgeries (RR 0.55, 95% CI: 0.45–0.67, $p = 0.0001$). Similarly, Lemans et al. [12] pooled 20 studies (2 RCTs and 18 observational studies) and showed that using preventive intrawound antibiotics and antiseptics also decreased the risk of deep SSIs in instrumented surgeries (RR 0.26, 95% CI: 0.17–0.51, $p < 0.0001$).

Surgical procedures with instrumentation have a higher risk of biofilm formation [1]. Therefore, our study focused exclusively on instrumented procedures in adult patient populations and yielded a result consistent with other systematic reviews

[9, 12]. Neither the meta-analysis of the five RCTs nor the meta-analysis of the three propensity-matched cohort studies showed the same significant reduction that occurred with the pooling of cohort studies. Many observational studies used a "before-and-after" study design that is prone to confounding bias, which may explain the greater effect size observed in non-propensity-matched studies [64]. The blinded RCT remains the methodological gold standard for proving the efficacy of therapeutic intervention; it is important that any future observational studies incorporate design and analytical methods to control for bias, such as propensity score adjustment [65].

TABLE 2: Summary of infection rates and methodology of studies of fracture repair.

Authors/year	Study design/ method of controlling for bias	No. of pts	Age range of pts	Diagnosis	Intervention	Wound infection rates in treatment group	Wound infection rates in control group
Bibbo and Patel 2006 [50]	PC/NR	44	17–59	Calcaneal fractures	Vancomycin/DBM-calcium sulfate bone graft substitute	0% (0/33)	0% (0/11)
Cichos et al. 2021 [51][a]	RC/multivariate analysis	789	18–89	Acetabular fractures	Vancomycin powder 1 g; Vancomycin 1 g and tobramycin 1.2 g	Vancomycin: 6.80% (20/294, 18 deep, 2 suprafascial) Vancomycin and tobramycin 9.47% (16/169, 12 deep, 4 suprafascial)	8.28% (27/ 326, 20 deep, 7 suprafascial)
Junker et al. 2019 [52]	PC/NR	285	18 or above	Rib fractures	Vancomycin 2 g and gentamicin 2.4 g PMMA	0% (0/8)	3.61% (10/ 277)
Keating et al. 1996 [53][‡]	RC/NR	79 (79 patients, 81 fractures)	16–88	Open tibial fractures	2.4 g Tobramycin-loaded pouch	3.77% (2/55)	16.0% (4/26)
Lawing et al. 2015 [54][*]	RC/logistic regression	351	"Excluded kids <10"	Open fractures	Aminoglycosides 2 mg/mL	9.52% (16/168, 10 deep, 6 superficial)	19.67% (36/ 183, 26 deep, 10 superficial)
Malizos et al. 2017 [55][*]	RCT/ randomization	253	20–99	Closed fractures	Antibiotic-loaded hydrogel 20–50 mg/ mL	0% (0/126)	4.72% (6/127)
Moehring et al. 2000 [56][‡,b]	RCT/ randomization	55 (treatment: 22 patients, 24 fractures; Control: 33 patients, 38 fractures)	16–76	Open fractures (primarily lower extremity)	2.4 g tobramycin-impregnated beads	9.09% (2/22)	6.06% (2/33)
O'Toole et al. 2021 [57][*,c]	RCT/ randomization	980	"Adult patients"	Tibial plateau and pilon fractures	Vancomycin powder 1 g	6.03% (29/481)	9.22% (46/ 499)
Ostermann et al. 1995 [58][*]	PC/NR	914 (1085 fractures)	14–99	Open fractures (primarily lower extremity)	Tobramycin-PMMA	3.67% (31/845)	12.08% (29/ 240)
Owen et al. 2017 [59][‡,*]	RC/stratification, logistic regression	140	19–65	Pelvic and acetabular fractures	Vancomycin 1 g and tobramycin 1.2 g powder	4.23% (3/71)	14.49% (10/ 69)
Prevost et al. 2019 [60][‡]	RC/NR	90	NR	Open tibial fractures	Vancomycin and tobramycin powder	16.67% (11/66)	25.0% (6/24)
Qadir et al. 2020 [61][*,‡,d]	RC/propensity-score matching, nearest-neighbor matching	105	16–85	Bicondylar tibial plateau, tibial pilon, and calcaneus fractures	Vancomycin powder 1 g	0% (0/35)	14.29% (10/ 70)
Singh et al. 2015 [62][‡]	RC/NR	93	"Adults"	Tibial plateau and pilon fractures	Vancomycin 1 g	10.00% (1/10)	16.87% (14/ 83)
Vaida et al. 2019 [63][‡]	RC/NR	457	NR	Open lower extremity fractures	Vancomycin powder	8.51% (4/47)	8.78% (36/ 410)

Abbreviations: No., number; pts, patients; RCT, randomized controlled trial; PC, prospective cohort; RC, retrospective cohort; NR, not reported; DBM, demineralized bone matrix; PMMA, polymethyl methacrylate. [a]We combined the two treatment groups into one intervention group in our analysis. [b]The treatment group received just antibiotic beads, and the control group received just parenteral antibiotics. Not included are the nonrandomized third cohort that received antibiotic beads + IV. This group of patients all had Grade 3 Gustilo–Anderson open fractures. [c]We included only deep SSI, which was the primary study outcome. Superficial SSI was excluded because the sample sizes for superficial SSI did not match those for deep SSI. [d]This study conducted analyses using two separate methods of matching: nearest-neighbor matching and propensity score matching. It also had both prospective and retrospective control cohorts. We included the data from propensity scores matching with the prospective control cohort. [‡]Only deep infections were reported in this study. [*]Studies showed a significant difference between the control and treatment groups.

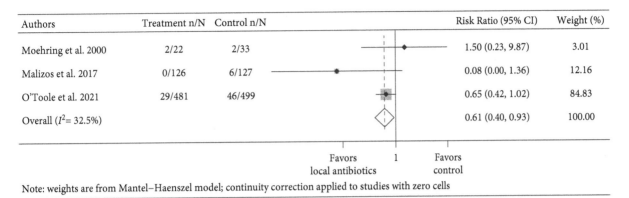

Authors	Treatment n/N	Control n/N		Risk Ratio (95% CI)	Weight (%)
Moehring et al. 2000	2/22	2/33		1.50 (0.23, 9.87)	3.01
Malizos et al. 2017	0/126	6/127		0.08 (0.00, 1.36)	12.16
O'Toole et al. 2021	29/481	46/499		0.65 (0.42, 1.02)	84.83
Overall (I^2= 32.5%)				0.61 (0.40, 0.93)	100.00

Favors local antibiotics — 1 — Favors control

Note: weights are from Mantel–Haenszel model; continuity correction applied to studies with zero cells

FIGURE 4: Forest plot of infection data of 3 fracture randomized controlled trials. Treatment n/N: number of infections in the treatment group/total number of patients in the treatment group. Control n/N: number of infections in the control group/total number of patients in the control group.

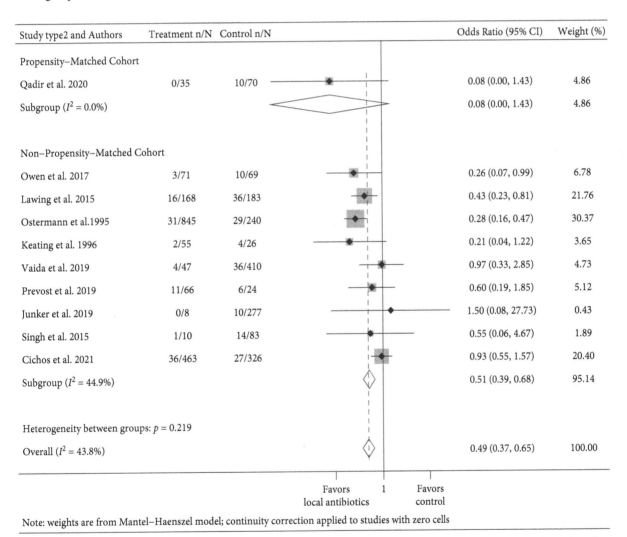

Study type2 and Authors	Treatment n/N	Control n/N		Odds Ratio (95% CI)	Weight (%)
Propensity–Matched Cohort					
Qadir et al. 2020	0/35	10/70		0.08 (0.00, 1.43)	4.86
Subgroup (I^2 = 0.0%)				0.08 (0.00, 1.43)	4.86
Non–Propensity–Matched Cohort					
Owen et al. 2017	3/71	10/69		0.26 (0.07, 0.99)	6.78
Lawing et al. 2015	16/168	36/183		0.43 (0.23, 0.81)	21.76
Ostermann et al.1995	31/845	29/240		0.28 (0.16, 0.47)	30.37
Keating et al. 1996	2/55	4/26		0.21 (0.04, 1.22)	3.65
Vaida et al. 2019	4/47	36/410		0.97 (0.33, 2.85)	4.73
Prevost et al. 2019	11/66	6/24		0.60 (0.19, 1.85)	5.12
Junker et al. 2019	0/8	10/277		1.50 (0.08, 27.73)	0.43
Singh et al. 2015	1/10	14/83		0.55 (0.06, 4.67)	1.89
Cichos et al. 2021	36/463	27/326		0.93 (0.55, 1.57)	20.40
Subgroup (I^2 = 44.9%)				0.51 (0.39, 0.68)	95.14
Heterogeneity between groups: p = 0.219					
Overall (I^2 = 43.8%)				0.49 (0.37, 0.65)	100.00

Favors local antibiotics — 1 — Favors control

Note: weights are from Mantel–Haenszel model; continuity correction applied to studies with zero cells

FIGURE 5: Forest plot of observational fracture studies. Treatment n/N: number of infections in the treatment group/total number of patients in the treatment group. Control n/N: number of infections in the control group/total number of patients in the control group.

4.2. Fracture Repair. Previous systematic reviews found that intrawound antibiotics in open fractures reduced the risk of SSIs. Craig et al. [16] evaluated the role of local antibiotic prophylaxis in open tibia fractures treated with intramedullary nails in their meta-analysis of seven articles (one RCT and six observational studies). For patients with Gustilo–Anderson (GA) type III fractures, those who received only parenteral antibiotics had an infection rate of 14.4% (95% CI: 10.5%–18.5%). In comparison, those who received local prophylactic antibiotics had an infection rate of

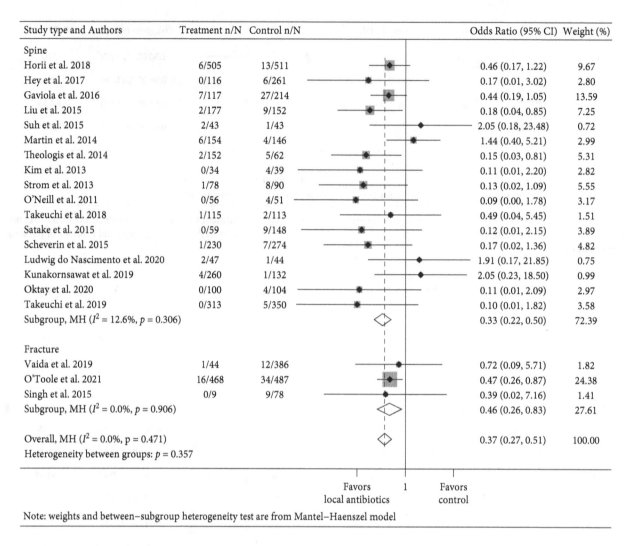

Study type and Authors	Treatment n/N	Control n/N		Odds Ratio (95% CI)	Weight (%)
Spine					
Horii et al. 2018	6/505	13/511		0.46 (0.17, 1.22)	9.67
Hey et al. 2017	0/116	6/261		0.17 (0.01, 3.02)	2.80
Gaviola et al. 2016	7/117	27/214		0.44 (0.19, 1.05)	13.59
Liu et al. 2015	2/177	9/152		0.18 (0.04, 0.85)	7.25
Suh et al. 2015	2/43	1/43		2.05 (0.18, 23.48)	0.72
Martin et al. 2014	6/154	4/146		1.44 (0.40, 5.21)	2.99
Theologis et al. 2014	2/152	5/62		0.15 (0.03, 0.81)	5.31
Kim et al. 2013	0/34	4/39		0.11 (0.01, 2.20)	2.82
Strom et al. 2013	1/78	8/90		0.13 (0.02, 1.09)	5.55
O'Neill et al. 2011	0/56	4/51		0.09 (0.00, 1.78)	3.17
Takeuchi et al. 2018	1/115	2/113		0.49 (0.04, 5.45)	1.51
Satake et al. 2015	0/59	9/148		0.12 (0.01, 2.15)	3.89
Scheverin et al. 2015	1/230	7/274		0.17 (0.02, 1.36)	4.82
Ludwig do Nascimento et al. 2020	2/47	1/44		1.91 (0.17, 21.85)	0.75
Kunakornsawat et al. 2019	4/260	1/132		2.05 (0.23, 18.50)	0.99
Oktay et al. 2020	0/100	4/104		0.11 (0.01, 2.09)	2.97
Takeuchi et al. 2019	0/313	5/350		0.10 (0.01, 1.82)	3.58
Subgroup, MH (I^2 = 12.6%, p = 0.306)				0.33 (0.22, 0.50)	72.39
Fracture					
Vaida et al. 2019	1/44	12/386		0.72 (0.09, 5.71)	1.82
O'Toole et al. 2021	16/468	34/487		0.47 (0.26, 0.87)	24.38
Singh et al. 2015	0/9	9/78		0.39 (0.02, 7.16)	1.41
Subgroup, MH (I^2 = 0.0%, p = 0.906)				0.46 (0.26, 0.83)	27.61
Overall, MH (I^2 = 0.0%, p = 0.471)				0.37 (0.27, 0.51)	100.00
Heterogeneity between groups: p = 0.357					

Favors   1   Favors
local antibiotics   control

Note: weights and between−subgroup heterogeneity test are from Mantel−Haenszel model

FIGURE 6: Forest plot of Gram-positive infection data of studies that used vancomycin with subgroup analysis for spine and fracture cases. Treatment n/N: number of infections in the treatment group/total number of patients in the treatment group. Control n/N: number of infections in the control group/total number of patients in the control group.

2.4% (95% CI: 0.0–9.4), with an OR of 0.17. A meta-analysis of eight articles (one RCT and seven observational studies) by Morgenstern et al. [15] showed a similar significant reduction in infection risk in open fractures (OR = 0.30, 95% CI: 0.22–0.40).

Our meta-analysis showed a pooled benefit of prophylactic intrawound antibiotics in both randomized and nonrandomized studies. Similar to our analysis of spine instrumentation studies, bias reduction from randomization revealed that the magnitude of the effect is likely to be smaller than previously thought yet trending towards a protective effect. Subgroup analysis by antibiotic type showed that local vancomycin reduced SSI in fracture repair, which is in line with the established coverage pattern of vancomycin and common infectious organisms. Larger studies and trials that combine vancomycin with agents with Gram-negative coverage may be required to achieve the precision and possible added magnitude of effect to prove the impact of local antibiotics for the prevention of SSI in this population.

4.3. Microbiology with the Use of Vancomycin Powder. Our meta-analyses assessed the microbiology of SSIs by pooling culture data from studies that used vancomycin powder. We specifically addressed vancomycin because of its widespread use and concern that its selective coverage of Gram-positive pathogens may increase the incidence of Gram-negative infection [1]. In a study of 2802 patients undergoing spinal surgery, Chotai et al. [11] observed a lower incidence of deep SSIs in the vancomycin group. However, there was a higher percentage of SSI caused by Gram-negative organisms in the vancomycin group than in the control group (28% vs. 12.5%).

We demonstrated that vancomycin reduces Gram-positive infection and has no effect on Gram-negative infection in both instrumented spinal procedures and fracture surgeries. The effectiveness of vancomycin against Gram-positive pathogens is consistent with its established antibacterial spectrum covering some of the most commonly cultured organisms in SSI of both instrumented spinal procedures and

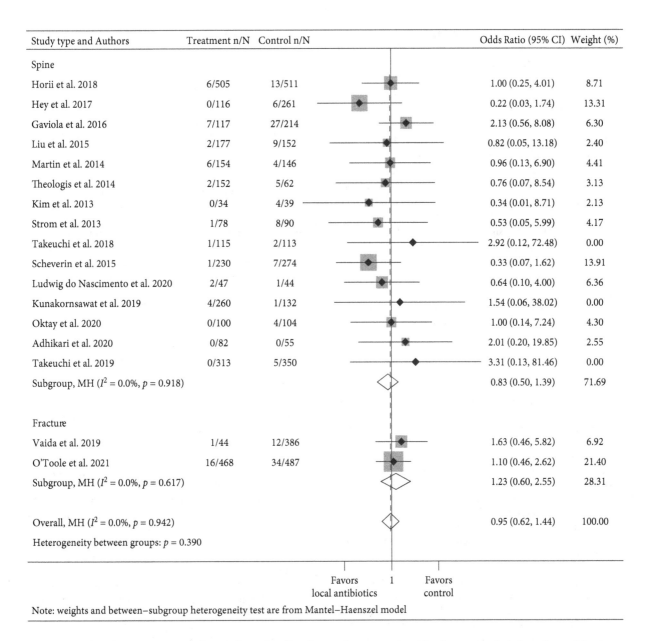

FIGURE 7: Forest plot of Gram-negative infection data of studies that used vancomycin with subgroup analysis for spine and fracture cases. Treatment n/N: number of infections in the treatment group/total number of patients in the treatment group. Control n/N: number of infections in the control group/total number of patients in the control group.

fractures, including *Staphylococcus aureus* [8, 10, 11]. Furthermore, our results are reassuring to orthopedic surgeons who are apprehensive about the potential for vancomycin to increase the incidence of Gram-negative infections.

4.4. Adverse Events. No studies reported any adverse events attributable to local antibiotics. The majority of the included studies had a single sentence denying side effects. Some studies explicitly reported that intrawound antibiotics did not impact the rates of nonunion, addressing the concern that topical antibiotics can impede bone healing [7, 31, 42, 50, 54, 57]. It is important to note that most of the

included studies were not powered to detect differences in pseudarthrosis.

5. Limitations

The primary limitation of this study is the pooling of cohort studies in the meta-analysis. We intentionally included both RCTs and observational studies because there are very few RCTs that investigate the prophylactic effect of intrawound antibiotics, but the RCTs and nonrandomized studies were analyzed separately. The majority of the current evidence is from observational studies. A high degree of heterogeneity in study design, outcome assessment, treatment protocols, and definition of SSI existed among the included studies. There was a hierarchy of study designs among observational studies across which differences in effect were identified.

6. Conclusion

Prophylactic topical antibiotics are associated with decreased risk of surgical site infection after both instrumented spine and fracture surgeries in much of the published literature on the topic. Although the effect is weak or absent in more rigorous study designs in the instrumented spinal fusion literature, pooling of fracture repair RCTs revealed that intrawound antibiotics significantly reduced SSIs. There is no evidence to suggest a higher incidence of Gram-negative infection or other adverse events among patients treated with local vancomycin, irrespective of study quality. These results do not support the use of local antibiotics in patients undergoing spinal fusion but suggest therapeutic efficacy in patients undergoing fracture repair.

References

[1] J. M. Cancienne, M. T. Burrus, D. B. Weiss, and S. R. Yarboro, "Applications of local antibiotics in orthopedic trauma," *Orthopedic Clinics of North America*, vol. 46, no. 4, pp. 495–510, 2015.

[2] O. G. Blam, A. R. Vaccaro, J. S. Vanichkachorn et al., "Risk factors for surgical site infection in the patient with spinal injury," *Spine*, vol. 28, no. 13, pp. 1475–1480, 2003.

[3] J. Redfern, S. M. Wasilko, M. E. Groth, W. D. Mcmillian, and C. S. Bartlett, "Surgical site infections in patients with type 3 open fractures: comparing antibiotic prophylaxis with cefazolin plus gentamicin versus piperacillin/tazobactam," *Journal of Orthopaedic Trauma*, vol. 30, no. 8, pp. 415–419, 2016.

[4] W. J. Metsemakers, R. Kuehl, T. F. Moriarty et al., "Infection after fracture fixation: current surgical and microbiological concepts," *Injury*, vol. 49, no. 3, pp. 511–522, 2018.

[5] Y. Chang, S. A. Kennedy, M. Bhandari et al., "Effects of antibiotic prophylaxis in patients with open fracture of the extremities: a systematic review of randomized controlled trials," *JBJS reviews*, vol. 3, no. 6, 2015.

[6] F. G. Barker, "Efficacy of prophylactic antibiotic therapy in spinal surgery: a meta-analysis," *Neurosurgery*, vol. 51, no. 2, pp. 391–401, 2002 Aug.

[7] C. R. Rathbone, J. D. Cross, K. V. Brown, C. K. Murray, and J. C. Wenke, "Effect of various concentrations of antibiotics on osteogenic cell viability and activity," *Journal of Orthopaedic Research*, vol. 29, no. 7, pp. 1070–1074, 2011.

[8] D. Campoccia, L. Montanaro, and C. R. Arciola, "The significance of infection related to orthopedic devices and issues of antibiotic resistance," *Biomaterials*, vol. 27, no. 11, pp. 2331–2339, 2006.

[9] V. Dodson, N. Majmundar, V. Swantic, and R. Assina, "The effect of prophylactic vancomycin powder on infections following spinal surgeries: a systematic review," *Neurosurgical Focus*, vol. 46, no. 1, pp. E11–E17, 2019.

[10] D. N. Gilbert, G. M. Eliopoulos, H. F. Chambers, M. S. Saag, and A. Pavia, *The Sanford Guide to Antimicrobial Therapy 2019*, Antimicrobial Therapy, Inc, Sperryville, VA, USA, 2019.

[11] S. Chotai, P. W. Wright, A. T. Hale et al., "Does intrawound vancomycin application during spine surgery create vancomycin-resistant organism?" *Neurosurgery*, vol. 80, no. 5, pp. 746–753, 2017.

[12] J. V. C. Lemans, S. P. J. Wijdicks, W. Boot et al., "Intrawound treatment for prevention of surgical site infections in instrumented spinal surgery: a systematic comparative effectiveness review and meta-analysis," *Global Spine Journal*, vol. 9, no. 2, pp. 219–230, 2019.

[13] S. D. Fernicola, M. J. Elsenbeck, P. D. Grimm, A. J. Pisano, and S. C. Wagner, "Intrasite antibiotic powder for the prevention of surgical site infection in extremity surgery," *Journal of the American Academy of Orthopaedic Surgeons*, vol. 28, 2019.

[14] R. Yao, T. Tan, J. W. Tee, and J. Street, "Prophylaxis of surgical site infection in adult spine surgery: a systematic review," *Journal of Clinical Neuroscience*, vol. 52, pp. 5–25, 2018.

[15] M. Morgenstern, A. Vallejo, M. A. McNally et al., "The effect of local antibiotic prophylaxis when treating open limb fractures," *Bone & Joint Research*, vol. 7, no. 7, pp. 447–456, 2018.

[16] J. Craig, T. Fuchs, M. Jenks et al., "Systematic review and meta-analysis of the additional benefit of local prophylactic antibiotic therapy for infection rates in open tibia fractures treated with intramedullary nailing," *International Orthopaedics*, vol. 38, no. 5, pp. 1025–1030, 2014.

[17] K. Krishnan, T. Chen, and B. Paster, "A practical guide to the oral microbiome and its relation to health and disease," *Oral Diseases*, vol. 23, no. 3, pp. 276–286, 2017.

[18] H. J. Newton, A. Editors, N. J. Cox, F. X. Diebold, J. M. Garrett, and M. Pagano, "A publication to promote communication among Stata users," *Stata Tech Bull*, 1998.

[19] N. Mantel and W. Haenszel, "Statistical aspects of the analysis of data from retrospective studies of disease," *Journal of the National Cancer Institute: Journal of the National Cancer Institute*, vol. 22, no. 4, pp. 719–748, 1959.

[20] P. Adhikari, V. N. Nabiyev, S. Bahadir et al., "Does the application of topical intrawound vancomycin powder affect deep surgical site infection and the responsible organisms after spinal surgery?: a retrospective case series with a historical control group," *Asian Spine Journal*, vol. 14, no. 1, pp. 72–78, 2020.

[21] C. Caroom, J. M. Tullar, E. G. Benton, J. R. Jones, and C. D. Chaput, "Intrawound vancomycin powder reduces surgical site infections in posterior cervical fusion," *Spine*, vol. 38, no. 14, pp. 1183–1187, 2013.

[22] M. C. Dewan, S. S. Godil, S. L. Zuckerman et al., "Comparative effectiveness and cost-benefit analysis of topical vancomycin powder in posterior spinal fusion for spine trauma and degenerative spine disease," *The Spine Journal*, vol. 13, no. 9, p. S56, 2013.

[23] A. P. Ehlers, S. Khor, N. Shonnard et al., "Intra-Wound antibiotics and infection in spine fusion surgery: a report from Washington state's SCOAP-CERTAIN collaborative," *Surgical Infections*, vol. 17, no. 2, pp. 179–186, 2016.

[24] O. Emohare, C. G. Ledonio, B. W. Hill, R. A. Davis, D. W. Polly, and M. M. Kang, "Cost savings analysis of intrawound vancomycin powder in posterior spinal surgery," *The Spine Journal*, vol. 14, no. 11, pp. 2710–2715, 2014.

[25] M. L. Gaviola, W. D. McMillian, S. E. Ames, J. A. Endicott, and W. K. Alston, "A retrospective study on the protective effects of topical vancomycin in patients undergoing multi-level spinal fusion," *Pharmacotherapy: The Journal of Human*

Pharmacology and Drug Therapy, vol. 36, no. 1, pp. 19–25, 2016.

[26] S. Haimoto, R. T. Schär, Y. Nishimura, M. Hara, T. Wakabayashi, and H. J. Ginsberg, "Reduction in surgical site infection with suprafascial intrawound application of vancomycin powder in instrumented posterior spinal fusion: a retrospective case-control study," *Journal of Neurosurgery: Spine*, vol. 29, no. 2, pp. 193–198, 2018.

[27] A. Heller, T. E. McIff, S.-M. Lai, and D. C. Burton, "Intrawound vancomycin powder decreases staphylococcal surgical site infections after posterior instrumented spinal arthrodesis," *Journal of Spinal Disorders & Techniques*, vol. 28, no. 10, pp. E584–E589, 2015.

[28] H. W. D. Hey, D. W. Thiam, Z. S. D. Koh, J. S. Thambiah, N. Kumar, and L. L. Lau, "Is intraoperative local vancomycin powder the answer to surgical site infections in spine surgery?" *Spine*, vol. 42, no. 4, pp. E267–E274, 2017.

[29] C. Horii, T. Yamazaki, H. Oka et al., "Does intrawound vancomycin powder reduce surgical site infection after posterior instrumented spinal surgery? A propensity score-matched analysis," *The Spine Journal*, vol. 18, no. 12, pp. 2205–2212, 2018.

[30] H. S. Kim, S. G. Lee, W. K. Kim, C. W. Park, and S. Son, "Prophylactic intrawound application of vancomycin powder in instrumented spinal fusion surgery," *Korean Journal of Spine*, vol. 10, no. 3, p. 121, 2013.

[31] S. Kunakornsawat, S. Sirikajohnirun, C. Piyaskulkaew et al., "Comparison between 1 g and 2 g of intrawound vancomycin powder application for prophylaxis in posterior instrumented thoracic or lumbosacral spine surgery: a preliminary report," *Asian journal of neurosurgery*, vol. 14, no. 3, pp. 710–714, 2019.

[32] J. Lemans, C. Oner, M. Ekkelenkamp, C. Vogely, and M. Kruyt, "Evaluation of intra-wound povidone-iodine irrigation and intra-woundVancomycin powder in the prevention ofSurgical site infection in spinal surgery," *Global Spine Journal*, vol. 19, pp. 87S-88S, 2017.

[33] N. Liu, K. B. Wood, J. H. Schwab, T. D. Cha, R. D. Puhkan, and P. M. Osler, "Comparison of intrawound vancomycin utility in posterior instrumented spine surgeries between patients with tumor and nontumor patients," *Spine*, vol. 40, no. 20, pp. 1586–1592, 2015.

[34] T. Ludwig do Nascimento, G. Finger, E. Sfreddo, A. Martins de Lima Cecchini, F. Martins de Lima Cecchini, and M. A. Stefani, "Double-blind randomized clinical trial of vancomycin in spinal arthrodesis: No effects on surgical site infection," *Journal of Neurosurgery: Spine*, vol. 32, no. 3, pp. 473–480, 2020.

[35] J. R. Martin, O. Adogwa, C. R. Brown et al., "Experience with intrawound vancomycin powder for spinal deformity surgery," *Spine*, vol. 39, no. 2, pp. 177–184, 2014.

[36] S. Ogihara, T. Yamazaki, M. Shiibashi et al., "Risk factors for deep surgical site infection following posterior instrumented fusion for degenerative diseases in the thoracic and/or lumbar spine: a multicenter, observational cohort study of 2913 consecutive cases," *European Spine Journal*, vol. 30, no. 6, pp. 1756–1764, 2021.

[37] K. Oktay, K. M. Özsoy, K. M. Ozsoy, N. E. Cetinalp, T. Erman, and A. Guzel, "Efficacy of prophylactic application of vancomycin powder in preventing surgical site infections after instrumented spinal surgery: a retrospective analysis of patients with high-risk conditions," *Acta Orthopaedica et Traumatologica Turcica*, vol. 55, no. 1, pp. 48–52, 2021.

[38] K. R. O'Neill, J. G. Smith, A. M. Abtahi, K. R. Archer, D. M. Spengler, and M. J. McGirt, "Reduced surgical site infections in patients undergoing posterior spinal stabilization of traumatic injuries using vancomycin powder," *The Spine Journal*, vol. 11, no. 7, pp. 641–646, 2011.

[39] K. Satake, T. Kanemura, H. Yamaguchi, and N. Segi, "Selective application of intrawound vancomycin powder with use of fiblin glue and/or intravenous daptmycin for open posterior thoracic/lumbar arthrodesis," *European Spine Journal*, vol. 24, no. 6, pp. S669–S710, 2015.

[40] N. Scheverin, A. Steverlynck, R. Castelli et al., "Prophylaxis of surgical site infection with vancomycin in 513 patients that underwent to lumbar fusion," *Coluna/Columna*, vol. 14, no. 3, pp. 177–180, 2015 Jul.

[41] R. G. Strom, D. Pacione, S. P. Kalhorn, and A. K. Frempong-Boadu, "Decreased risk of wound infection after posterior cervical fusion with routine local application of vancomycin powder," *Spine*, vol. 38, no. 12, pp. 991–994, 2013.

[42] R. G. Strom, D. Pacione, S. P. Kalhorn, and A. K. Frempong-Boadu, "Lumbar laminectomy and fusion with routine local application of vancomycin powder: decreased infection rate in instrumented and non-instrumented cases," *Clinical Neurology and Neurosurgery*, vol. 115, no. 9, pp. 1766–1769, 2013.

[43] B.-K. Suh, S.-H. Moon, T.-H. Kim et al., "Efficacy of antibiotics sprayed into surgical site for prevention of the contamination in the spinal surgery," *Asian Spine Journal*, vol. 9, no. 4, pp. 517–521, 2015.

[44] F. A. Sweet, M. Roh, and C. Sliva, "Intrawound application of vancomycin for prophylaxis in instrumented thoracolumbar fusions," *Spine*, vol. 36, no. 24, pp. 2084–2088, 2011.

[45] M. Takeuchi, N. Wakao, M. Kamiya, A. Hirasawa, K. Murotani, and M. Takayasu, "A double-blind randomized controlled trial of the local application of vancomycin versus ampicillin powder into the operative field for thoracic and/or lumbar fusions," *Journal of Neurosurgery: Spine*, vol. 29, no. 5, pp. 553–559, 2018.

[46] H. Takeuchi, I. Oda, S. Oshima, M. Suzuki, and M. Fujiya, "Is the administration of vancomycin to operative field effective? Studying from operative wound drainage tube culture," *European Journal of Orthopaedic Surgery and Traumatology*, vol. 30, no. 2, pp. 215–219, 2020.

[47] A. A. Theologis, G. Demirkiran, M. Callahan, M. Pekmezci, C. Ames, and V. Deviren, "Local intrawound vancomycin powder decreases the risk of surgical site infections in complex adult deformity reconstruction," *Spine*, vol. 39, no. 22, pp. 1875–1880, 2014.

[48] K. Tofuku, H. Koga, M. Yanase, and S. Komiya, "The use of antibiotic-impregnated fibrin sealant for the prevention of surgical site infection associated with spinal instrumentation," *European Spine Journal*, vol. 21, no. 10, pp. 2027–2033, 2012.

[49] V. R. Tubaki, S. Rajasekaran, and A. P. Shetty, "Effects of using intravenous antibiotic only versus local intrawound vancomycin antibiotic powder application in addition to intravenous antibiotics on postoperative infection in spine surgery in 907 patients," *Spine*, vol. 38, no. 25, pp. 2149–2155, 2013.

[50] C. Bibbo and D. V. Patel, "The effect of demineralized bone matrix-calcium sulfate with vancomycin on calcaneal fracture healing and infection rates: a prospective study," *Foot & Ankle International*, vol. 27, no. 7, pp. 487–493, 2006.

[51] K. H. Cichos, C. A. Spitler, J. H. Quade, B. A. Ponce, G. McGwin, and E. S. Ghanem, "Intrawound antibiotic powder in acetabular fracture open reduction internal fixation does not reduce surgical site infections," *Journal of Orthopaedic Trauma*, vol. 35, no. 4, pp. 198–204, 2021.

[52] M. S. Junker, A. Kurjatko, M. C. Hernandez, S. F. Heller, B. D. Kim, and H. J. Schiller, "Salvage of rib stabilization hardware with antibiotic beads," *The American Journal of Surgery*, vol. 218, 2019.

[53] J. F. Keating, P. A. Blachut, P. J. O'Brien, R. N. Meek, and H. Broekhuyse, "Reamed nailing of open tibial fractures: does the antibiotic bead pouch reduce the deep infection rate?" *Journal of Orthopaedic Trauma*, vol. 10, no. 5, pp. 298–303, 1996.

[54] C. R. Lawing, F. C. Li, and L. E. Dahners, "Local injection of aminoglycosides for prophylaxis against infection in open fractures," *Journal of Bone and Joint Surgery*, vol. 97, no. 22, pp. 1844–1851, 2014.

[55] K. Malizos, M. Blauth, A. Danita et al., "Fast-resorbable antibiotic-loaded hydrogel coating to reduce post-surgical infection after internal osteosynthesis: a multicenter randomized controlled trial," *Journal of Orthopaedics and Traumatology*, vol. 18, no. 2, pp. 159–169, 2017.

[56] H. D. Moehring, C. Gravel, M. W. Chapman, and S. A. Olson, "Comparison of antibiotic beads and intravenous antibiotics in open fractures," *Clinical Orthopaedics and Related Research*, vol. 372, pp. 254–261, 2000.

[57] R. V. O'Toole, M. Joshi, A. R. Carlini, C. K. Murray, L. E. Allen, and Y. Huang, "Effect of intrawound vancomycin powder in operatively treated high-risk tibia fractures: a randomized clinical trial," *JAMA Surgery*, vol. 156, no. 5, 2021.

[58] P. Ostermann, D. Seligson, and S. Henry, "Local antibiotic therapy for severe open fractures. A review of 1085 consecutive cases," *The Journal of Bone and Joint Surgery. British volume*, vol. 77-B, no. 1, pp. 93–97, 1995.

[59] M. T. Owen, E. M. Keener, Z. B. Hyde et al., "Intraoperative topical antibiotics for infection prophylaxis in pelvic and acetabular surgery," *Journal of Orthopaedic Trauma*, vol. 31, no. 11, pp. 589–594, 2017.

[60] M. A. Prevost, W. Cutchen, P. G. Young, and P. S. Barousse, *Infection Rates in Open Tibia Fractures with the Use Of Intraoperative Topical Vancomycin/Tobramycin Powder*- Orthopaedic Trauma Association, Rosemont, IL, USA, 2019.

[61] R. Qadir, T. Costales, M. Coale et al., "Vancomycin powder use in fractures at high risk of surgical site infection," *Journal of Orthopaedic Trauma*, vol. 35, no. 1, pp. 23–28, 2021.

[62] K. Singh, J. M. Bauer, G. Y. LaChaud, J. E. Bible, and H. R. Mir, "Surgical site infection in high-energy peri-articular tibia fractures with intra-wound vancomycin powder: a retrospective pilot study," *Journal of Orthopaedics and Traumatology*, vol. 16, no. 4, pp. 287–291, 2015.

[63] J. Vaida, D. A. Bravin, and M. Bramer, *Evaluating the Efficacy of Topical Vancomycin Powder in the Treatment of Open Lower-Extremity Fractures*Orthopaedic Trauma Association, Rosemont, IL, USA, 2019.

[64] S. Barton, "Which clinical studies provide the best evidence?" *BMJ*, vol. 321, no. 7256, pp. 255-256, 2000.

[65] P. R. Rosenbaum and D. B. Rubin, "The central role of the propensity score in observational studies for causal effects," *Biometrika*, vol. 70, no. 1, pp. 41–55, 1983.

3

Balanced Suspension versus Pillow on Preoperative Pain for Proximal Femur Fractures

Varah Yuenyongviwat ⓘD, Chonthawat Jiarasrisatien, Khanin Iamthanaporn ⓘD, Theerawit Hongnaparak, and Boonsin Tangtrakulwanich

Department of Orthopedics, Faculty of Medicine, Prince of Songkla University, Songkhla 90110, Thailand

Correspondence should be addressed to Varah Yuenyongviwat; varahortho@gmail.com

Academic Editor: Allen L. Carl

Introduction. To evaluate the efficacy of a balanced suspension system, using the Thomas splint, with Pearson attachment, compared with a pillow for preoperative pain in patients with proximal femoral fractures. *Materials and Methods.* Sixty patients with proximal femur fractures were randomized into two groups: a balanced suspension group and a pillow group. In the first group, a balanced suspension was applied after length adjustment, to match the patient's leg and thigh. In the pillow group, a pillow was placed below the patient's leg, to position the patient's hip in a semiflexion and external rotation position. Preoperative pain severity, by using a verbal numerical rating scale (VNRS), the amount of morphine consumed, and complication were recorded. *Results.* There were no differences in patient characteristics between the groups. The mean VNRS for pain was not statistically different between the groups, from the start of the study up to 48 hours. The mean of morphine consumption was not different between the groups at the start of the study, on day 1, and on day 2 ($p = 0.25$, 0.89, and 0.053, respectively). *Conclusions.* A balanced suspension did not improve patient outcome to the same level as other tractions in previous studies. Hence, other methods for reducing pain, while waiting for definite operations, should be focused on. The clinical trial is registered with TCTR20150514002.

1. Introduction

A fracture at the proximal femur usually occurs in the elderly because of osteoporosis [1]. Patients who have had these types of fractures have increased mortality rates of 8.4% to 36% in the first year after the fracture [2]. Complications of these fractures are pressure sore, pneumonia, and deep vein thrombosis, due to the immobility of the patient [3]. Surgical treatment with internal fixation or hip arthroplasty is the standard treatment for early ambulation [4]. However, in some conditions, patients are not able to have an operation on the same day of injury, due to underlying diseases that require preoperative management, or the operation must be delayed because of long operative schedules in some hospitals.

There are many options for preoperative intervention for patients with proximal femur fractures, such as skin traction, skeletal traction, or simple placement of a pillow under the injured limb [5–10]. However, none of these techniques have shown to have any superior effect of pain relief among other techniques [6].

The balanced suspension system is familiar to practitioners in clinical practice. This technique is an immobilization technique, which allows the proximal and distal parts of the fractured limb to float above the bed [11]. A balanced suspension supports the extremity and allows movement of the injured limb, along with the patient's body, when the patient moves. Therefore, patients should, theoretically, have less pain compared with other immobilization methods.

Therefore, the primary outcome of this study was the evaluation on the efficacy of balanced suspension, using the Thomas splint with Pearson attachment, on preoperative pain compared with a pillow while patients are waiting for an operation.

2. Materials and Methods

The inclusion criteria were patients aged 60 or above, with closed femoral neck fractures or intertrochanteric fractures. The excluded patients were those with multiple fractures, pathological fracture from the neoplasm and abnormal neurological system, patients allergic to the medications in this study, and patients who had cognitive impairment or could not communicate. Finally, all patients provided written informed consent.

This trial was approved by the Ethics Committee and Institutional Review Board. The procedures in this study were in accordance with the Declaration of Helsinki on ethical principles for medical research involving human subjects.

This was a prospective randomized controlled trial. Blocks of four, using a computer-generated random number, were used to randomize the patients into two groups. Allocation concealment was performed by opaque, sealed envelopes. The patients were randomized at the time of admission in the ward. Each group had 30 patients. In the first group, the fracture was immobilized by using a balanced suspension (a Thomas splint with a Pearson attachment), for the fractured limb. In other group, a polyester pillow (size: $45 \times 13 \times 62$ centimeters, weight: 1200 grams) was placed under the fractured limb.

Balanced suspension was applied after length adjustment to match the patient's leg and thigh. The proximal part was placed for support of the thigh, whilst the distal part supported the leg. The joint position of the splint was placed at the knee joint. The proximal and distal parts of the splint were hung separately with metal weights. Each part was hung with 1/12 of the patient's body weight (Figure 1). After applying the weight, the patient's ischial tuberosity floated above the bed at 1-2 centimeters. In this study, the patient's hip was placed at a 45 degree angle of flexion, and the leg was floating parallel to the bed. In the pillow group, a pillow was placed below the patient's leg, so as to position the patient's hip in a semiflexion and external rotation position.

All patients were continuously on either a balanced suspension or a pillow, from admission until hip surgery was performed. All patients received a 500 mg paracetamol tablet every six hours for pain control. Intravenous morphine (2 mg) or fentanyl (20 μg) was used as rescue medication, if the level of pain via the verbal numeric rating scale (VNRS, 0 (no pain) to 10 (worst imaginable pain)) was 4 or higher or if the patient required additional analgesics. All patients had an inserted urinary catheter, which was connected to a drainage bag in the operative room. The catheters were removed on the day after the operation.

Pain scores were recorded using the verbal numeric rating scale (VNRS), which is the standard scale for pain evaluation. Scores were validated in another study [12]. The pain scores were recorded before and immediately after positioning the patient in either the balanced suspension or by placement of the pillow and, then, subsequently at 15 mins and every 8 hr. The pain score and morphine consumption were recorded by a nurse. Both the pain score and morphine consumption from the start of the study to 48 hours were analyzed.

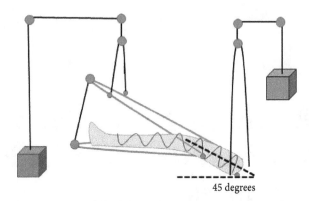

45 degrees

FIGURE 1: Setup of the balanced suspension, using the Thomas splint with the Pearson attachment.

R version 3.1.0 software (R Foundation for statistical computing, Vienna, Austria) was used for the data analyses. Patient demographic data, in terms of age, were compared by Student's t-test. The gender, injured side, American Society of Anesthesiologists (ASA) classification, and type of fracture were analyzed by the Chi-squared test. Body weight and time to surgery were evaluated using the Wilcoxon rank-sum test. The pain score and morphine consumption were compared by Student's t-test. Complications, such as pressure ulcer, urinary tract infection, pneumonia, deep vein thrombosis, and delirium, were analyzed using Fisher's exact test. The primary outcome was analyzed on the intention-to-treat.

The sample size was estimated from a previous study [7]. Twenty-seven patients, per study group, were required to detect 2 score differences in the VNRS for pain between the groups, with a significance level set at 0.05 and power set at 0.9.

3. Results

Sixty-four patients were recruited in this study, with four patients being excluded due to exclusion criteria. Finally, 60 patients were included into the study and were analyzed (Figure 2).

Differences in the demographic data, for example, age, gender, ASA classification, weight, the type of fracture, and the side of injury, were not statistically significant between the groups (Table 1).

The mean VNRS for pain was not different between the groups at the start of the study, immediately after the applied intervention, or at 15 mins, 1 hr, 8 hrs, 16 hrs, 24 hrs, 32 hrs, and 40 hrs or until 48 hours had lapsed ($p = 0.58$, 0.35, 0.55, 0.9, 0.9, 0.35, 0.78, 0.51, 0.73, and 0.23, respectively) (Figure 3).

The means of morphine consumption were not different between the groups at the start of the study (pillow group: 0.3 mg (SD, 0.6) versus the balanced suspension group: 0.6 mg (SD, 1.3), $p = 0.25$), on day 1 (pillow group: 1.8 mg (SD, 2.3) versus the balanced suspension group: 1.9 mg (SD, 3.1), $p = 0.89$), and on day 2 (pillow group: 0.9 mg (SD, 1.2) versus the balanced suspension group: 2 mg (SD, 2.5), $p = 0.053$).

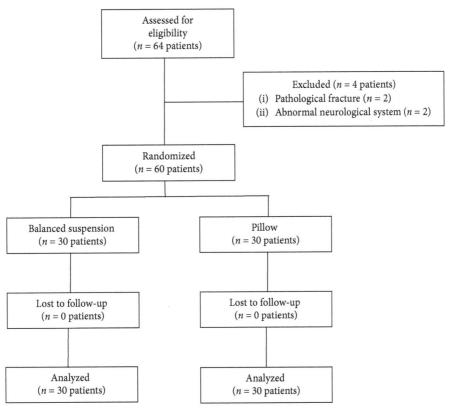

FIGURE 2: Flow study diagram.

TABLE 1: Demographic data.

Demographic data	Balanced suspension $n = 30$	Pillow $n = 30$	p value
Age (years)	79.3 (7.9)*	81.4 (7.9)*	0.30
Gender (male:female)	7 : 23	9 : 21	0.77
Weight (kg)	50 (45,55.8)**	50.5 (42,57.8)**	0.85
Side (right:left)	16 : 14	16 : 14	1.00
ASA classification (II : III)	21 : 9	19 : 11	0.58
Type of fracture			0.12
(i) Intertrochanteric fracture	13	20	
(Evan's stable/unstable)	(6/7)	(12/8)	
(ii) Femoral neck fracture	17	10	
(Garden's III/IV)	(7/10)	(4/6)	
Time to surgery (hours)	69 (44.5,93.2)**	59 (24.8,96.2)**	0.40
Treatment			0.12
(i) Internal fixation	13	20	
(ii) Hip replacement	17	10	

*Mean (SD); **Median (IQR).

The incidence of complications was higher in the pillow group (1 pulmonary embolism, 2 urinary tract infections, 1 pneumonia, 1 delirium, and 1 atelectasis) compared with the balanced suspension group (1 delirium). The incidence of complications was statistically different between the groups ($p = 0.04$).

4. Discussion

Proximal femur fractures are painful and can cause complications while the patient is waiting for definitive surgery. There are many interventions to either immobilize or adjust a limb, so

as to reduce pain in patients with skeletal fractures, for example, skin traction and a pillow, but none of them show superiority to the others [5–7]. Balanced suspension is an intervention that can reduce the gravitational load on the extremity. It was reported for use in postoperative treatment of hip fractures, as well as arthroplasties of patients [11]. This method is a preoperative option for patients who are not suitable for an early operation, due to unstable medical conditions or long operating room waiting lists in some hospitals. Therefore, the authors evaluated the efficacy of the balanced suspension technique, using the Thomas splint with the Pearson attachment, on preoperative pain compared with a pillow.

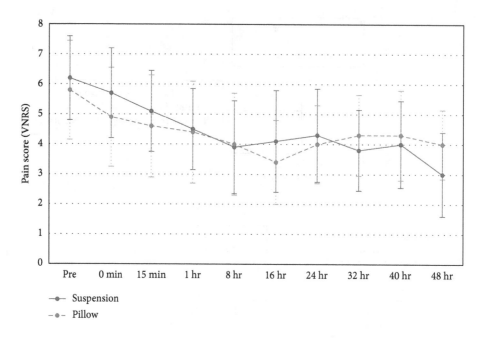

FIGURE 3: Means of the verbal numeric rating scale (VNRS) for pain by time.

Preoperative pain was not different between the balanced suspension group and the pillow group in this study. This was similar with previous randomized control studies. Anderson et al. reported no differences in terms of pain levels in patients with proximal femur fractures, as compared with skin traction and nursed free in bed [13]. Saygi et al. studied the efficacy of skin traction using 2 kg of weights, skin traction without weights, and pillow placement under the affected limb [14]. They found that patients treated with skin traction using 2 kg of weights compared with patients in a pillow group were not statistically different in terms of pain. However, patients who had skin traction applied without weights had a statistically significant reduction in pain, which they stated was possibly due to the placebo effect.

In this study, morphine consumption was not different between the balanced suspension group and the pillow group, over a period of 0 to 48 hrs. A randomized study by Yip et al. reported that the analgesic requirements were not different in patients with skin traction or a pillow below the limb, from day 0 to day 7 [15].

Complications in the balanced suspension group were statistically lower than those in the pillow group in this study. These results were contrary to a previous study by Anderson et al. who reported the same rates of complications in skin traction and nursed free in bed [13]. However, the complication rate in our study was a total complication rate, which could not be compared separately for each complication, due to the limit of the sample size. Our results might have happened by chance, or it might be possibly because the patients in the balanced suspension group could move their bodies or limbs more than those in the pillow group. Balanced suspension can, theoretically, support their limbs so as to move along with their body. Further studies with a larger number of patients would be able to evaluate complications in more detail.

This study had a number of limitations. First, our study could not blind the patients from the intervention. Second, the assessor was also not blinded to the groups of patients, due to the need to record data frequently, while the patient was on the bed with the intervention. However, the assessor was not involved with the study. Third, post hoc analysis found that this study was underpowered, due to the lower-than-expected differences in pain scores. The number of participants to detect differences in pain at 48 hours, after fracture, with a significance level set at 0.05, and power set at 0.8 should be 104 patients per group. Although there were some limitations, we believe that our study was a pilot study that provides useful information, suggesting further study in this topic.

5. Conclusions

This study found no differences in either pain scores or morphine consumption between balanced suspension and pillow groups, from the start of the study up to 48 hours. The balanced suspension did not improve patient outcome to the same level as other tractions used in previous studies. Therefore, other methods for reducing pain, while waiting for a definite operation, should be focused on.

Acknowledgments

The authors wish to thank Andrew Jonathan Tait, from the International Affairs Department, for his assistance in proofreading the English of this report. This study was funded by the Faculty of Medicine, Prince of Songkla University, Songkhla, Thailand (grant no. 58-039-11-1).

References

[1] J. A. Kanis, A. Odén, A. Odén et al., "A systematic review of hip fracture incidence and probability of fracture worldwide," *Osteoporosis International*, vol. 23, no. 9, pp. 2239–2256, 2012.

[2] B. Abrahamsen, T. van Staa, R. Ariely, M. Olson, and C. Cooper, "Excess mortality following hip fracture: a systematic epidemiological review," *Osteoporosis International*, vol. 20, no. 10, pp. 1633–1650, 2009.

[3] S. Hansson, O. Rolfson, K. Åkesson, S. Nemes, O. Leonardsson, and C. Rogmark, "Complications and patient-reported outcome after hip fracture. a consecutive annual cohort study of 664 patients," *Injury*, vol. 46, no. 11, pp. 2206–2211, 2015.

[4] N. Simunovic, P. J. Devereaux, S. Sprague et al., "Effect of early surgery after hip fracture on mortality and complications: systematic review and meta-analysis," *Canadian Medical Association Journal*, vol. 182, no. 15, pp. 1609–1616, 2010.

[5] J. Endo, S. Yamaguchi, M. Saito et al., "Efficacy of preoperative skin traction for hip fractures: a single-institution prospective randomized controlled trial of skin traction versus no traction," *Journal of Orthopaedic Science*, vol. 18, no. 2, pp. 250–255, 2013.

[6] M. J. Parker and H. H. G. Handoll, "Pre-operative traction for fractures of the proximal femur in adults," *The Cochrane Database of Systematic Reviews*, vol. 3, no. 3, Article ID CD000168, 2006.

[7] J. E. Rosen, F. S. Chen, R. Hiebert, and K. J. Koval, "Efficacy of preoperative skin traction in hip fracture patients: a prospective, randomized study," *Journal of Orthopaedic Trauma*, vol. 15, no. 2, pp. 81–85, 2001.

[8] V. Finsen, M. Børset, G. E. Buvik, and I. Hauke, "Preoperative traction in patients with hip fractures," *Injury*, vol. 23, no. 4, pp. 242–244, 1992.

[9] S. Resch and K. G. Thorngren, "Preoperative traction for hip fracture: a randomized comparison between skin and skeletal traction in 78 patients," *Acta Orthopaedica Scandinavica*, vol. 69, no. 3, pp. 277–279, 1998.

[10] M. Needoff, P. Radford, and R. Langstaff, "Preoperative traction for hip fractures in the elderly: a clinical trial," *Injury*, vol. 24, no. 5, pp. 317-318, 1993.

[11] T. R. Sprenger, "The Amsterdam suspension. Balanced suspension after hip surgery," *Clinical Orthopaedics and Related Research*, vol. 132, pp. 55-56, 1978.

[12] R. Daoust, P. Beaulieu, C. Manzini, J. M. Chauny, and G. Lavigne, "Estimation of pain intensity in emergency medicine: a validation stud," *Pain*, vol. 138, no. 3, pp. 565–570, 2008.

[13] G. Anderson, W. Harper, C. Connolly, J. Badham, N. Goodrich, and P. Gregg, "Preoperative skin traction for fractures of the proximal femur. a randomised prospective trial," *The Journal of Bone and Joint Surgery*, vol. 75, no. 5, pp. 794–796, 1993.

[14] B. Saygi, K. Ozkan, E. Eceviz, C. Tetik, and C. Sen, "Skin traction and placebo effect in the preoperative pain control of patients with collum and intertrochanteric femur fractures," *Bulletin of the NYU Hospital for Joint Diseases*, vol. 68, no. 1, pp. 15–17, 2010.

[15] D. Yip, C. Chan, P. Chiu, J. Wong, J. Kong, and J. K. F. Kong, "Why are we still using pre-operative skin traction for hip fractures?" *International Orthopaedics*, vol. 26, no. 6, pp. 361–364, 2002.

4

Challenges in the Diagnosis and Treatment of Aneurysmal Bone Cyst in Patients with Unusual Features

Ziyad M. Mohaidat [ID],[1,2] Salah R. Al-gharaibeh,[3] Osama N. Aljararhih,[3] Murad T. Nusairat,[3] and Ali A. Al-omari[1,2]

[1]Orthopedic & Spine Surgeon, King Abdullah University Hospital, Irbid 22110, Jordan
[2]Assistant Professor, Orthopedic Surgery Division, Special Surgery Department, Faculty of Medicine, Jordan University of Science and Technology, Irbid 22110, Jordan
[3]Orthopedic Surgery Resident, King Abdullah University Hospital, Jordan University of Science and Technology, Irbid 22110, Jordan

Correspondence should be addressed to Ziyad M. Mohaidat; zmmohaidat@just.edu.jo

Academic Editor: Andreas K. Demetriades

Objectives. Aneurysmal bone cyst (ABC) is a benign but locally aggressive tumor. It has several challenging features. The aim of this study is to identify challenges in the diagnosis and treatment of ABC especially in patients with unusual features. *Methods.* This retrospective study involved medical record review of primary ABC patients with one or more of the following features: unusual clinical presentation with a mass or a pathological fracture especially at an unusual age, rare locations, radiological findings suggesting other diagnoses especially sarcoma, and a nondiagnostic histopathology of biopsy samples. *Results.* 25 patients (17 males and 8 females) were included. Most patients were either younger than 10 or older than 20 years. 10 patients presented with a mass or a pathological fracture. Unusual locations include the scapula, the olecranon, the hamate, the calcaneus, and the first metatarsal bone. Extension into the epiphysis occurred in 2 patients with proximal fibula and olecranon ABCs. Two separate synchronous cysts existed in the proximal epiphysis and middiaphysis of one humerus. Radiological imaging suggested other primary diagnoses in 8 patients. Core needle biopsy was diagnostic in only 2 of 7 patients. The main treatment was intralesional resection/curettage with bone grafting. Wide resection was performed in 4 patients. Recurrence rate was 28%. Recurrence risk factors included the following: age less than 10 years, male gender, and proximal femur location. Late recurrence occurred in 3/7 patients. One patient with asymptomatic radiological recurrence showed subsequent spontaneous resolution one year later. *Conclusions.* This study presented multiple unusual features of ABC including: unusual age, rare locations, and nondiagnostic radiological and histopathological findings. These features can complicate the diagnosis and management. Given these features, especially with pathological fractures, a well-planned incision, the use of frozen section examination, and the application of either external fixation or plate osteosynthesis for fracture fixation can be recommended.

1. Introduction

Cystic lesion of the bone is one of the common challenges that might be encountered by orthopedic surgeons. Aneurysmal bone cyst (ABC) is a major differential diagnosis in such lesions. Although first described in 1942 by Jaffe and Leichstein [1, 2], the true etiology is still unknown [3].

ABC is a benign expansile osteolytic lesion that typically affects the metaphysis of long bones in young patients during their second decade of life [4–8]. Although benign, it can be locally aggressive. The radiological features can mimic both benign and malignant tumors [2].

ABC can be either primary with no preexisting lesions or secondary to other underlying pathologies [9]. This adds to the challenge in ABC diagnosis since it may be confused even after histopathological examination with more serious diagnosis especially telangiectatic osteosarcoma [10]. Cytogenetic studies can be used to confirm the diagnosis of primary ABC since specific translocations of the ubiquitin-specific protease (USP) 6 gene has been identified only in primary ABCs [4, 11, 12].

Several ABC treatment modalities had been utilized including wide resection [2, 13–15], intralesional resection/curettage with or without different adjuvants [6, 15–19], radiation [20], curopsy [21], embolization [22–24], intralesional sclerotherapy [25, 26], and more recently denosumab [27]. These methods have been reported with variable risk of recurrence, a major concern when treating ABC.

In this cohort, we present a group of patients who had one or more of the unusual features of ABC. In addition, the diagnostic and management considerations of these patients with such unusual features are presented.

2. Patients and Methods

This retrospective study involved review of the medical records of patients with primary ABC diagnosis who were treated at King Abdullah University hospital from January 2009 to June 2018. Patients included in this cohort have one or more of the following features: the less common clinical presentation with a palpable mass or with a pathological fracture especially at an unusual age, the cyst presented at rare locations, the radiological findings suggestive of other differential diagnoses especially sarcoma, and the histopathological examination, after either open or needle biopsy, suggested other diagnoses or could not exclude an underlying more serious pathology.

The management approach, outcome, and follow-up were reviewed for patients considered to have one or more of these unusual ABC features. This study was approved by the University Research Committee.

3. Results

A total of 25 patients were included as having one or more of the unusual features of ABC. There were 17 males and 8 females. Their average age at the time of diagnosis was 12.8 years (3 to 32 years). 12 patients were younger than 10 years, among which 7 patients were 5 or less years of age. While 7 patients presented during the second decade, 6 patients were older than 20 years.

Regarding clinical presentation, most patients (15/25) presented with localized pain. Four patients had a palpable mass as their initial complaint (Figure 1(a)). While three patients had their initial presentation with a pathological fracture (Figure 2(a)), another three patients were referred with a pathological fracture at the time of recurrence.

The anatomical location of the reported cysts included long and flat bones (Figure 3). The involved flat bones were the scapula, the hamate, the calcaneus, and the iliac bones. Although confined within the cortices of the hamate and calcaneus, the cysts involving the iliac bone and the scapulae had a periosteal location (Figure 1(b)). Within long bones, about half of the patients (13/25) had the cyst confined to the metaphysis. However, in one patient with distal tibial metaphyseal ABC (Figure 4), the cyst had extracortical extension into the surrounding soft tissue. The cyst was

located in the diaphysis in two patients with humerus and distal femur ABCs (Figure 2(a)). Epiphyseal extension occurred in two patients with fibular and olecranon ABCs (Figures 5(a) and 5(b)). In one patient with humerus ABC, two synchronous separate cysts existed in the proximal epiphysis and middiaphysis (Figure 6).

Radiological workup included primarily X-ray imaging. CT, MRI, and bone scan were done selectively. The radiological evaluation suggested ABC as the primary differential diagnosis in 17/25 patients. Sarcoma was the primary radiological diagnosis in two patients (Figures 1(b) and 4). Giant cell tumor of bone was the primary differential diagnosis in three patients with proximal fibula, iliac bone, and one scapular cyst. In 3 patients with proximal femur cyst; fibrous dysplasia was suggested in one cyst while unicameral bone cyst was the main radiological diagnosis in the other two cysts.

All patients in this study had a final pathological diagnosis of primary ABC among which two patients with distal humerus (Figure 7(a)) and distal tibia cysts (Figure 4) showed the histologic solid variant of ABC. In 15 patients, no biopsy prior to definitive surgery was obtained. However, frozen section examination was used in 6 patients before proceeding with further intralesional resection/curettage. Among these 15 patients, one patient, with proximal femur cyst (Figure 8(a)), was diagnosed with benign fibrous histiocytoma. However, 2 years later, he presented with a pathological fracture due to recurrence (Figure 8(b)). Histopathology at this time confirmed the diagnosis of ABC.

Biopsy methods included open and core needle biopsy in 3 and 7 patients, respectively. While open biopsy confirmed ABC diagnosis in 2 patients, a more serious pathology could not be excluded in the third patient. Core needle biopsy provided the diagnosis in 2 patients while it was inadequate in 2 other patients. In the remaining 3 patients, the diagnoses were unicameral bone cyst, nonossifying fibroma, and giant cell tumor of bone.

As for treatment, wide resection was performed in 4 patients. Intralesional resection/curettage with bone grafting was done in the rest of the patients. No adjuvants were added after curettage in 10 patients. Different adjuvants including bone cement, liquid nitrogen, and hydrogen peroxide were used in 1, 3, and 7 patients, respectively. Different bone graft options including demineralized bone matrix (DBM), allograft chips, autograft, and tricalcium phosphate were used either alone or in combination. Different orthopedic hardware options were used including plates (Figure 2(b)), external fixators (Figure 8(c)), and intramedullary nails.

The follow-up period of these patients after treatment ranged from 12 months to more than 120 months with an average of 55.2 months. While none of the patients who had wide resection as their treatment developed a recurrence, 7 of the 21 patients who were treated with intralesional resection/curettage and bone grafting developed at least one recurrence (Table 1). Their first recurrence occurred at an average of 29 months after surgery. Three patients presented with a pathological fracture at the time of recurrence. Subsequent management of the recurrent ABCs involved mainly recurettage with bone grafting. Elastic intramedullary

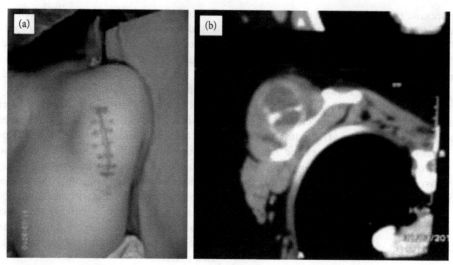

FIGURE 1: (a) Posterior Scapular mass with broad scar after resection attempt. (b) Axial CT showing soft tissue mass extending posterior to the scapula.

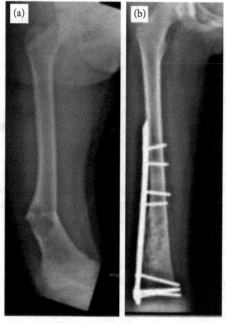

FIGURE 2: (a) AP X-ray with pathological fracture through a diaphyseal ABC. (b) AP X-ray after intralesional resection/curettage followed by fracture fixation with plate and screws.

nails, plate with screws, and external fixators were used to fix the concurrent pathological fractures. However, the distal humerus ABC received no treatment since the patient was asymptomatic with almost complete healing of the cyst on radiographs repeated one year later (Figure 7(b)).

4. Discussion

This study investigates the different unusual clinical, radiological, and histopathological features of ABC that can reflect significantly on the management approach.

In this study, most patients (18/25) were either younger than 10 years of age or older than 20 years. This age can represent an unusual age since the peak incidence of ABC occurs in the second decade of life [7, 8, 23, 28, 29]. ABC might not be included in the initial differential diagnosis especially in older patients given that more than 90% of ABC occurs before the age of 20 years [30, 31]. In addition, the younger age can complicate the management with increased risk of recurrence [32].

ABC most commonly presents with a localized pain [13, 31, 33]. However, the less common presentation as a palpable mass or with a pathological fracture can further complicate the diagnosis and treatment [2, 6, 13, 23, 31, 34, 35]. Pathological fracture as an initial ABC presentation, as in 3 patients in this series, has been reported with variable rates and controversial management approaches by different series [2, 6, 14, 31, 34–39]. In addition, ABC presentation with a palpable mass especially at an older age or unusual location for ABC may be confused with more common pathologies. For instance, one patient with a scapular ABC (Figure 1(a)) was referred after an attempted excisional biopsy of what was thought to be a possible lipoma overlying the scapula.

The unusual ABC locations in this study include the scapula, the olecranon, the hamate, the calcaneus, and the first metatarsal bone [2, 8, 40–42]. In these locations, ABC diagnosis might not be considered. ABC typically affects the metaphysis of long bones [9]. Hence, when a cyst is located in the diaphysis or extending into the epiphysis, other diagnoses can be considered more typical. Also, as was observed in one patient, when two separate synchronous cysts exist in a single bone (Figure 6), ABC diagnosis can be excluded since multicentric ABC is extremely rare [43, 44].

ABC has a variable radiological appearance with no pathognomonic radiological features [2, 4, 45]. Although in most patients (17/25), the radiological diagnosis was concordant with the final histopathological diagnosis of ABC, other diagnoses were suggested in the remaining patients. This can complicate the radiological and histopathological

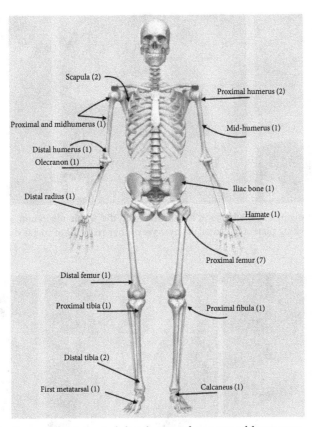

FIGURE 3: Anatomical distribution of aneurysmal bone cysts.

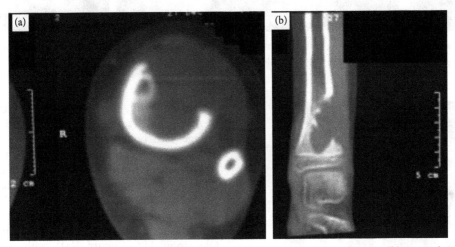

FIGURE 4: (a) Axial CT showing destruction of the anterior tibial cortex with extension into soft tissue. (b) Coronal CT showing ill-defined distal tibial lesion with cortical destruction.

correlation especially when sarcoma is suggested due to cortical destruction or soft tissue extension (Figures 1(b) and 4). In such situations, cytogenetic studies, although not performed in this study, can be suggested to confirm the diagnosis of primary rather than secondary ABC.

The role of image guided needle biopsy prior to the definitive surgery is debated [2, 4]. Core needle biopsies done in 7 patients were diagnostic in only 2 patients. This might be explained by the fact that the tissue obtained might not be adequate or representative of the whole lesion.

Although frozen section histopathology did not provide the definitive diagnosis in patients included in this cohort, it was helpful to confirm the benign nature of the lesion. Therefore, it can be a reasonable step prior to proceeding with more definitive surgery.

The optimal treatment of ABC is controversial [13, 33], which can be related to different experiences of the treating physicians in different centers (Table 2). Due to the continuously evolving treatment options of ABC, selective arterial embolization as a less invasive treatment modality can

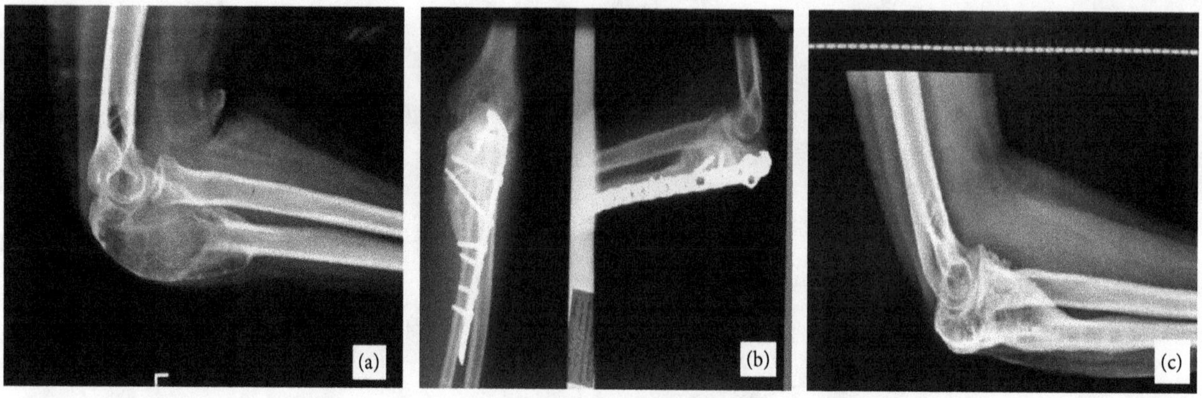

FIGURE 5: (a) Lateral elbow X-ray showing expansile cystic lesion involving the whole olecranon. (b) AP and lateral elbow X-rays after surgery with olecranon anatomical locking plate. (c) Lateral X-ray 4 years after removal of metal showing complete healing of the lesion.

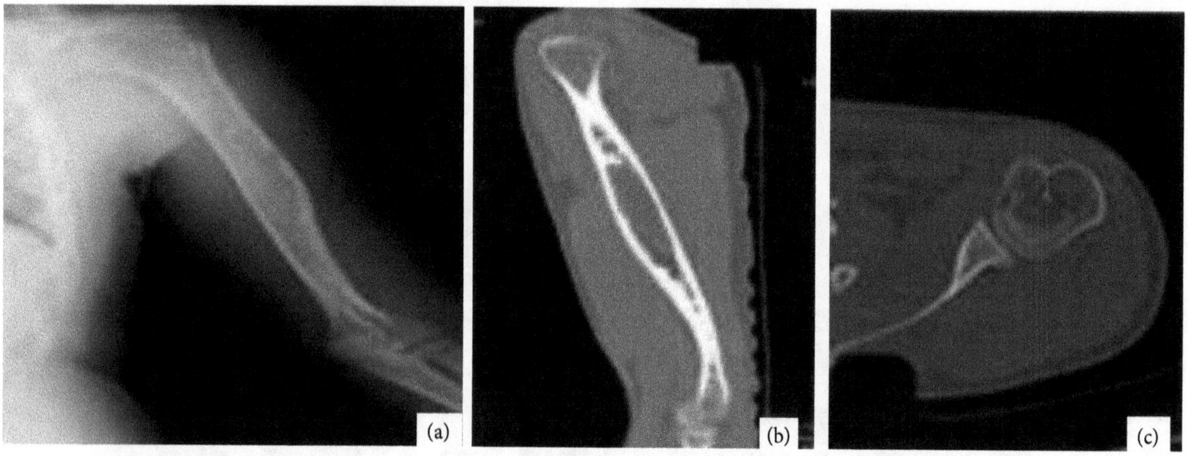

FIGURE 6: (a) AP X-ray of the humerus showing cystic lesions involving the proximal and midhumerus. (b, c) Sagittal and axial CT for the same patient showing expansile cysts of the mid and proximal humerus, respectively.

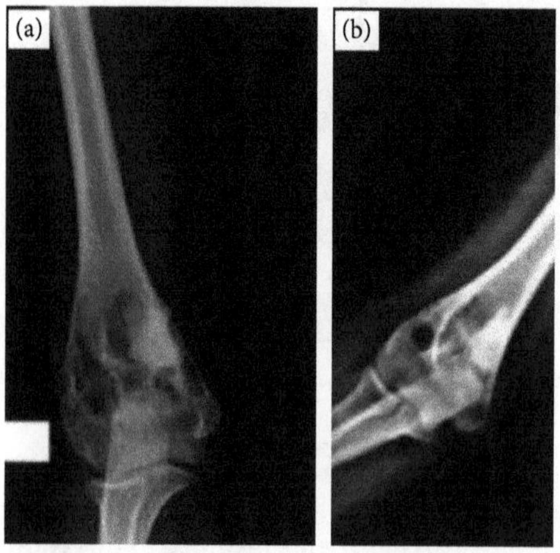

FIGURE 7: (a) AP X-ray of the distal humerus solid variant ABC about 4 years after surgery showing signs of recurrence. (b) X-ray repeated one year later with no further intervention showing almost complete healing and remodeling of the cyst.

be considered a suitable initial option especially with the encouraging results of the more recent large series of ABC treatment with embolization [22, 23]. Similar to other several studies [2, 4, 6, 8, 15, 19, 46–48], the main treatment of ABC in this series involved intralesional resection/curettage with bone graft. However, the unusual locations added to the therapeutic challenge. In the distal humerus ABC, the anatomy of the distal humeral metaphysis made it difficult to adequately curette cyst walls especially using single anteromedial approach. Also, in the patient with the double humerus ABCs, the cysts were approached by two separate bone windows through deltopectoral approach. Olecranon ABC (Figure 5(a)), with almost complete involvement of the articular surface, did add to the management challenge since failure to preserve the joint can be associated with significant morbidity. Adding tricortical iliac crest graft held with a locking plate (Figure 5(b)) was helpful to support the articular surface and preserve the joint (Figure 5(c))

Wide resection of ABC can be associated with significant morbidity. However, it can be indicated especially in expandable locations in which significant functional deficit is not expected after resection [4, 49, 50]. In this study, wide excision was performed for ABCs involving the scapula, the iliac bone, and the proximal fibular epiphysis. Scapular ABC patients presented at an older age for ABC. In addition, their MRI scans

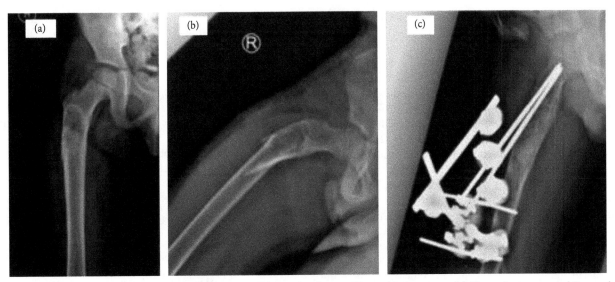

FIGURE 8: (a) AP Femur X-ray with proximal femur cyst diagnosed as benign fibrous histiocytoma. (b) The patient presented 2 years later with a pathological fracture. Final pathology revealed ABC. (c) Lateral X-ray of proximal femur with external fixator showing partial healing of the cyst and a well-maintained fracture reduction about 6 weeks after surgery.

TABLE 1: Clinical and management features of the 7 recurrent ABC patients.

Location	Age (years)	Sex	Adjuvant	Bone graft	Time to first recurrence (months)
Distal Humerus[S]	8	F	NO	Chips, Vitoss	48
Proximal Humerus	4	M	H_2O_2	Chips	24
Distal Tibia[S]	8	M	LN	Chips	6
Proximal Femur[P]	13	M	Cement	BC	55
Proximal Femur[P]	3	M	No	DBM	24
Proximal Femur	5	M	LN	DBM, chips	12
Proximal Humerus[P]	8	M	No	DBM	37

M: male; F: female; H_2O_2: hydrogen peroxide; LN: liquid nitrogen; BC: bone cement; DBM: demineralized bone matrix; chips: allograft chips; Vitoss: calcium triphosphate bone graft substitute. [S]Solid ABC variant. [P]Pathological fracture.

TABLE 2: ABC treatment modalities and their recurrence rates reported by different series.

Authors	Year	Main treatment	Patients (N)	Recurrence rate (%)
Vergel De dios et al. [6]	1992	Curettage and bone graft	124	21.8
Marcove et al. [15]	1995	Curettage and cryosurgery	51	17.6
Marcove et al. [15]	1995	Curettage and bone graft	44	59
Mankin et al. [2]	2005	Curettage and allograft	101	21
Rastogi et al. [25]	2006	Sclerotherapy	72	2.7
Varshney et al. [26]	2010	Sclerotherapy	45	6.7
Rossi et al. [23]	2010	Selective arterial embolization	36	39
Steffner et al. [16]	2011	Curettage, burring, and argon beam coagulation	40	7.5
Reddy et al. [21]	2014	Curopsy	102	18.6
Erol et al. [14]	2015	Curettage, burring, and graft	59	7
Terzi et al. [24]	2017	Selective arterial embolization	23	26
Rossi et al. [22]	2017	Selective arterial embolization	88	18.2
Zhu et al. [20]	2017	Radiation	12	0
Palmerini et al. [27]	2018	Denosumab	9	22.2
Aiba et al. [17]	2018	Endoscopic curettage	30	10
Syvänen et al. [18]	2018	Curettage and bioactive glass	18	11

showed heterogenous soft tissue mass which was also demonstrated in the iliac bone ABC. Needle biopsy of the ABC involving the proximal fibular epiphysis suggested giant cell tumor of bone rather than ABC. Given these features together with the fact that ABC can be associated with an underlying

sarcoma, wide excision in such expandable locations can be the treatment of choice.

As for pathological fractures treatment, several authors had suggested that a formal histopathological diagnosis should be obtained prior to further interventions [36–38]. Since a more serious pathology may not be excluded at least initially even after an open or a needle biopsy of a suspected ABC, our treatment included a planned surgical approach to avoid further tissue planes contamination. This can make wide resection still possible should the final pathology show an underlying primary sarcoma. In addition, we used frozen section examination before proceeding with further definitive intralesional resection/curettage. Also, we used either external fixation (Figure 8(c)) or plate osteosynthesis (Figure 2(b)) rather than intramedullary devices for fracture fixation so as to minimize further contamination of the medullary canal.

Recurrence rates after different therapeutic approaches vary widely, ranging from 0% to more than 59% [2, 4, 8, 15, 19, 29, 35, 49–52]. Recurrence rate in this study was 28%. In this study, most patients with recurrence were males and were less than 10 years of age. The proximal femur was the most frequent location involved while ABC in the unusual locations including the scapula, the olecranon, the hamate, the calcaneus, and the first metatarsal bone showed no recurrence during follow-up. These risk factors are similar to what is reported by other studies [2, 32]. It is worth mentioning that none of the patients who had wide resection had a recurrence. However, one third of patients treated with intralesional resection/curettage and bone graft (Table 1) developed a recurrence. Based on these findings, it may be recommended that whenever possible, wide resection be considered as the first option. Also, a closer follow-up can be recommended when treating a young male with ABC especially in the proximal femur. Additionally, a pathological fracture at the site of a previous treated ABC can be considered a sign of recurrence.

The rare atypical solid variant of ABC has been reported by several authors to have a better prognosis with lower recurrence risk compared to the usual ABC [31, 53–55]. However, Johnson and Caracciolo [56] reported increased recurrence risk of the solid ABC variant. In this study, both solid ABC patients developed a recurrence (Table 1). This can be explained by the inadequate curettage especially in the distal humerus ABC as already mentioned. In addition, both patients were younger than 10 years of age.

Late recurrence, more than 3 years after treatment (Table 1), was observed in 3 patients. This can represent an unusual feature given that most recurrences occur during the first 2 years after treatment [6, 33]. Long-term follow-up might be warranted given the possibility of late recurrence. Interestingly, the distal humerus ABC patient showed an unusual asymptomatic radiological recurrence more than 4 years after surgery which resolved one year later with no further treatment (Figure 7). This might represent the atypical ABC behavior of spontaneous resolution [57].

5. Conclusions

This study presented multiple unusual features of ABC including unusual age, rare locations, and nondiagnostic radiological and histopathological findings. These features can complicate both the diagnosis and management of ABC. Given these features, especially with pathological fractures, a well-planned incision, the use of frozen section examination, and the application of either external fixation or plate

osteosynthesis for fracture fixation can be recommended. Recurrence is common especially in young males with proximal femur cyst. Closer follow-up can be warranted.

Authors' Contributions

ZM was responsible for data collection, analysis, study design, and manuscript writing; SA contributed to data collection and manuscript writing; MN was responsible for study design, data collection, and manuscript writing; and OA and AA analyzed the data and wrote the manuscript.

References

[1] H. L. Jaffe and L. Lichtenstein, "Solitary unicameral bone cyst: with emphasis on the roentgen picture, the pathologic appearance and the pathogenesis." *Archives of Surgery*, vol. 44, no. 6, pp. 1004–1025, 1942.

[2] H. J. Mankin, F. J. Hornicek, E. Ortiz-Cruz, J. Villafuerte, and M. C. Gebhardt, "Aneurysmal bone cyst: a review of 150 patients," *Journal of Clinical Oncology*, vol. 23, no. 27, pp. 6756–6762, 2005.

[3] H. Sasaki, S. Nagano, H. Shimada et al., "Diagnosing and discriminating between primary and secondary aneurysmal bone cysts," *Oncology Letters*, vol. 13, no. 4, pp. 2290–2296, 2017.

[4] H. Y. Park, S. K. Yang, W. L. Sheppard et al., "Current management of aneurysmal bone cysts," *Current Reviews in Musculoskeletal Medicine*, vol. 9, no. 4, pp. 435–444, 2016.

[5] T. B. Rapp, J. P. Ward, and M. J. Alaia, "Aneurysmal bone cyst," *Journal of the American Academy of Orthopaedic Surgeons*, vol. 20, no. 4, pp. 233–241, 2012.

[6] A. M. Vergel De Dios, J. R. Bond, T. C. Shives, R. A. McLeod, and K. K. Unni, "Aneurysmal bone cyst. A clinicopathologic study of 238 cases," *Cancer*, vol. 69, no. 12, pp. 2921–2931, 1992.

[7] A. Leithner, R. Windhager, S. Lang, O. A. Haas, F. Kainberger, and R. Kotz, "Aneurysmal bone cyst. A population based epidemiologic study and literature review," *Clinical Orthopaedics and Related Research*, vol. 363, pp. 176–179, 1999.

[8] H. W. B. Schreuder, R. P. H. Veth, M. Pruszczynski, J. A. M. Lemmens, H. S. Koops, and W. M. Molenaar, "Aneurysmal bone cysts treated by curettage, cryotherapy and bone grafting," *Journal of Bone and Joint Surgery. British volume*, vol. 79, no. 1, pp. 20–25, 1997.

[9] M. J. Kransdorf and D. E. Sweet, "Aneurysmal bone cyst: concept, controversy, clinical presentation, and imaging," *American Journal of Roentgenology*, vol. 164, no. 3, pp. 573–580, 1995.

[10] N. A. Sangle and L. J. Layfield, "Telangiectatic osteosarcoma," *Archives of Pathology & Laboratory Medicine*, vol. 136, no. 5, pp. 572–576, 2012.

[11] C. Galant, P.-L. Docquier, G. Ameye, Y. Guiot, J. Malghem, and H. A. Poirel, "Aneurysmal bone cystic lesions: value of genomic studies," *Acta Orthopaedica Belgica*, vol. 82, no. 4, pp. 768–778, 2016.

[12] A. M. Oliveira, A. R. Perez-Atayde, C. Y. Inwards et al., "USP6 and CDH11 oncogenes identify the neoplastic cell in primary aneurysmal bone cysts and are absent in so-called secondary aneurysmal bone cysts," *The American Journal of Pathology* vol. 165, no. 5, pp. 1773–1780, 2004.

[13] P. Tsagozis and O. Brosjö, "Current strategies for the treatment of aneurysmal bone cysts," *Orthopedic Reviews*, vol. 7, no. 4, p. 6182, 2015.

[14] B. Erol, M. O. Topkar, E. Caliskan, and R. Erbolukbas, "Surgical treatment of active or aggressive aneurysmal bone cysts in children," *Journal of Pediatric Orthopaedics B*, vol. 24, no. 5, pp. 461–468, 2015.

[15] R. C. Marcove, D. S. Sheth, S. Takemoto, and J. H. Healey, "The treatment of aneurysmal bone cyst," *Clinical Orthopaedics and Related Research*, vol. 311, pp. 157–163, 1995.

[16] R. J. Steffner, C. Liao, G. Stacy et al., "Factors associated with recurrence of primary aneurysmal bone cysts: is argon beam coagulation an effective adjuvant treatment?," *Journal of Bone and Joint Surgery-American Volume*, vol. 93, no. 21, pp. e122(1)–e122(9), 2011.

[17] H. Aiba, M. Kobayashi, Y. Waguri-Nagaya et al., "Treatment of aneurysmal bone cysts using endoscopic curettage," *BMC Musculoskeletal Disorders*, vol. 19, no. 1, p. 268, 2018.

[18] J. Syvänen, Y. Nietosvaara, I. Kohonen et al., "Treatment of aneurysmal bone cysts with bioactive glass in children," *Scandinavian Journal of Surgery*, vol. 107, no. 1, pp. 76–81, 2018.

[19] E. H. M. Wang, M. L. Marfori, M. V. T. Serrano, and D. A. Rubio, "Is curettage and high-speed burring sufficient treatment for aneurysmal bone cysts?," *Clinical Orthopaedics and Related Research*, vol. 472, no. 11, pp. 3483–3488, 2014.

[20] S. Zhu, K. E. Hitchcock, and W. M. Mendenhall, "Radiation therapy for aneurysmal bone cysts," *American Journal of Clinical Oncology*, vol. 40, no. 6, pp. 621–624, 2017.

[21] K. I. A. Reddy, F. Sinnaeve, C. L. Gaston, R. J. Grimer, and S. R. Carter, "Aneurysmal bone cysts: do simple treatments work?," *Clinical Orthopaedics and Related Research*, vol. 472, no. 6, pp. 1901–1910, 2014.

[22] G. Rossi, A. F. Mavrogenis, G. Facchini et al., "How effective is embolization with N-2-butyl-cyanoacrylate for aneurysmal bone cysts?," *International Orthopaedics*, vol. 41, no. 8, pp. 1685–1692, 2017.

[23] G. Rossi, E. Rimondi, T. Bartalena et al., "Selective arterial embolization of 36 aneurysmal bone cysts of the skeleton with N-2-butyl cyanoacrylate," *Skeletal Radiology*, vol. 39, no. 2, pp. 161–167, 2010.

[24] S. Terzi, A. Gasbarrini, M. Fuiano et al., "Efficacy and safety of selective arterial embolization in the treatment of aneurysmal bone cyst of the mobile spine," *SPINE*, vol. 42, no. 15, pp. 1130–1138, 2017.

[25] S. Rastogi, M. K. Varshney, V. Trikha, S. A. Khan, B. Choudhury, and R. Safaya, "Treatment of aneurysmal bone cysts with percutaneous sclerotherapy using polidocanol," *Journal of Bone and Joint Surgery. British Volume*, vol. 88, no. 9, pp. 1212–1216, 2006.

[26] M. K. Varshney, S. Rastogi, S. A. Khan, and V. Trikha, "Is sclerotherapy better than intralesional excision for treating aneurysmal bone cysts?," *Clinical Orthopaedics and Related Research®*, vol. 468, no. 6, pp. 1649–1659, 2010.

[27] E. Palmerini, P. Ruggieri, A. Angelini et al., "Denosumab in patients with aneurysmal bone cysts: a case series with preliminary results," *Tumori Journal*, vol. 104, no. 5, pp. 344–351, 2018.

[28] S. Sharma, P. Gupta, S. Sharma, M. Singh, and D. Singh, "Primary aneurysmal bone cyst of talus," *Journal of Research in Medical Sciences*, vol. 17, no. 12, pp. 1192–1194, 2012.

[29] A. R. Ramírez and R. P. Stanton, "Aneurysmal bone cyst in 29 children," *Journal of Pediatric Orthopaedics*, vol. 22, no. 4, pp. 533–539, 2002.

[30] J. Cottalorda and S. Bourelle, "Modern concepts of primary aneurysmal bone cyst," *Archives of Orthopaedic and Trauma Surgery*, vol. 127, no. 2, pp. 105–114, 2007.

[31] E. Mascard, A. Gomez-Brouchet, and K. Lambot, "Bone cysts: unicameral and aneurysmal bone cyst," *Orthopaedics & Traumatology: Surgery & Research*, vol. 101, no. 1, pp. S119–S127, 2015.

[32] H. Zehetgruber, B. Bittner, D. Gruber et al., "Prevalence of aneurysmal and solitary bone cysts in young patients," *Clinical Orthopaedics and Related Research*, vol. 439, pp. 136–143, 2005.

[33] O. Hauschild, M. Lüdemann, M. Engelhardt et al., "Aneurysmal bone cyst (ABC): treatment options and proposal of a follow-up regime," *Acta Orthopaedica Belgica*, vol. 82, no. 3, pp. 474–483, 2016.

[34] J. Cottalorda, R. Kohler, F. Chotel et al., "Recurrence of aneurysmal bone cysts in young children: a multicentre study," *Journal of Pediatric Orthopaedics B*, vol. 14, no. 3, pp. 212–218, 2005.

[35] C. P. Gibbs, M. C. Hefele, T. D. Peabody, A. G. Montag, V. Aithal, and M. A. Simon, "Aneurysmal bone cyst of the extremities. Factors related to local recurrence after curettage with a high-speed burr," *Journal of Bone & Joint Surgery*, vol. 81, no. 12, pp. 1671–1678, 1999.

[36] F. Canavese, A. Samba, and M. Rousset, "Pathological fractures in children: diagnosis and treatment options," *Orthopaedics & Traumatology: Surgery & Research*, vol. 102, no. 1, pp. S149–S159, 2016.

[37] W. F. M. Jackson, T. N. Theologis, C. L. M. H. Gibbons, S. Mathews, and G. Kambouroglou, "Early management of pathological fractures in children," *Injury*, vol. 38, no. 2, pp. 194–200, 2007.

[38] C. B. R. De Mattos, O. Binitie, and J. P. Dormans, "Pathological fractures in children," *Bone & Joint Research*, vol. 1, no. 10, pp. 272–280, 2012.

[39] E. J. Ortiz, M. H. Isler, J. E. Navia, and R. Canosa, "Pathologic fractures in children," *Clinical Orthopaedics and Related Research*, vol. 432, pp. 116–126, 2005.

[40] O. E. Aycan, İ. Y. Çamurcu, D. Özer, Y. Arıkan, and Y. S. Kabukçuoğlu, "Unusual localizations of unicameral bone cysts and aneurysmal bone cysts: a retrospective review of 451 cases," *Acta Orthopaedica Belgica*, vol. 81, no. 2, pp. 209–212, 2015.

[41] Y. Kabukcuoglu, F. Kabukcuoglu, M. Kucukkaya, and U. Kuzgun, "Aneurysmal bone cyst in the hamate," *The American Journal of Orthopedics*, vol. 32, no. 2, pp. 101-102, 2003.

[42] A. F. Mavrogenis, G. Rossi, E. Rimondi, and P. Ruggieri, "Aneurysmal bone cyst of the acromion treated by selective arterial embolization," *Journal of Pediatric Orthopaedics B*, vol. 20, no. 5, pp. 354–358, 2011.

[43] S. Scheil-Bertram, E. Hartwig, S. Brüderlein et al., "Metachronous and multiple aneurysmal bone cysts: a rare variant of primary aneurysmal bone cysts," *Virchows Archiv*, vol. 444, no. 3, pp. 293–299, 2004.

[44] M. Sundaram, D. J. McDonald, C. K. Steigman, and T. Bocchini, "Metachronous multiple aneurysmal bone cysts," *Skeletal Radiology*, vol. 26, no. 9, pp. 564–567, 1997.

[45] A. Mahnken, C. Nolte-Ernsting, J. Wildberger et al., "Aneurysmal bone cyst: value of MR imaging and conventional radiography," *European Radiology*, vol. 13, no. 5, pp. 1118–1124, 2002.

[46] W. M. Mendenhall, R. A. Zlotecki, C. P. Gibbs, J. D. Reith, M. T. Scarborough, and N. P. Mendenhall, "Aneurysmal bone cyst," *American Journal of Clinical Oncology*, vol. 29, no. 3, pp. 311–315, 2006.

[47] B. Kececi, L. Küçük, A. Isayev, and D. Sabah, "Effect of adjuvant therapies on recurrence in aneurysmal bone cysts," *Acta Orthopaedica et Traumatologica Turcica*, vol. 48, no. 5, pp. 500–506, 2014.

[48] M. Campanacci, R. Capanna, and P. Picci, "Unicameral and aneurysmal bone cysts," *Clinical Orthopaedics and Related Research*, vol. 204, pp. 25–36, 1986.

[49] P. Flont, M. Kolacinska-Flont, and K. Niedzielski, "A comparison of cyst wall curettage and en bloc excision in the treatment of aneurysmal bone cysts," *World Journal of Surgical Oncology*, vol. 11, no. 1, p. 109, 2013.

[50] J. E. Cummings, R. A. Smith, and R. K. Heck, "Argon beam coagulation as adjuvant treatment after curettage of aneurysmal bone cysts: a preliminary study," *Clinical Orthopaedics and Related Research®*, vol. 468, no. 1, pp. 231–237, 2010.

[51] S. P. Peeters, I. C. M. Van der Geest, J. W. J. de Rooy, R. P. H. Veth, and H. W. B. Schreuder, "Aneurysmal bone cyst: the role of cryosurgery as local adjuvant treatment," *Journal of Surgical Oncology*, vol. 100, no. 8, pp. 719–724, 2009.

[52] J. P. Dormans, B. G. Hanna, D. R. Johnston, and J. S. Khurana, "Surgical treatment and recurrence rate of aneurysmal bone cysts in children," *Clinical Orthopaedics and Related Research*, vol. 421, pp. 205–211, 2004.

[53] A. Singh, A. Majeed, S. Mallick, S. A. Khan, and A. R. Mridha, "Solid variant of aneurysmal bone cyst masquerading as malignancy," *Journal of Clinical and Diagnostic Research*, vol. 11, no. 7, pp. ED35–ED36, 2017.

[54] F. Bertoni, P. Bacchini, R. Capanna et al., "Solid variant of aneurysmal bone cyst," *Cancer*, vol. 71, no. 3, pp. 729–734, 1993.

[55] K. Sato, H. Sugiura, S. Yamamura, M. Takahashi, T. Nagasaka, and T. Fukatsu, "Solid variant of an aneurysmal bone cyst (giant cell reparative granuloma) of the 3rd lumbar vertebra," *Nagoya Journal of Medical Science*, vol. 59, no. 3-4, pp. 159–165, 1996.

[56] E. M. Johnson and J. T. Caracciolo, "Solid variant aneurysmal bone cyst in the distal fibular metaphysis: radiologic and pathologic challenges to diagnosis," *Radiology Case Reports*, vol. 12, no. 3, pp. 555–559, 2017.

[57] D. Louahem, P. Kouyoumdjian, I. Ghanem et al., "Active aneurysmal bone cysts in children: possible evolution after biopsy," *Journal of Children's Orthopaedics*, vol. 6, no. 4, pp. 333–338, 2012.

5

The Results of Unstable Intertrochanteric Femur Fracture Treated with Proximal Femoral Nail Antirotation-2 with respect to Different Greater Trochanteric Entry Points

Sharan Mallya,[1] **Surendra U. Kamath** ⓘ**,**[1] **Rajendra Annappa,**[1] **Nithin Elliot Nazareth,**[2] **Krithika Kamath,**[3] **and Pragya Tyagi**[3]

[1]Department of Orthopaedics, Kasturba Medical College, Mangalore, Manipal Academy of Higher Education, Manipal, India
[2]Department of Orthopaedics, Father Muller Medical College Hospital, Mangalore, India
[3]Kasturba Medical College, Mangalore, Manipal Academy of Higher Education, Manipal, India

Correspondence should be addressed to Surendra U. Kamath; surendra.kamath@manipal.edu

Academic Editor: Benjamin Blondel

Background. Proximal femoral nail antirotation-2 (PFNA-2) has been widely used to treat intertrochanteric fractures with varied outcomes in the previous studies. The entry point of the nail plays an important role in achieving acceptable reduction, stable fixation, and avoiding implant related complications. This study was proposed to determine the optimal greater trochanteric entry point for PFNA-2 in unstable intertrochanteric femur fractures. *Methods.* We conducted an observational study on 40 patients with unstable intertrochanteric fracture treated with PFNA-2 implant in a tertiary care hospital. The patients were grouped into two based on the entry point: group L for lateral and group M for medial entry. Randomization was carried out by assigning the patients to the group by alternate allocation. The quality of reduction, tip apex distance, Cleveland index, and all the complications were noted. The final follow-up was conducted at six months. The functional outcome was evaluated using modified Harris hip score. The data analysis was performed using Student's *t*-test, chi square test, and Mann–Whitney test. A *P* value below 0.05 was considered significant. *Results.* Forty patients with 20 patients treated with medial entry point were included in group M and 20 patients in group L with lateral entry point. The group L had an average tip apex distance of 20.53 and group M had 20.02 (*P* = 0.8). The complication of screw back out was seen in 3 out of 4 patients with poor reduction in group L. As per the Cleveland index, 6 patients in each group had suboptimal position and 4 out of 6 patients in group L with suboptimal position had screw back out. The lateral cortex impingement was seen in 14 patients of group L and 6 patients in group M with significant comparison (*P* = 0.01). Three patients in group L had varus collapse with screw back out. Also, none in group M (0.05). The average modified Harris hip score in group L at six months follow-up was 71.94 and 76.8 in group M (*P* = 0.84). *Conclusion.* Overall, to achieve good quality of fixation and reducing damage to gluteus medius entry point for PFNA-2 should be 5 mm medial to the greater trochanter tip.

1. Introduction

Intertrochanteric femur fracture is more common among elderly patients with osteoporosis and surgically fixing the fracture has been the accepted method to gain reduction and early mobilization [1]. Literature suggests that intra-medullary nailing is one of the best choices for surgical fixation and has better clinical outcomes when compared to arthroplasty [2–4]. Proximal femoral nail antirotation-2

(PFNA-2) is the newer design and has been widely used to treat this fracture [5]. The results obtained with this implant in previous studies had varied outcome [6, 7]. This may be attributed to many factors like old age, fracture type, implant design, quality of reduction, and fixation. The entry point plays an important role in acceptable reduction, stable fixation, and avoiding implant-related complications [8, 9]. It has been suggested in a study that lateral entry point causes damage to the gluteus muscle tendon while reaming of intramedullary nail insertion. The study on anatomy of greater trochanter has concluded that entry point should be at the rear tip to accommodate the implant in proximal femoral medullary canal curvature [10]. This study was proposed to determine the optimal greater trochanteric entry point for PFNA-2 in unstable intertrochanteric femur fractures. The study was accepted by Institutional Ethics Committee.

2. Materials and Methods

An observational study was conducted on 40 patients with intertrochanteric femur fracture operated with PFNA-2 implant in the Department of Orthopaedics, Government Wenlock Hospital, Kasturba Medical College, and its allied hospitals in Mangalore between January 2017 and July 2018. Patients with Type A31A2 and A31A3 (unstable intertrochanteric femur fracture) as per AO classification [11] and age more than 50 years were included. Patients with a stable type of fracture, expired before final follow-up, less than 50 years, and previous implant in the injured hip were excluded. The patients were divided into two groups: group M for medial entry (5 mm medial to the greater trochanter tip) and group L for lateral entry point over greater trochanter based on anteroposterior view of the X-ray. On lateral view of the X-ray, the entry point was in the centre (Figure 1). Randomization was carried out by assigning the patients to the group by alternate allocation.

The quality of reduction was noted by taking the difference of neck shaft angle between operated and normal hip. The difference of less than $5°$ was graded as excellent, between 5 and $10°$ as good, and $>10°$ as poor [12]. The quality of fixation was evaluated using tip apex distance (T-A distance) [13]. The position of the compression screw was noted using the Cleveland index [14]. To avoid bias, the values were measured using MB ruler in the hospital's computed radiographic system by two trained orthopaedic surgeons.

All the complications were noted. Final follow-up was conducted at 6 months with modified Harris hip score (HHS) [15]. The study was permitted by the Institutional ethics Committee.

2.1. Data Analysis. The results were assessed using Student's *t*-test, chi square test, and Mann–Whitney test. A *P* value less than 0.05 was considered significant. The results were entered in MS Excel spreadsheet, and statistical analysis was performed using Statistical Package for Social Sciences (SPSS) version 16.0.

3. Results

Forty patients with unstable intertrochanteric femur fracture, operated with PFNA-2, were enrolled in the study. Twenty patients treated with lateral entry point were included in group L (Figure 2), and group M included 20 patients with medial entry point (Figure 3). The average age of the patients in group L was 69.6 and group M was 69.85 (Table 1). The difference in age distribution was not significant between two groups ($P = 0.23$). The group L had 12 female and 8 male patients, whereas group M had 8 female and 12 male patients ($P = 0.1$). As per AO classification, group L had 13 patients with A2 type and 7 patients with A3 type. Group M had 11 patients with A2 type and 9 patients with A3 type of fracture ($P = 0.37$) (Table 1).

3.1. Radiographic Parameters (Table 2). The group L had average tip apex distance of 20.53 and group M had 20.02 ($P = 0.8$). 4 in group L and 5 in group M had tip apex distance >25 mm ($P = 0.5$) (Table 2). 3 out of 4 patients in group L with TAD more than 25 mm had screw back out. 3 patients of group L and 6 patients of group M had good reduction ($5–10°$) as per the neck shaft angle difference. 4 patients of group L had poor reduction ($>10°$). There were no patients with poor reduction in group M ($P = 0.08$) (Table 2). The complication of screw back out was seen in 3 out of 4 patients with poor reduction in group L. As per the Cleveland index, 6 patients each in both groups had suboptimal position ($P = 0.63$) (Table 2). Four out of 6 patients in group L with suboptimal position had screw back out.

3.2. Complications (Table 3). The lateral cortex impingement was seen in 14 patients of group L and 6 patients in group M with significant comparison ($P = 0.01$) (Figure 4). Three patients in group L had varus collapse with screw back out and none in group M ($P = 0.05$) (Figure 5). Screw back only was seen in one patient of group L. Subtrochanteric femur fracture was seen in 1 patient with lateral entry of the nail (Table 3). Out of three patients with varus collapse and screw back out, 2 were treated with exchange nailing and 1 with arthroplasty. The only case with screw back out was treated with implant removal (Figure 4).

3.3. Functional Outcome (Table 4 and Figure 6). The modified Harris hip score (average) for group L at 6 months was 71.94 and group M was 76.8 ($P = 0.84$). In group L, excellent results were seen in 2 patients, 4 had good, 6 had fair, and 8 had poor results. In group M, 2 patients had excellent, 9 had good, 4 had fair, and 5 had poor results. When results of both the groups were correlated, there was no significance ($P = 0.84$) (Table 4 and Figure 6).

4. Discussion

Entry point of the nail is more important as it will play a vital role in improving the quality of reduction and fixation and thus leading to good functional outcome without complications. The unstable intertrochanteric femur fracture in elderly needs good reduction and stable fixation, for early mobilisation [1]. Our aim was to figure out the optimal entry point for PFNA-2 which is widely being used at present in Asian population. There were no discrepancies in age distribution difference between the groups.

The tip apex distance was >25 mm in 4 patients with lateral entry. Three had screw back out. These 3 patients with screw back out had lateral cortex impingement. TAD was

The Results of Unstable Intertrochanteric Femur Fracture Treated with Proximal Femoral Nail Antirotation-2...

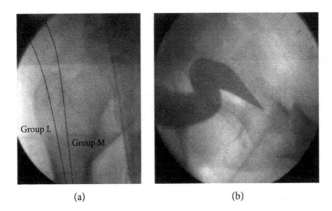

(a)   (b)

FIGURE 1: Entry points over the greater trochanter.

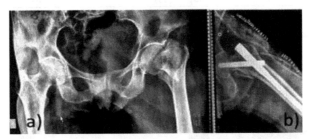

FIGURE 2: PFNA-2 with medial entry point.

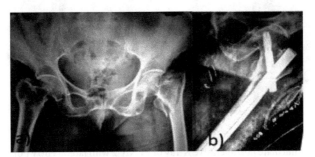

FIGURE 3: PFNA-2 with lateral entry point.

TABLE 1: Demographic statistics.

$n = 40$	Group L (20)	Group M (20)	P value
Age (average)	69.6	69.85	0.23
Sex			
Male	8	12	0.1
Female	12	8	
Fracture type			
31. A2	13	11	0.37
31. A3	7	9	

more than 25 mm in 5 patients in medial entry group and none showed any complications. There was no significance when TAD of both groups were compared. This supports the hypothesis of Kane et al. [16] that the position of the screw in the head and neck is more important than the tip apex distance.

This has also been concluded in the study by Nikoloski et al. [17] that a tip apex distance <25 mm is not a reliable indicator for PFNA. In their study on PFNA in elderly patients, Karapinar et al. [12] measured difference in neck shaft angle between surgically operated and normal hip. They found that 93% patients had good/acceptable reduction

TABLE 2: Radiographic parameters.

$n = 40$	Group L (20)	Group M (20)	P value
Tip apex distance (more than 25 mm)	4	5	0.5
Average tip apex distance	20.53	20.02	0.8
Mean and SD	6.2	6.63	
Neck shaft angle (difference between operated and normal side)			
<5° good	13	14	
5°–10° acceptable	3	6	0.08
>10° poor	4	0	
Cleveland index			
Suboptimal position	6	6	0.63
Ideal position	14	14	

TABLE 3: Complications.

$n = 40$	Group L (20)	Group M (20)	P value
Varus collapse + screw back out	3	0	0.05
Screw back out	1	0	
Lateral cortex impingement	14	6	0.01
Subtrochanteric fracture	1	0	

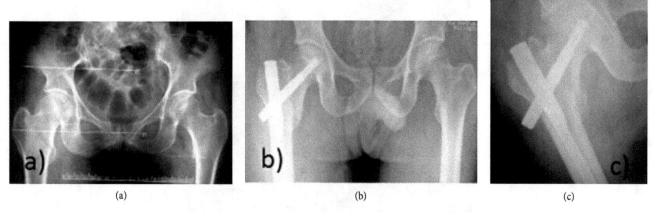

(a) (b) (c)

FIGURE 4: (a) Preoperative X-ray. (b) Immediate postoperative X-ray of PFNA-2 with lateral entry point showing lateral cortex impingement with gap at fracture site. (c) Follow-up at 6 months. Fracture union was seen at 6 months but with screw back out.

and 85.9% had ideal implant position. Out of 88% patients with neck shaft angle >120°, 12% had varus collapse. In a study by Radaideh et al. [18], 3 out of 4 patients with a neck shaft angle difference of more than 10° in the lateral entry group had screw back out. These three patients had varus reduction (<125°) of fracture which eventually led to loss of reduction and screw back out. The patients in the medial entry group had good/acceptable reduction as measured by the neck shaft angle. The reduction quality can be improved with entry point being just medial to the greater trochanter tip.

The ideal position of the screw was found to be in lower-centre and centre-centre position in the study by Kane et al. [16], and this resulted in stable fixation. As per the Cleveland index in present study, 4 out of 6 patients with suboptimal position in lateral entry group and none in medial entry group had screw back out. When results of both group were compared, there was no significance.

All three radiological parameters, when compared between the groups, had no significance. The complications were seen mainly in the lateral entry group and none in medial entry group. Hence, entry point of the nail is suggested to be the most important factor.

PFNA has been advised in elderly patients, and studies have found it to be a better implant and has given satisfactory functional and radiological results with minimal complications [18–20]. We got satisfactory results with PFNA-2, and there was no considerable difference between 2 groups in terms of functional outcome.

The varus collapse was seen in 12% [18], 5.8% [21], and 4.9% [22] of cases in previous studies. We got 15% cases with varus collapse with screw back out in the lateral entry group. There were no cases of varus collapse in the medial entry group. PFNA-2 had minimized lateral cortex impingement in unstable peritrochanteric fractures as concluded in a study by Macheras et al. [23]. We encountered lateral cortex

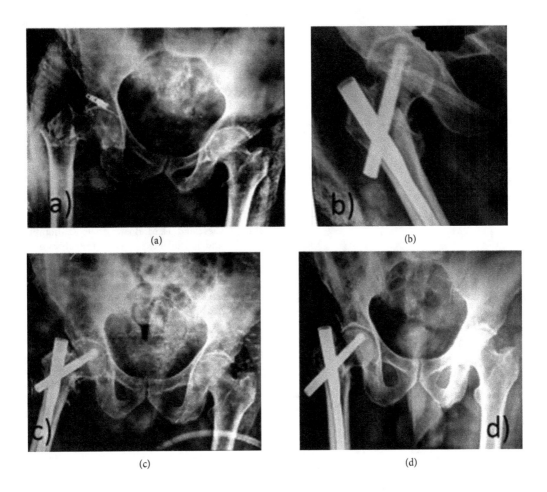

FIGURE 5: (a) Preoperative X-ray. (b) Immediate postoperative X-ray with lateral entry showing varus reduction, (c) at 6 weeks and (d) at final follow-up showing screw back out.

TABLE 4: Functional outcome at 6 months.

$n = 40$	Group L (20)	Group M (20)	P value
Modified Harris hip score at six months (Mean and SD)	71.94 14.81	76.8 14.15	0.84

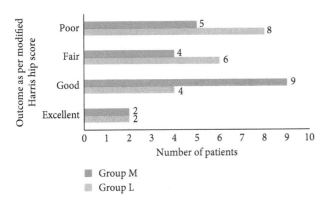

FIGURE 6: Functional outcome at 6 months.

impingement in 70% patients of group L and 30% patients of group M with unstable intertrochanteric femur fracture. Nail shaft axis was described by Jiamton et al. as a potential risk factor for failed osteosynthesis due to its association with secondary varus displacement [24]. Tao et al. [25] emphasized that regardless of the implant choice and its characteristics, the inserting technique is the key factor for stable fixation without complications. Hence, we recommend the entry point for PFNA-2 should be 5 mm medial to the greater trochanter tip for achieving adequate fixation and thus minimizing complications. More damage to the gluteus medius insertion has been described by McConnell et al. [26]. An average of 27% tendon damage might occur during reaming of entry point which could be a cause of postoperative morbidity. The placement of the trochanteric entry point is difficult to precisely locate intraoperatively by image intensifier. High degree of variability existed with respect to trochanteric entry point according to Streubel et al., and they concluded preoperative templating was an accurate way of obtaining ideal entry point [27]. The limitation of our study was short follow-up period of six months.

5. Conclusion

Both the entry points gave equivocal functional results at final follow-up ($P = 0.8445$). More complications were encountered with lateral entry point compared to medial entry ($P = 0.05$). The lateral entry point showed more cases with lateral cortex impingement as compared to medial entry ($P = 0.01$). The outcome can be good when the TAD is less than 25 mm, neck shaft angle difference is less than 5°, and the Cleveland index is in an optimal position (centre-centre or inferior-centre). Overall, to achieve good quality of fixation and minimal damage to the gluteus medius, the entry point for PFNA-2 should be 5 mm medial to the greater trochanter tip.

Acknowledgments

The authors are grateful for the help and support from KMC Mangalore and Manipal Academy of Higher Education (MAHE) for performing this study.

References

[1] S. Babhulkar, "Management of trochanteric fractures," *Indian Journal of Orthopaedics*, vol. 40, no. 4, pp. 210–218, 2006.

[2] A. C. Dhamangaonkar, "Management options and treatment algorithm in intertrochanteric fractures," *Trauma International*, vol. 1, no. 1, pp. 12–16, 2015.

[3] S.-Y. Kim, Y. G. Kim, and J. K. Hwang, "Cementless calcar-replacement hemiarthroplasty compared with intramedullary fixation of unstable intertrochanteric fractures," *The Journal of Bone and Joint Surgery (American)*, vol. 87, no. 10, pp. 2186–2192, 2005.

[4] U. Bhakat and R. Bandyopadhayay, "Comparative study between proximal femoral nailing and dynamic hip screw in intertrochanteric fracture of femur," *Open Journal of Orthopaedics*, vol. 3, no. 7, pp. 291–295, 2013.

[5] Y. Endo, G. B. Aharonoff, J. D. Zuckerman, K. A. Egol, and K. J. Koval, "Gender differences in patients with hip fracture: a greater risk of morbidity and mortality in men," *Journal of Orthopaedic Trauma*, vol. 19, no. 1, pp. 29–35, 2005.

[6] W. L. Loo, S. Y. J. Loh, and H. C. Lee, "Review of proximal nail antirotation (PFNA) and PFNA-2—our local experience," *Malaysian Orthopaedic Journal*, vol. 5, no. 2, pp. 1–5, 2011.

[7] S. J. Hu, S. M. Chang, Z. Ma, S. C. Du, L. P. Xiong, and X. Wang, "PFNA-II protrusion over greater trochanter in the Asian population used in proximal femoral fractures," *Indian Journal of Orthopaedics*, vol. 50, no. 6, pp. 641–646, 2016.

[8] G. Anastopoulos, D. Chissas, J. Dourountakis et al., "Computer-assisted three-dimensional correlation between the femoral neck-shaft angle and the optimal entry point for antegrade nailing," *Injury*, vol. 41, no. 3, pp. 300–305, 2010.

[9] C. M. Ansari Moein, H. J. Ten Duis, P. L. Oey, G. A. de Kort, W. van der Meulen, and C. van der Werken, "Intramedullary femoral nailing through the trochanteric fossa versus greater trochanter tip: a randomized controlled study with in-depth functional outcome results," *European Journal of Trauma and Emergency Surgery*, vol. 37, no. 6, pp. 615–622, 2011.

[10] K. Farhang, R. Desai, J. H. Wilber, D. R. Cooperman, and R. W. Liu, "An anatomical study of the entry point in the greater trochanter for intramedullary nailing," *The Bone & Joint Journal*, vol. 96-B, no. 9, pp. 1274–1281, 2014.

[11] I. B. Schipper, E. W. Steyerberg, R. M. Castelein, and A. B. van Vugt, "Reliability of the AO/ASIF classification for pertrochanteric femoral fractures," *Acta Orthopaedica Scandinavica*, vol. 72, no. 1, pp. 36–41, 2001.

[12] L. Karapinar, M. Kumbaraci, A. Kaya, A. Imrci, and M. Incesu, "Proximal femoral nail antirotation (PFNA) to treat peritrochnteric fracture in elderly patients," *European Journal of Orthopaedic Surgery & Traumatology*, vol. 22, no. 3, pp. 237–243, 2012.

[13] M. R. Baumgaertner, S. L. Curtin, D. M. Lindskog, and J. M. Keggi, "The value of the tip apex distance in predicting failure of fixation of peritrochanteric fractures of the hip," *The Journal of Bone & Joint Surgery*, vol. 77, no. 7, pp. 1058–1064, 1995.

[14] M. Cleveland, D. M. Bosworth, F. R. Thompson, H. J. Wilson Jr., and T. Ishizuka, "A ten-year analysis of intertrochanteric fractures of the femur," *The Journal of Bone & Joint Surgery*, vol. 41-A, pp. 1399–1408, 1959.

[15] K. Vishwanathan, K. Akbari, and A. J. Patel, "Is the modified Harris hip score valid and responsive instrument for outcome assessment in the Indian population with pertrochanteric fractures?" *Journal of Orthopaedics*, vol. 15, no. 1, pp. 40–46, 2018.

[16] P. Kane, B. Vopat, W. Heard et al., "Is tip apex distance as important as we think? a biomechanical study examining optimal lag screw placement," *Clinical Orthopaedics and Related Research®*, vol. 472, no. 8, pp. 2492–2498, 2014.

[17] A. N. Nikoloski, A. L. Osbrough, and P. J. Yates, "Should the tip-apex distance (TAD) rule be modified for the proximal femoral nail antirotation (PFNA)? a retrospective study," *Journal of Orthopaedic Surgery and Research*, vol. 8, p. 35, 2013.

[18] A. M. Radaideh, H. A. Qudah, Z. A. Audat, R. A. Jahmani, I. R. Yousef, and A. A. A. Saleh, "Functional and radiological results of proximal femoral nail antirotation (PFNA) osteosynthesis in the treatment of unstable pertrochanteric fractures," *Journal of Clinical Medicine*, vol. 7, no. 4, p. 78, 2018.

[19] A. Sharma, A. Mahajan, and B. John, "A comparison of the clinico-radiological outcomes with proximal femoral nail (PFN) and proximal femoral nail antirotation (PFNA) in fixation of unstable intertrochanteric fractures," *Journal of Clinical and Diagnostic Research*, vol. 11, no. 7, pp. RC05-RC09, 2017.

[20] G. N. K. Kumar, G. Sharma, K. Khatri et al., "Treatment of unstable intertrochanteric fractures with proximal femoral nail antirotation II: our experience in Indian patients," *The Open Orthopaedics Journal*, vol. 9, pp. 456–459, 2015.

[21] H. Zhang, X. Zhu, G. Pei et al., "A retrospective analysis of the InterTan nail and proximal femoral nail anti-rotationin in the treatment of intertrochanteric fractures in elderly patients with osteoporosis: a minimum follow-up of 3 years," *Journal of Orthopaedic Surgery and Research*, vol. 12, no. 1, p. 147, 2017.

[22] W. Yu, X. Zhang, X. Zhu, J. Hu, and Y. Liu, "A retrospective analysis of the InterTan nail and proximal femoral nail anti-rotation-Asia in the treatment of unstable intertrochanteric femur fractures in the elderly," *Journal of Orthopaedic Surgery and Research*, vol. 11, no. 1, p. 10, 2016.

[23] G. A. Macheras, S. D. Koutsostathis, S. Galanakos, K. Kateros, and S. A. Papadakis, "Does PFNA II avoid lateral cortex impingement for unstable peritrochanteric fractures?" *Clinical Orthopaedics and Related Research®*, vol. 470, no. 11, pp. 3067–3076, 2012.

[24] C. Jiamton, K. Boernert, R. Babst et al., "The nail–shaft-axis of the

the of proximal femoral nail antirotation (PFNA) is an important prognostic factor in the operative treatment of intertrochanteric fractures," *Archives of Orthopaedic and Trauma Surgery*, vol. 138, no. 3, pp. 339–349, 2018.

[25] Y. Tao, Z. Ma, and S. Chang, "Does PFNA II avoid lateral cortex impingement for unstable peritrochanteric fractures?" *Clinical Orthopaedics and Related Research®*, vol. 471, no. 4, pp. 1393-1394, 2013.

[26] T. McConnell, P. Tornetta, E. Benson, and J. Manuel, "Gluteus medius tendon injury during reaming for gamma nail insertion," *Clinical Orthopaedics and Related Research*, vol. 407, pp. 199–202, 2003.

[27] P. N. Streubel, A. H. Wong, W. M. Ricci, and M. J. Gardner, "Is there a standard trochanteric entry site for nailing of subtrochanteric femur fractures?" *Journal of Orthopaedic Trauma*, vol. 25, no. 4, pp. 202–207, 2011.

6

A Safe Method for Early Rehabilitation of Articular Fracture at the Base of Thumb Metacarpal Bone

Yunus Oc ⓘ,[1] Bekir Eray Kilinc ⓘ,[2] Ali Varol ⓘ,[3] and Adnan Kara ⓘ[4]

[1]Medilife Health Group, Bagcilar Hospital, Department of Orthopaedics and Traumatology, Istanbul, Turkey
[2]Health Science University Istanbul Fatih Sultan Mehmet Training and Research Hospital,
 Department of Orthopaedics and Traumatology, Istanbul, Turkey
[3]Health Ministry, Silopi State Hospital, Department of Orthopaedics and Traumatology, Sirnak, Turkey
[4]Medipol University Istanbul, Department of Orthopaedics and Traumatology, Istanbul, Turkey

Correspondence should be addressed to Bekir Eray Kilinc; dreraykilinc@gmail.com

Academic Editor: Benjamin Blondel

Background. To evaluate the clinical and radiological results of closed reduction, distraction using an external fixator, and percutaneous fixation in patients with Bennet and Rolando fractures. *Methods.* Patients over 18 years of age, who had isolated fracture at the base of the first metacarpal bone, had no previous functional limitations and pain complaints, were regularly followed up, and had fixation using K-wire combined with an external fixator, were included. Arthrosis was evaluated according to Eaton and Littler classification. Pain intensity was evaluated using the visual analogue scale (VAS) on a 0–10 scale. Furthermore, patients were questioned regarding limitations in their daily activities and hobbies. Pinch and grasp strengths were evaluated. *Results.* Thirteen of the patients were male and five were female, with a mean age of 31.5 ± 12.5 years. The surgical procedure was performed on the right extremity in 12 patients and left extremity in six patients. Twelve patients were found to have Bennet fractures, whereas six patients had Rolando fractures. The mean follow-up period of the patients was found to be 29.6 ± 5.4 months. The VAS score was rated as 2 in one patient and 1 in one patient. Other patients had a pain VAS score of 0. The mean Quick-DASH score was calculated to be 1.20. No statistical difference was found in pinch strength between the two extremities ($p > 0.05$). No difference was observed in terms of the range of motion ($p > 0.05$). *Conclusion.* Fixation using K-wire combined with an external fixator has more benefits than its disadvantages and is superior to other methods in the intra-articular fractures of the first metacarpal bone.

1. Introduction

The thumb is an essential part of hand function in dexterity, particularly for pinching and grasping. The trapeziometacarpal (TMC) joint serves as a pivot point in the thumb column and allows simple and complex movements to be performed.

Proximal metacarpal fractures usually occur due to exposure to a moderate trauma, and their incidence is higher in the working adult population. These injuries can present as both extra- and intra-articular injuries, both causing problems with stability at the fracture level [1, 2]. Since these fractures are generally displaced at the time of presentation, they are risky in terms of stiffness, instability, and progression to arthrosis in the carpometacarpal joint.

Intra-articular fractures of the first metacarpal proximal end, which are generally referred to as Rolando and Bennet fractures, account for 1.4% of hand fractures [3, 4]. Treatment of these fractures is still controversial. In addition to conservative treatment, many different surgical treatment modalities have been defined. The common goal of all treatment methods is the high-quality restoration of the articular surface [1, 2].

The hypothesis of the present study is that the initiation of movement at the same time in the first carpometacarpal joint restored by distraction and percutaneous pinning method with an external fixator will not create functional restrictions during the treatment process and will reduce posttreatment complications.

This study aimed to evaluate the clinical and radiological results of closed reduction, distraction using an external fixator, and percutaneous fixation in patients with intra- and extra-articular fractures at the base of the first metacarpal bone.

2. Materials and Methods

This retrospective study conducted over a two-year period included all Bennett-type or Rolando-type intra-articular fractures at the base of the first metacarpal bone. Analysis of patient records revealed that mainly young males suffered these fractures. The study was conducted at a single institution between 2018 and 2020. This study was conducted with the approval of the Institutional Review Board and was in line with the ethical principles of the Declaration of Helsinki. The reference number for the ethics committee approval was 2020/344-67.

Patients over 18 years of age, who had isolated fracture at the base of the first metacarpal bone, had no previous functional limitations and pain complaints, and were regularly followed up, were included.

Patients were evaluated with standard anteroposterior (AP) and lateral radiographs of the hand. The thumb column was placed parallel to the antepulsion-retropulsion axis in the AP view and the flexion-extension axis in the lateral view.

2.1. Surgical Technique. General anaesthesia was induced in all patients. Closed reduction was achieved under fluoroscopy with longitudinal traction of the thumb combined with abduction-extension maneuver and metacarpal pronation. Two Schanz pins were applied in the trapezium and two Schanz pins to the distal of the first metacarpal bone. Then, alignment was achieved by placing an external fixator. Using the ligamentotaxis effect of the fixator (Unilateral finger fixator, Design Med, Turkey), a 2 mm distraction was applied to the joint. The joint restoration was ensured with Kirschner wires (K-wire) of 1.4 mm in the appropriate configuration according to the intra-articular fracture fragment of each patient. Intra-articular step-off was accepted as 1 mm. Thumb movements were examined under fluoroscopy to check the stability of the fixation (Figure 1).

Rehabilitation was started on the first postoperative day. The patients were evaluated in the 1st, 3rd, 6th, and 24th months. The K-wires and fixator were removed under local anaesthesia since the consolidation was seen in the control graph taken in the first month. Wound healing and functional healing were evaluated at the third- and fifth-month controls. Patients were evaluated in terms of pain and function at the 24th month. Pain intensity was evaluated using the visual analogue scale (VAS) on a 0–10 scale. Furthermore, patients were questioned regarding limitations in their daily activities and hobbies. Pinch and grasp strengths were evaluated using a Hand Dynamometer and Pinch Gauge (Fabrication Enterprises Inc., New York, NY, USA).

The values of the operated and healthy sides of the patients were compared to measure the pinch and grasp strengths. A difference of 20% with the dominant hand was considered significant [5].

In radiographs, posttraumatic arthrosis was evaluated according to van Niekerk and Owens modification of the Eaton and Littler classification: Stage I: no clear arthritic changes, Stage II: osteophytes smaller than 2 mm, Stage III: osteophytes larger than 2 mm or joint narrowing, and Stage IV: joint space more or less disappeared [6, 7]. Statistical analyses were performed using Statistical Package for Social Sciences (SPSS) version 14.0. A nonparametric Mann–Whitney test was used to compare the functional results between the injured and noninjured hand.

General anaesthesia was induced in all patients. All patients were hospitalized for one day following the operation, and the external fixator was kept in place for six weeks in all patients. At the sixth week, fixators and K-wires were extracted under local anaesthesia under polyclinic conditions. Outpatient clinic controls were made in all patients at the third, sixth, 12th, and 24th weeks. At the 24-week controls, VAS was applied to all patients to measure the pain intensity, and the shortened version of the disabilities of the arm, shoulder, and hand questionnaire (Quick-DASH) was performed to evaluate physical functions subjectively.

3. Results

A total of 18 patients meeting the study criteria, who had proximal end intra-articular extension fracture at the first metacarpal bone and were treated with an external fixator and percutaneous pinning between 2016 and 2019, were included in the study. Thirteen of the patients were male and five were female, with a mean age of 31.5 ± 12.5 years. The surgical procedure was performed on the right extremity in 12 patients and left extremity in six patients. The affected extremity was the dominant extremity in 14 patients. The mechanism of injury was occupational accidents in five patients, traffic accident in four patients, battery in two patients, and simply falling in seven patients. Twelve patients were found to have Bennet fractures (according to the Gedda classification: five patients had type 1, six patients had type 2, and one patient had type 3), whereas six patients had Rolando fractures. The mean follow-up period of the patients was found to be 29.6 ± 5.4 months (Table 1).

The pain VAS score was rated as 2 in one patient and 1 in one patient. Other patients had a pain VAS score of 0. The mean Quick-DASH score of the patients was calculated to be 1.20. The pinch and grasp strengths of the patients were measured by evaluating the opposite (nonaffected) extremity, and the mean pinch strength was found to be 94% whereas the mean grasp strength was 98%. There was no statistical difference between the two extremities ($p > 0.05$). No difference was observed between the operated and nonoperated sides in terms of the range of motion (ROM) ($p > 0.05$). Similarly, there was no difference between the affected and nonaffected sides in terms of ROM ($p > 0.05$).

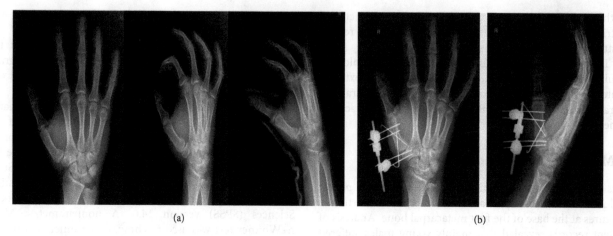

(a)   (b)

FIGURE 1: (a) Preop AP/lateral and oblique X-ray views of Bennet fracture. (b) Postop AP/lateral X-ray views of Bennet fracture.

TABLE 1: Demographic data of the patients.

Patient	Age	Sex	Side	Type of fracture	Injury type	f/u	Complication	VAS	Quick-dash	Pinch %	Grasp	Eaton–Littler classification
1	28	M	R	Bennet	İA	26	—	0	0	96	96	Stage 1
2	26	M	R	Bennet	TA	27	—	0	0	96	100	Stage 1
3	38	M	L	Rolando	Fall	30	—	1	6, 8	90	96	Stage 2
4	44	F	R	Bennet	DT	26	PTE	0	0	98	100	Stage 1
5	36	M	R	Rolando	İA	24	—	0	0	94	98	Stage 1
6	29	F	R	Bennet	Fall	28	—	0	0	94	100	Stage 1
7	34	M	L	Bennet	TA	32	—	0	0	94	96	Stage 1
8	40	M	R	Bennet	İA	31	—	0	0	96	98	Stage 1
9	26	F	R	Rolando	DT	34	—	0	0	94	100	Stage 1
10	42	M	R	Bennet	Fall	28	—	0	0	94	98	Stage 1
11	30	M	L	Bennet	Fall	32	—	0	0	96	100	Stage 1
12	26	M	R	Rolando	İA	24	PTE	0	0	94	98	Stage 1
13	19	F	L	Bennet	Fall	34	—	0	0	96	100	Stage 1
14	24	M	R	Rolando	TA	27	—	0	0	94	100	Stage 1
15	21	M	R	Bennet	TA	35	—	0	0	94	96	Stage 1
16	39	F	L	Bennet	Fall	36	—	0	0	96	98	Stage 1
17	41	M	R	Rolando	İA	28	—	2	11, 4	88	90	Stage 2
18	25	M	L	Bennet	Fall	32	—	0	0	96	100	Stage 1

İA: industrial accident, TA: traffic accident, DT: direct trauma, PTE: pin Tract infection.

Full opening was observed in the interphalangeal (IP), metacarpophalangeal (MCP), and carpometacarpal (CMC) joints.

Joint arthrosis was evaluated in the radiographs taken at the 24th week. According to Eaton and Littler's classification [8], 16 patients had stage I arthrosis and two had stage II arthrosis. Two patients were observed to have pin tract infection, which regressed with one-week antibiotic treatment (Figure 2).

4. Discussion

Distraction using an external fixator and K-wire fixation provide safe stability for early postoperative rehabilitation of the fractures at the base of the first metacarpal bone. These methods are useful in early rehabilitation of the joint movements and full recovery of functional capacity. The high bone union rates and low rate of joint degeneration

obtained by the method applied in the present study indicate that this method is effective.

Since the time when Rolando and Bennet fractures were first identified, various treatment modalities from conservative treatment to open reduction and fixation and even arthroscopic-assisted fixation have been presented for these fractures. Reduction of proximal fractures of the 1stmetacarpal bone with intra-articular extension and maintaining the reduction are difficult due to the complexity of the forces acting on the joint [9]. Therefore, various treatment modalities are used in the treatment of fractures at the base of the first metacarpal bone. The most common ones among these treatment modalities are closed reduction and plaster cast application; closed reduction and pinning; closed reduction and external fixator application; open reduction and fixation with plate or screw; and closed reduction, external fixator application, and pinning [9–12]. Closed reduction and plaster cast application is not preferred since it does not allow early mobilization and fails to prevent arthrosis in the

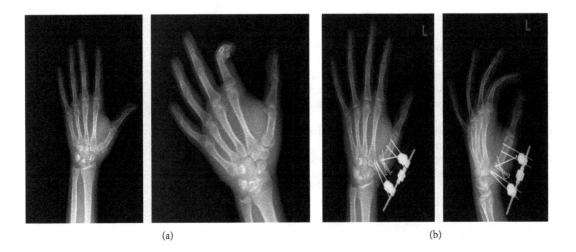

FIGURE 2: (a) Preop AP and oblique X-ray views of Rolando fracture. (b) Postop AP/lateral X-ray views of Rolando fracture.

joint. Since closed reduction and external fixator application alone is not sufficient for joint surface restoration, the possibility of arthrosis development in the joint is higher in the long term. Kontakis et al. [13] performed closed reduction and external fixator application in 11 patients and reported that there was joint arthrosis in four of these patients and one of them was severe. Open reduction and plate fixation is a preferred treatment modality since it provides early mobilization and stable fixation. Development of soft tissue problems, devascularization of fracture fragments, and collateral ligament and tendon injuries are more common in this method. In a study by Mumtaz et al. [14], the implant was required to be removed in four of nine patients, who underwent open reduction and plate osteosynthesis, due to local tenderness and pain, and soft tissue problem and superficial infection were reported in two patients. Closed reduction and external fixator and pinning is presented as a much safer method for fractures of this region in terms of both joint restoration and early mobilization. In a case series by Houshain and Jing [12] involving 16 patients, two pin tract infections were reported as a complication, and the authors reported that they achieved excellent results in 12 of the 16 patients and good results in four. In the present study, change was observed in VAS scores and joint arthritis in only two of the patients. The fixation preferred in the current study is reliable enough to allow early mobilization without causing loss of reduction. Thus, complications such as joint stiffness and future arthrosis can be minimized. No limitation was observed in joint movements of the patients included in this study. Achieving better and safer results with the reduction of the fractures of this area through the effect of ligamentotaxis and restoration using K-wires in the joint, compared to others, will make it to be preferred more often.

The small number of patients and its retrospective design are among the limitations of the present study. The sample size of the present study determined using power analysis is strong, which is compatible with the literature. Another limitation is the absence of a control group. We believe that it will be difficult to create a control group since there are various options in the treatment of the first metacarpal basis fractures. Therefore, there is a need for a large prospective series with long-term follow-up to determine optimal treatment guidelines.

Compared to the traditional treatment methods, such as fixation with a splint or K-wire fixation, fixation using K-wire combined with an external fixator is superior in maintaining anatomic reduction of displaced and severely communated fractures [12, 13]. The surgical method used in the present study eliminates the need for large soft tissue in cases where open reduction and internal fixation is indicated and prevents dissection for the fixation of the fractured part and complications such as avascular necrosis. We can recommend this method as a primary and definitive treatment in cases where conservative treatments and other surgical interventions fail.

The following are among the main advantages of this method: providing good functional results, causing fewer complications, allowing early mobilization, and not requiring neither reoperation nor physical therapy. Living with an external fixator though for a short time and pin tract infections are the disadvantages of this method.

5. Conclusions

We believe that this method, which has more benefits than its disadvantages, is superior to other methods in the intra-articular fractures of the first metacarpal bone.

References

[1] K. R. Carter and S. V. Nallamothu, *Bennett Fracture. Treasure Island (FL)*, StatPearls Publishing, Treasure Island, FL, USA, 2020.

[2] J. R. Kang, A. W. Behn, J. Messana, and A. L. Ladd, "A biomechanical model and relevant ligamentous anatomy," *Journal of Hand Surgery (American Volume)*, vol. 44, no. 2, p. 154, 2019.

[3] L. M. Hove, "Fractures of the hand," *Scandinavian Journal of*

Plastic and Reconstructive Surgery and Hand Surgery, vol. 27, no. 4, pp. 317–319, 1993.

[4] S. Rolando, "Fracture de la bas edu premier metacarpien et principalment sur une variete von encore decrite," *Clinical Orthopaedics and Related Research*, vol. 327, pp. 4–8, 1996.

[5] C. A. Crosby, M. A. Wehbé, and B. Mawr, "Hand strength: normative values," *The Journal of Hand Surgery*, vol. 19, no. 4, pp. 665–670, 1994.

[6] C. Obry, "Fracture de la base du premier métacarpien," *Annales de Chirurgie*, vol. 43, pp. 80–87, 1989.

[7] I. A. Kapandji, "Radiographie spécifique de l'articulation trapézo-métacarpienne," *Traité de la chirurgie de la main*, vol. 2, pp. 497–511, 1984.

[8] R. G. Eaton and J. W. Littler, "Ligament reconstructionfor the painful thumb carpometacarpal joint," *Journal of Bone and Joint Surgery*, vol. 51, pp. 1655–1666, 1969.

[9] A. Byrne, S. Kearns, S. Morris, and E. Kelly, ""S" quattro external fixation for complex intra-articular thumb fractures," *Journal of Orthopaedic Surgery*, vol. 16, no. 2, pp. 170–174, 2008.

[10] S. Uludag, Y. Ataker, A. Seyahi, O. Tetik, and E. Gudemez, "Early rehabilitation after stable osteosynthesis of intra-articular fractures of the metacarpal base of the thumb," *Journal of Hand Surgery (European Volume)*, vol. 40, no. 4, pp. 370–373, 2015.

[11] M. Lutz, R. Sailer, R. Zimmermann, M. Gabl, H. Ulmer, and S. Pechlaner, "Closed reduction transarticular Kirschner wire fixation versus open reduction internal fixation in the treatment of Bennett's fracture dislocation," *Journal of Hand Surgery (Edinburgh, Scotland)*, vol. 28, no. 2, pp. 142–147, 2003.

[12] S. Houshian and S. S. Jing, "Treatment of Rolando fracture by capsuloligamentotaxis using mini external fixator: a report of 16 cases," *Hand Surgery*, vol. 18, no. 1, pp. 73–78, 2013.

[13] G. M. Kontakis, P. G. Katonis, and K. A. Steriopoulos, "Rolando's fracture treated by closed reduction and external fixation," *Archives of Orthopaedic and Trauma Surgery*, vol. 117, no. 1-2, pp. 84-85, 1998.

[14] M. U. Mumtaz, F. Ahmad, A. A. Kawoosa, and I. Hussain, "Wani I treatment of Rolando fractures by open reduction and internal fixation using mini T-plate and screws," *Journal of Hand and Microsurgery*, vol. 8, no. 2, pp. 80–85, 2016.

7

The Role of Fibular Fixation in Distal Tibia-Fibula Fractures

Chengxin Li,[1] Zhizhuo Li,[1] Qiwei Wang,[1] Lijun Shi,[2] Fuqiang Gao,[3] and Wei Sun ⓘ[3]

[1]Department of Orthopedics, Peking University China-Japan Friendship School of Clinical Medicine,
 2 Yinghuadong Road, Chaoyang District, Beijing 100029, China
[2]Department of Orthopedics, Graduate School of Peking Union Medical College,
 China-Japan Friendship Institute of Clinical Medicine, 2 Yinghuadong Road, Chaoyang District, Beijing 100029, China
[3]Beijing Key Laboratory of Immune Inflammatory Disease, China-Japan Friendship Hospital,
 2 Yinghuadong Road, Chaoyang District, Beijing 100029, China

Correspondence should be addressed to Wei Sun; cjfhsunw@163.com

Academic Editor: Francesco Liuzza

Objectives. The necessity of fibular fixation in distal tibia-fibula fractures remains controversial. This study aimed to assess its impact on radiographic outcomes as well as rates of nonunion and infection. *Methods.* A systematic search of the electronic databases of PubMed, Embase, and Cochrane library was performed to identify studies comparing the outcomes of reduction and internal fixation of the tibia with or without fibular fixation. Radiographic outcomes included malalignment and malrotation of the tibial shaft. Data regarding varus/valgus angulation, anterior/posterior angulation, internal/external rotation deformity, and the rates of nonunion and infection were extracted and then polled. A meta-analysis was performed using the random-effects model for heterogeneity. *Results.* Additional fibular fixation was statistically associated with a decreased rate of rotation deformity (OR = 0.13; 95% CI 0.02–0.82, $p = 0.03$). However, there was no difference in the rate of malreduction between the trial group and the control group (OR = 0.86; 95% CI 0.27–2.74, $p = 0.80$). There was also no difference in radiographic outcomes of varus-valgus deformity rate (OR = 0.17; 95% CI 0.03–1.00, $p = 0.05$) or anterior-posterior deformity rate (OR = 0.76; 95% CI 0.02–36.91, $p = 0.89$) between the two groups. Meanwhile, statistical analysis showed no significant difference in the nonunion rate (OR = 0.62; 95% CI 0.37–1.02, $p = 0.06$) or the infection rate (OR = 0.81; 95% CI 0.18–3.67, $p = 0.78$) between the two groups. *Conclusions.* Additional fibular fixation does not appear to reduce the rate of varus-valgus deformity, anterior-posterior deformity, or malreduction. Meanwhile, it does not appear to impair the union process or increase the odds of infection. However, additional fibular fixation was associated with decreased odds of rotation deformity compared to controls.

1. Introduction

Combined distal tibia and fibula fractures are one of the most common diaphyseal fractures among all long bones. These injuries are caused mainly by high-energy trauma such as motor vehicle accidents or low-energy torsional trauma. With the widespread use of high-speed transport, the incidence of this injury is still increasing [1]. Today, the use of intramedullary (IM) nailing to treat the tibial fracture has been well defined because of the development of newer intramedullary implants and the associated reduction in complications [2]. However, the role of fibular fixation in addition to tibial IM nailing in distal extraarticular tibia-fibular fractures remains controversial [3, 4]. Several studies exploring the effects of fibular fixation on distal tibial fractures have been carried out [5–7]. Studies supporting fibular fixation found that it is related to a better anatomical alignment and better control over rotation while also introducing stability and restoring limb length [8–10]. Additionally, it has been reported that there are significantly higher rates of loss of reduction in distal tibia fractures treated with an IM nail without plate stabilization of the combined fibula fracture [11]. Moreover, after fibula fixation, the biomechanical structure is considered to be more similar to that present before the injury, which will reduce by 1/6 the total load applied to the knee joint [12] and between 6% and 7% of the total load transmitted through both the tibia and fibula [13, 14]. Conversely, the opposing view is that fibular fixation may result in delayed union or nonunion because it inhibits cyclic loading on the tibial fracture site [15, 16]. Meanwhile, high-energy fractures of the distal tibia are often accompanied with a high incidence of soft tissue trauma leading to a high incidence of wound infections and necrosis [17]. Consequently, the open reduction and internal fixation of the fibula required often increases the rate of wound complications [18]. Present, there is no clear consensus on the optimum management of combined distal third tibia and fibula fractures. Our aim was to assess whether combined distal third tibia and fibula fractures will benefit from concurrent fibular fixation.

2. Materials and Methods

2.1. Search Strategy. A systematic search of PubMed, Embase, and Cochrane library was conducted to identify studies comparing the outcomes with or without fibular fixation in addition to tibial reduction and internal fixation in distal extraarticular tibia-fibular fractures. The following keywords or corresponding Medical Subject Headings (MeSH) were used: "distal tibia and fibular fracture," "extra-articular fracture," "fibula fixation," and "tibia fixation." The systematic search of medical reference libraries occurred between August 1 through August 15, 2020. Reference lists of related publications (especially reviews and meta-analyses) mentioning the role of fibular fixation were also carefully screened to identify studies that were not captured in our initial database search. There were no language or data restrictions.

2.2. Involvement Inclusion and Exclusion Criteria. An article was considered eligible when it concerned (1) distal extra-articular tibia and fibula fractures, (2) fibular fixation versus lack of fibula fixation, (3) closed or open fractures, and (4) radiographic outcomes, nonunion, and infection rate as well as other clinical variables provided as endpoints. Exclusion criteria of this investigation were (1) intraarticular fractures; (2) cadaver studies, animal studies, and other biomechanical studies; (3) case reports, study protocols, letters, correspondence, conference presentations, and noncomparative studies; and (4) studies that did not report on the primary outcomes, radiographic, and/or functional outcomes. We first removed redundant and unrelated records by reading the titles and abstracts. Then, full texts of the remaining articles were downloaded to confirm their eligibility based on the above criteria.

2.3. Data Extraction. Two reviewers reviewed and extracted data from studies that fulfilled all inclusion and exclusion criteria. The following variables were extracted from each study: author's name, year of study, type of study, level of evidence, demographic data, and type of surgery.

2.4. Patient and Public Involvement. No patients were involved in this study.

2.5. Assessment of Methodological Quality and Risk of Bias of the Study. The assessments of each of the studies selected for the final analysis were performed independently by two reviewers. A 12-item scale [19] was used to assess the methodological quality of each included study. The 12-item scale consisted of the following: adequate randomization, concealment of allocation, patient blinding, care provider blinding, outcome assessor blinding, dropout rate, intention-to-treat (ITT) analysis, avoidance of selective reporting, similarity of baseline characteristics, similarity or absence of cofactors, patient compliance, and similarity of timing. Any disagreement was resolved by discussion and consensus.

2.6. Statistical Analysis. Statistical analyses were performed using the random-effects model with inverse variance weighting. Meta-analyses and forest plots were constructed with the statistical software Review Manager (RevMan) ((computer program) Version 5.3. Copenhagen: The Nordic Cochrane Centre, The Cochrane Collaboration, 2014). For binary data, pooled odds ratios (OR) as well as related 95% confidence intervals (CIs) were adopted, and a pooled 95% CI not covering 1 indicated a significant difference between the two groups; meanwhile, pooled weighted mean difference (WMD) or standardized mean difference (SMD), as well as related 95% CIs, were used to evaluate continuous data, and a 95% CI not covering 0 revealed a significant difference. Heterogeneity was evaluated between individual studies with a Q statistic and I^2 value for each meta-analysis. I^2 heterogeneity less than 25% generally indicates consistent results and homogenous studies, while 25–75% indicates moderate heterogeneity and greater than 75% indicates severe heterogeneity. If I^2 was >50%, sensitivity analyses were conducted by omitting one study at a time to examine the influence of each.

3. Results

3.1. Description of Included Studies. Overall, the initial search yielded 119 potentially relevant articles: 86 from PubMed and 33 from Embase. Of these, 30 duplicates were removed using Endnote software. After reading the titles and abstracts of the 89 remaining articles, 82 were excluded. Therefore, seven studies [20–26] fulfilled all inclusion and exclusion criteria and were included in this systematic review and meta-analysis. The inclusion processes and reasons for exclusion are depicted in Figure 1. Three [22, 24, 25] studies were randomized controlled trials, another three [20, 21, 26] of the seven were retrospective studies, and only one [23] was a prospective cohort study. All patients, both in the trial and control groups, were treated with interlocking IM nail or plate fixation for tibia fracture, and patients in the trial group additionally underwent fixation with a 3.5 mm dynamic compression plate (DCP) for fibula fracture. Two studies [22, 23] excluded patients with open fractures, leaving all patients included with closed fractures. All patients were followed up for more than 6 months (from 6 to 21 months)

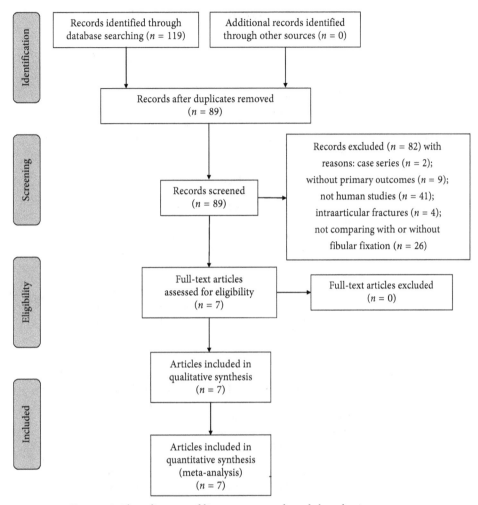

FIGURE 1: Flow diagram of literature research and the selection process.

with valgus/varus and posterior/anterior angulations and nonunion, and the infection rates of most patients were assessed. Two studies [23, 24] mentioned the functional outcomes or the range of movements at the ankle. Two studies [20, 21] only reported the nonunion rate or union of time. The main characteristics of the selected studies are listed in Table 1.

As for the risk of bias (RoB) of the included articles, only if the method of randomizing was explicitly described and the dropout rate was <20%, was the study given a score of "1;" otherwise, the score was "0." For ITT, only if all randomized participants were analyzed in the group, were they allocated to the study and received a "1" score. If the studies met at least 6 of the 12 criteria, the study was regarded as having low RoB. If five or fewer of the 12 criteria were met, the study was labeled as high RoB. Results of the RoB assessment are summarized in Table 2.

3.2. Quantitative Analysis

3.2.1. Nonunion Rate at 6 Months after Surgery. Radiographic union was defined as cortical bridging on three or more cortices on orthogonal radiographic views.

Nonunion was defined as a fracture with no radiographic progression toward healing at 9 months after surgery on consecutive radiographs over a minimum 2-month period accompanied by clinical symptoms of nonunion (pain, inability to bear weight). Delayed union was defined using the same definition, but for fractures between 6 and 9 months.

Based on six comparative studies, the statistical results (OR = 0.62; 95% CI 0.37–1.02, $p = 0.06$; $I^2 = 0\%$, p for heterogeneity = 0.94) suggested no differences in the nonunion rate at 6 months after surgery between the trial group and the controls (Figure 2).

3.2.2. Varus-Valgus Deformity. Varus-valgus deformity was measured on the anteroposterior projections by determining the angle formed by the intersection between the perpendicular lines drawn from the tibial plateau and the tibia plafond. Varus-valgus deformity was defined as coronal plane deviation >5° on final radiographs. From five comparative studies, there was no difference in varus-valgus deformity rates between patients in the trial group and controls (OR = 0.17; 95% CI 0.03–1.00, $p = 0.05$; $I^2 = 87\%$, $p < 0.00001$ for heterogeneity) (Figure 3).

TABLE 1: The main characteristics of selected studies.

Author	Years	Type of design	Case	Average	Open fracture: closed fracture	Type of surgery	Average follow-up	Assessment
Francesco et al. [23]	2018	Prospective cohort study	Fibular fixation: 49 No fibular fixation: 38	Fibular fixation: 56.4 No fibular fixation: 59.8	No open fractures	Interlocking intramedullary nail for tibia and plating fixation for fibular	18 months	Rotational alignment and valgus/varus and posterior/anterior angulations
Michael et al. [21]	2017	Retrospective study	Fibular fixation: 166 No fibular fixation: 174	Fibular fixation: 166 No fibular fixation: 174	Fibular fixation: 93 : 73 No fibular fixation: 95 : 79	Interlocking intramedullary nail for tibia and plating fixation for fibular	21 months	Time to union, delayed union, and nonunion
Mohammad et al. [22]	2017	Randomized controlled study	Fibular fixation: 24 No fibular fixation: 25	Fibular fixation: 36.9 No fibular fixation: 34.8	No open fractures	Interlocking intramedullary nail for tibia and 3.5 mm DCP fixation for fibula	9 months	Valgus/varus and posterior/anterior angulations and nonunion
Benjamin et al. [26]	2015	Retrospective study	Fibular fixation: 15 No fibular fixation: 83	Fibular fixation: 42.8 No fibular fixation: 40.3	Fibular fixation: 1 : 14 No fibular fixation: 30 : 53	Interlocking intramedullary nail for tibia and plating fixation for fibular	117 months	Valgus/varus and posterior/anterior angulations and nonunion
Berlusconi et al. [20]	2014	Retrospective study	Fibular fixation: 26 No fibular fixation: 34	Fibular fixation: 47.12 No fibular fixation: 44	Fibular fixation: 9 : 17 No fibular fixation: 10 : 24	Interlocking intramedullary nail for tibia and plating fixation for fibular	>6 months	Nonunion
Manish et al. [24]	2013	Randomized controlled study	Fibular fixation: 30 No fibular fixation: 30	NA	Fibular fixation: 14 : 16 No fibular fixation: 12 : 18	Interlocking intramedullary nail for tibia and 3.5 mm DCP fixation for fibula	18 months	Rotational alignment and valgus/varus and posterior/anterior angulations
Rouhani et al. [25]	2012	Randomized controlled study	Fibular fixation: 24 No fibular fixation: 29	Fibular fixation: 24.2 No fibular fixation: 28.6	Fibular fixation: 11 : 13 No fibular fixation: 17 : 12	Interlocking intramedullary nail for tibia and 3.5 mm DCP fixation for fibula	6 months	Valgus/varus and posterior/anterior angulations and nonunion

NA, not available.

3.2.3. Anterior-Posterior Deformity. Anterior-posterior deformity was defined as sagittal plane deviation >10° on the final radiograph. From two comparative studies, the pooled results (OR = 0.76; 95% CI 0.02–36.91, $p = 0.89$; $I^2 = 80\%$, $p = 0.03$ for heterogeneity) showed no significant difference in anterior-posterior deformity rates between patients in the trial group and controls (Figure 4).

3.2.4. Rotational Deformity. By standing at the foot end of the patient, the rotation of the ankle was determined by measuring the angle subtended by a plumb line with a line passing through the midpoint of the knee, the line joining the midpoint of the ankle (intermalleolar distance) and the second toe. Rotation deformity was defined as an internal/external rotation deformity >10° compared to the normal contralateral limb.

The pooled results (OR = 0.13; 95% CI 0.02–0.82, $p = 0.03$; $I^2 = 43\%$, $p = 0.019$ for heterogeneity) of two comparative studies suggested that fibular fixation was associated with decreased odds of rotational deformity (Figure 5).

3.2.5. Malreduction. Malreduction was defined as coronal or sagittal plane deviation of >5° on immediate postoperative

TABLE 2: Results of the risk of bias assessment.

Study	Randomized adequately	Allocation concealed	Patient blinded	Care provider blinded	Outcome assessor blinded	Acceptable dropout rate	ITT analysis	Avoided selective reporting	Similar baseline	Similar on avoided cofactor	Patient compliance	Similar timing	Total score	Risk of bias
Francesco et al. [23]	0	0	0	0	0	1	0	1	1	1	1	1	6	Low
Michael et al. [21]	0	0	0	0	0	1	0	1	1	1	1	1	6	Low
Mohammad et al. [22]	1	0	0	0	0	1	0	1	1	1	1	1	7	Low
Benjamin et al. [26]	0	0	0	0	0	1	0	1	1	1	1	1	6	Low
Berlusconi et al. [20]	0	0	0	0	0	1	0	1	1	1	1	1	6	Low
Manish et al. [24]	1	1	0	0	0	1	0	1	1	1	1	1	8	Low
Rouhani et al. [25]	1	1	0	0	0	1	0	1	1	1	1	1	8	Low

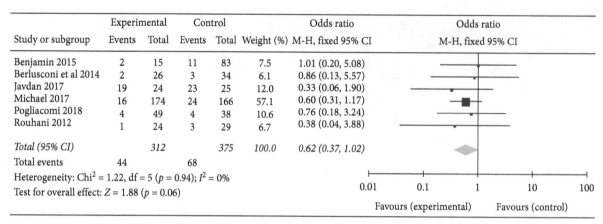

Study or subgroup	Experimental Events	Experimental Total	Control Events	Control Total	Weight (%)	Odds ratio M-H, fixed 95% CI
Benjamin 2015	2	15	11	83	7.5	1.01 (0.20, 5.08)
Berlusconi et al 2014	2	26	3	34	6.1	0.86 (0.13, 5.57)
Javdan 2017	19	24	23	25	12.0	0.33 (0.06, 1.90)
Michael 2017	16	174	24	166	57.1	0.60 (0.31, 1.17)
Pogliacomi 2018	4	49	4	38	10.6	0.76 (0.18, 3.24)
Rouhani 2012	1	24	3	29	6.7	0.38 (0.04, 3.88)
Total (95% CI)		312		375	100.0	0.62 (0.37, 1.02)
Total events	44		68			

Heterogeneity: Chi^2 = 1.22, df = 5 (p = 0.94); I^2 = 0%
Test for overall effect: Z = 1.88 (p = 0.06)

FIGURE 2: Nonunion rate at 6 months after surgery.

Study or subgroup	Experimental Events	Experimental Total	Control Events	Control Total	Weight (%)	Odds ratio M-H, random, 95% CI
Manish 2013	6	30	30	30	15.0	0.00 (0.00, 0.08)
Michael 2017	11	174	10	166	24.0	1.05 (0.43, 2.55)
Poliacomi 2018	14	49	33	38	23.1	0.06 (0.02, 0.19)
Rouhani 2012	0	23	4	26	14.7	0.11 (0.01, 2.09)
Taylor 2015	8	15	42	83	23.2	1.12 (0.37, 3.36)
Total (95% CI)		291		343	100.0	0.17 (0.03, 1.00)
Total events	39		119			

Heterogeneity: Tau^2 = 3.15; Chi^2 = 30.28, df = 4 (p < 0.00001); I^2 = 87%
Test for overall effect: Z = 1.96 (p = 0.05)

FIGURE 3: Varus-valgus deformity.

Study or subgroup	Experimental Events	Experimental Total	Control Events	Control Total	Weight (%)	Odds ratio M-H, random, 95% CI
Taylor 2015	2	15	3	83	54.4	4.10 (0.62, 26.96)
Rouhani 2012	0	24	4	26	45.6	0.10 (0.01, 2.00)
Total (95% CI)		39		109	100.0	0.76 (0.02, 36.91)
Total events	2		7			

Heterogeneity: Tau^2 = 6.29; Chi^2 = 4.90, df = 1 (p = 0.03); I^2 = 80%
Test for overall effect: Z = 0.14 (p = 0.89)

FIGURE 4: Anterior-posterior deformity.

Study or subgroup	Experimental Events	Experimental Total	Control Events	Control Total	Weight (%)	Odds ratio M-H, random, 95% CI
Manish 2013	0	30	10	30	27.8	0.03 (0.00, 0.58)
Poliacomi 2018	7	49	16	38	72.2	0.23 (0.08, 0.64)
Total (95% CI)		79		68	100.0	0.13 (0.02, 0.82)
Total events	7		26			

Heterogeneity: Tau^2 = 0.92; Chi^2 = 1.75, df = 1 (p = 0.19); I^2 = 43%
Test for overall effect: Z = 2.18 (p = 0.03)

FIGURE 5: Rotational deformity.

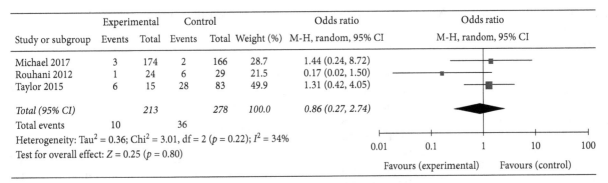

| Study or subgroup | Experimental | | Control | | | Odds ratio | Odds ratio |
	Events	Total	Events	Total	Weight (%)	M-H, random, 95% CI	M-H, random, 95% CI
Michael 2017	3	174	2	166	28.7	1.44 (0.24, 8.72)	
Rouhani 2012	1	24	6	29	21.5	0.17 (0.02, 1.50)	
Taylor 2015	6	15	28	83	49.9	1.31 (0.42, 4.05)	
Total (95% CI)		213		278	100.0	0.86 (0.27, 2.74)	
Total events	10		36				

Heterogeneity: Tau^2 = 0.36; Chi^2 = 3.01, df = 2 (p = 0.22); I^2 = 34%

Test for overall effect: Z = 0.25 (p = 0.80)

FIGURE 6: Malreduction.

| Study or subgroup | Experimental | | Control | | | Odds ratio | Odds ratio |
	Events	Total	Events	Total	Weight (%)	M-H, random, 95% CI	M-H, random, 95% CI
Javdan 2017	0	24	2	25	16.3	0.19 (0.01, 4.21)	
Manish 2013	6	30	0	30	17.5	16.18 (0.87, 301.62)	
Michael 2017	11	174	20	166	44.7	0.49 (0.23, 1.96)	
Rouhani 2012	1	24	2	29	21.6	0.59 (0.05, 6.90)	
Total (95% CI)		252		250	100.0	0.81 (0.18, 3.67)	
Total events	18		24				

Heterogeneity: Tau^2 = 1.18; Chi^2 = 6.07, df = 3 (p = 0.11); I^2 = 51%

Test for overall effect: Z = 0.28 (p = 0.78)

FIGURE 7: Rate of infection.

radiographs. The pooled results (OR = 0.86; 95% CI 0.27–2.74, p = 0.80; I^2 = 34%, p = 0.22 for heterogeneity) of three comparative studies suggested that there was no significant difference in malreduction rates between patients in the trial group and controls (Figure 6).

3.2.6. Rate of Infection. Six of the studies mentioned the adverse event of infection, but only five provided data and one of the studies noted that there were no infection cases in either of the groups. The results (OR = 0.81; 95% CI 0.18–3.67, p = 0.78; I^2 = 51%, p = 0.11 for heterogeneity) of the other four studies showed that there was no significant difference in infection rates between patients in the trial group and controls (Figure 7).

4. Discussion

With the frequent occurrence of traffic accidents, fractures of the distal tibia and fibula are common in this population. Most patients who suffer from this high-energy injury need surgical intervention. However, as a result of the low soft tissue coverage and poor blood supply of the distal tibia, the incidences of delayed union or nonunion and other complications are high. To reduce these complications and improve prognosis, the surgical options to treat distal tibia and fibular fractures have significantly evolved over the past several decades. In 1969, a precedent for fixation of the fibula associated with distal tibia intraarticular fractures was established by Ruedi and Allgower [27]. They advocated that

internal fixation was feasible for distal tibiofibular fractures within 10 cm of the ankle joint. However, the need for fibular fixation in distal tibia extraarticular fractures is not clear.

Cadaveric biomechanical experiments designed to investigate the value of adjunctive fibular fixation with tibial fixation have vastly contributed to this subject. Strauss et al. [6] conducted a laboratory experiment to compare IM nails with locked plates in the treatment of tibia fractures with concurrent same level fibula fractures. They found that an imperfect fibula achieved by osteotomy significantly increased the risk of construct displacement, regardless of which type of fixation was used. Therefore, the authors concluded that an intact fibula may improve the fracture fixation stability of the distal tibia. Another cadaveric study designed by Kumar et al. [3] investigated the effect of fibular plate fixation on axial rotation of simulated distal fractures of the tibia and fibula. They created a 5 mm transverse segmental defect which was 7 cm proximal to the ankle joint at the same level in the tibia and fibula and then used a 9 mm Russell-Taylor IM nail to fix the tibia. They also found that additional fibular plate fixation decreased axial rotation and increased the rotational stability, but did not increase rotational stiffness. However, Weber et al. [5] reported that the effect of fibular plate fixation on stability was weakened if the tibia was fixed with an IM nail.

According to our results, there were no significant differences in varus-valgus deformity, anterior-posterior deformity, and malreduction rate, and only the rotation deformity rate was significantly reduced. Usually, studies assessed distal tibia fibular fracture malalignment after IM nailing with and without fibular stabilization at two different times: immediately after surgery and again at regular follow-up after surgery. The initial alignment immediately after surgery represents the result of reduction. There were no significant differences regarding the malreduction in our study, which indicated that fibular fixation does not affect the surgery of the tibia. However, during the follow-up, the rate of rotation deformities was significantly reduced, which suggested that instability was associated with the lack of fibular fixation. Several groups of studies have reported that fibular fixation preserved the reduction of the tibia in the same level in combined tibial and fibular fractures and have suggested concurrent fibular fixation [11]. Kumar et al. reported that fibular plate fixation increased the initial rotational stability after distal tibial fracture in comparison with patients that were treated by tibial IM nailing alone, which correlated with our findings. Others have also mentioned that the highest rate of complications was seen in fibular distal fractures without fibular additional plating and recommended fibular fixation in combined tibial and fibular fractures [13, 14]. Regarding tibiofibular stability, fibular fixation is advisable to avoid rotational deformity. All seven studies included in this study involved a fibular fixation treatment group and a control group. To evaluate union, we adopted the nonunion rate at 6 months to assess the results. All studies reported the outcomes, and the incidence of nonunion ranged from 0 to 79% in the treatment group and from 0 to 92% in the control group. The pooled results (OR = 0.62; 95% CI 0.37–1.02; $p = 0.06$) suggested no significant differences in the nonunion rate at 6 months.

Sensitivity analysis showed that there was no change in the results with the removal of any set of data. We also examined the rate of infection, which is another complication that may relate to the surgery. The results (OR = 0.81; 95% CI 0.18–3.67; $p = 0.78$) also do not support the theory that supplementary fibular fixation increases the rate of infection. There have been previous reports that additional surgical procedures can destroy surrounding tissues and blood supply, which play important roles in fracture healing [15, 16]. However, the fact of the combined fracture itself suggests relatively high-energy trauma and a high incidence of complications such as delayed union and infection. The results of two studies which excluded patients with open fractures are similar to our meta-analysis. These results do not support the hypothesis that adjunctive fibular fixation can increase the rate of nonunion and infection. Additionally, the malalignment rate is another series of outcomes that we intend to compare.

To our knowledge, this is the first meta-analysis comparing tibia fixation with or without fibular fixation. However, there are also some limitations as follows. First, as only three RCTs in this area have been identified, our study included four non-RCTs, which inevitably involved selection, recall, and interviewer bias, thus eventually weakening our results. Second, patients were enrolled in every study according to different criteria; some excluded all open fractures, while some included both open and closed fractures, creating significant heterogeneity in wound healing and infection rates. Moreover, there is a lack of a uniform

method to treat tibia fractures or fibula fractures. None of the studies noted the reason for the choice of IM nailing or plate, which can influence the clinical outcomes. Finally, the follow-up duration was relatively short, preventing examination of long-term outcomes, especially postoperative function.

5. Conclusions

According to our systematic review and meta-analysis, we can conclude that additional fibular fixation does not appear to reduce the rates of varus-valgus deformity, anterior-posterior deformity, or malreduction. Moreover, neither does it appear to impair the union process or increase the odds of infection. However, additional fibular fixation was associated with decreased odds of rotation deformity compared to controls.

Authors' Contributions

LCX and LZZ contributed equally to this work; SW contributed to the conception of the study; LCX and LZZ contributed significantly to literature search, data extraction, quality assessment, data analyses, and manuscript preparation; WQW contributed improving the article for language and style and protocol preparation; SLJ and GFQ helped perform the analysis with constructive discussions; SW revised the manuscript and approved the final version.

Acknowledgments

This work was supported by the and 7182146), National Natural Science Foundation of China (81672236, 81802224, and 81871830), Graduate Innovation Foundation of Peking Union Medical College (2019-1002-91).

References

[1] D. Torino and S. Mehta, "Fibular fixation in distal tibia fractures: reduction aid or nonunion generator?" *Journal of Orthopaedic Trauma*, vol. 30, no. 4, pp. S22–S25, 2016.

[2] R. Schnettler, M. Borner, and E. Soldner, "Results of interlocking nailing of distal tibial fractures," *Unfallchirurg*, vol. 93, no. 11, pp. 534–537, 1990.

[3] A. Kumar, S. J. Charlebois, E. Lyle Cain, R. A. Smith, A. U. Daniels, and J. M. Crates, "Effect of fibular plate fixation on rotational stability of simulated distal tibial fractures treated with intramedullary nailing," *Journal of Bone and Joint Surgery*, vol. 85, no. 4, pp. 604–608, 2003.

[4] R. Varsalona and G. T. Liu, "Distal tibial metaphyseal fractures: the role of fibular fixation," *Strategies in Trauma & Limb Reconstruction*, vol. 1, no. 1, pp. 42–50, 2006.

[5] T. G. Weber, R. M. Harrington, M. B. Henley, and A. F. Tencer, "The role of fibular fixation in combined fractures of the tibia and fibula: a biomechanical investigation," *Journal of Orthopaedic Trauma*, vol. 11, no. 3, pp. 206–211, 1997.

[6] E. J. Strauss, D. Alfonso, F. J. Kummer, K. A. Egol, and N. C. Tejwani, "The effect of concurrent fibular fracture on the fixation of distal tibia fractures: a laboratory comparison of

intramedullary nails with locked plates," *Journal of Orthopaedic Trauma*, vol. 21, no. 3, pp. 172–177, 2007.

[7] P. M. Morin, R. Reindl, E. J. Harvey, L. Beckman, and T. Steffen, "Fibular fixation as an adjuvant to tibial intramedullary nailing in the treatment of combined distal third tibia and fibula fractures: a biomechanical investigation," *Canadian Journal of Surgery*, vol. 51, no. 1, pp. 45–50, 2008.

[8] T. Rüedi, "Fractures of the lower end of the tibia into the ankle joint: results 9 years after open reduction and internal fixation," *Injury*, vol. 5, no. 2, pp. 130–134, 1973.

[9] R. Attal, V. Maestri, H. K. Doshi et al., "The influence of distal locking on the need for fibular plating in intramedullary nailing of distal metaphyseal tibiofibular fractures," *Bone & Joint Journal*, vol. 96-B, no. 3, p. 385, 2014.

[10] G. N. Duda, F. Mandruzzato, M. Heller et al., "Mechanical boundary conditions of fracture healing: borderline indications in the treatment of unreamed tibial nailing," *Journal of Biomechanics*, vol. 34, no. 5, pp. 639–650, 2001.

[11] A. F. De Giacomo and P. Tornetta, "Alignment after intramedullary nailing of distal tibia fractures without fibula fixation," *Journal of Orthopaedic Trauma*, vol. 30, no. 10, pp. 561–567, 2016.

[12] K. L. Lambert, "The weight-bearing function of the fibula," *Journal of Bone & Joint Surgery*, vol. 53, no. 3, pp. 507–513, 1971.

[13] K. Takebe, A. Nakagawa, H. Minami, H. Kanazawa, and K. Hirohata, "Role of the fibula in weight-bearing," *Clinical Orthopaedics and Related Research*, vol. 184, no. 184, pp. 289–292, 1984.

[14] J. C. Goh, A. M. Mech, E. H. Lee, E. J. Ang, P. Bayon, and R. W. Pho, "Biomechanical study on the load-bearing characteristics of the fibula and the effects of fibular resection," *Clinical Orthopaedics & Related Research*, vol. 279, no. 279, p. 223, 1992.

[15] A. M. Whorton and M. B. Henley, "The role of fixation of the fibula in open fractures of the tibial shaft with fractures of the ipsilateral fibula: indications and outcomes," *Orthopedics*, vol. 21, no. 10, pp. 1101–1105, 1998.

[16] J. L. Marsh, S. Bonar, J. V. Nepola, T. A. Decoster, and S. R. Hurwitz, "Use of an articulated external fixator for fractures of the tibial plafond," *Journal of Bone and Joint Surgery*, vol. 77, no. 10, pp. 1498–1509, 1995.

[17] T. P. Rüedi and M. Allgöwer, "The operative treatment of intra-articular fractures of the lower end of the tibia," *Orthopedic Trauma Directions*, vol. 9, no. 1, pp. 23–25, 2011.

[18] T. M. Williams, J. L. Marsh, J. V. Nepola, T. A. DeCoster, S. R. Hurwitz, and S. B. Bonar, "External fixation of tibial plafond fractures: is routine plating of the fibula necessary?" *Journal of Orthopaedic Trauma*, vol. 12, no. 1, pp. 16–20, 1998.

[19] A. D. Furlan and V. C. Pennick, "2009 updated method guidelines for systematic reviews in the Cochrane Back Review Group," *Spine*, vol. 34, no. 18, pp. 1929–1941, 2009.

[20] M. Berlusconi, L. Busnelli, F. Chiodini, and N. Portinaro, "To fix or not to fix? the role of fibular fixation in distal shaft fractures of the leg," *Injury*, vol. 45, no. 2, pp. 408–411, 2014.

[21] M. Githens, J. Haller, J. Agel, and R. Firoozabadi, "Does concurrent tibial intramedullary nailing and fibular fixation increase rates of tibial nonunion? a matched cohort study," *Journal of Orthopaedic Trauma*, vol. 31, no. 6, pp. 316–320, 2017.

[22] M. Javdan, M. A. Tahririan, and M. Nouri, "The role of fibular fixation in the treatment of combined distal tibia and fibula fracture: a randomized, control trial," *Advanced Biomedical Research*, vol. 6, p. 48, 2017.

[23] F. Pogliacomi, S. Paolo, C. Filippo, C. Francesco, and V. Enrico, "When is indicated fibular fixation in extra-articular fractures of the distal tibia?" *Acta BioMedica*, vol. 89, no. 4, pp. 558–563, 2019.

[24] M. Prasad, S. Yadav, A. Sud, N. C Arora, N. Kumar, and S. Singh, "Assessment of the role of fibular fixation in distal-third tibia-fibula fractures and its significance in decreasing malrotation and malalignment," *Injury*, vol. 44, no. 12, pp. 1885–1891, 2013.

[25] A. Rouhani, A. Elmi, H. Akbari Aghdam, F. Panahi, and Y. Dokht Ghafari, "The role of fibular fixation in the treatment of tibia diaphysis distal third fractures," *Orthopaedics & Traumatology: Surgery & Research*, vol. 98, no. 8, pp. 868–872, 2012.

[26] B. C. Taylor, B. R. Hartley, N. Formaini, and T. J. Bramwell, "Necessity for fibular fixation associated with distal tibia fractures," *Injury*, vol. 46, no. 12, pp. 2438–2442, 2015.

[27] P. L. Ramsey and W. Hamilton, "Changes in tibiotalar area of contact caused by lateral talar shift," *Journal of Bone and Joint Surgery*, vol. 58, no. 3, pp. 356–357, 1976.

8

Fractures around Trochanteric Nails: The "Vergilius Classification System"

Giuseppe Toro [iD],[1,2] Antimo Moretti [iD],[1] Daniele Ambrosio [iD],[3] Raffaele Pezzella [iD],[4]
Annalisa De Cicco [iD],[1] Giovanni Landi [iD],[1] Nicola Tammaro [iD],[1] Pasquale Florio [iD],[3]
Antonio Benedetto Cecere [iD],[1] Adriano Braile [iD],[1] Antonio Medici [iD],[5] Antonio Siano [iD],[6]
Bruno Di Maggio [iD],[7] Giampiero Calabrò [iD],[8] Nicola Gagliardo [iD],[9] Ciro Di Fino [iD],[10]
Gaetano Bruno [iD],[11] Achille Pellegrino [iD],[12] Giacomo Negri [iD],[3] Vincenzo Monaco [iD],[13]
Michele Gison [iD],[14] Antonio Toro [iD],[14] Alfredo Schiavone Panni [iD],[1]
Umberto Tarantino [iD],[2] and Giovanni Iolascon [iD][1]

[1]Department of Medical and Surgical Specialties and Dentistry, University of Campania "Luigi Vanvitelli", Naples, Italy
[2]Department of Clinical Sciences and Translational Medicine, University of Rome Tor Vergata, Rome, Italy
[3]Unit of Orthopaedics and Traumatology, Evangelical Hospital Betania, Naples, Italy
[4]Department of Life Health & Environmental Sciences, University of L'Aquila, Unit of Orthopaedics and Traumatology, L'Aquila, Italy
[5]Unit of Orthopaedics and Traumatology, AORN S. Giuseppe Moscati, Avellino, Italy
[6]Unit of Orthopaedics and Traumatology, Santa Maria Della Speranza Hospital, Battipaglia, Italy
[7]Unit of Orthopaedics and Traumatology, "Ave Gratia Plena" Civil Hospital, Piedimonte Matese, Italy
[8]Unit of Orthopaedics and Traumatology, San Francesco D'Assisi Hospital, Oliveto Citra, Italy
[9]Unit of Orthopaedics and Traumatology, San Giuliano Hospital, Giugliano, Italy
[10]Unit of Orthopaedics and Traumatology, AOR San Carlo, Potenza, Italy
[11]Unit of Orthopaedics and Traumatology, AORN Sant'Anna e San Sebastiano, Caserta, Italy
[12]Unit of Orthopaedics and Traumatology, San Giuseppe Moscati Hospital, Aversa, Italy
[13]Unit of Orthopaedics and Traumatology, Santa Maria Incoronata Dell'Olmo Hospital, Cava de' Tirreni, Italy
[14]Unit of Orthopaedics and Traumatology, Villa Malta Hospital, Sarno, Italy

Correspondence should be addressed to Giuseppe Toro; giusep.toro@gmail.com

Academic Editor: Panagiotis Korovessis

Introduction. The fractures that occurred around trochanteric nails (perinail fractures, PNFs) are becoming a huge challenge for the orthopaedic surgeon. Although presenting some specific critical issues (i.e., patients' outcomes and treatment strategies), these fractures are commonly described within peri-implant ones and their treatment was based on periprosthetic fracture recommendations. The knowledge gap about PNFs leads us to convene a research group with the aim to propose a specific classification system to guide the orthopaedic surgeon in the management of these fractures. *Materials and Methods.* A steering committee, identified by two Italian associations of orthopaedic surgeons, conducted a comprehensive literature review on PNFs to identify the unmet needs about this topic. Subsequently, a panel of experts was involved in a consensus meeting proposing a specific classification system and formulated treatment statements for PNFs. *Results and Discussion.* The research group considered four PNF main characteristics for the classification proposal: (1) fracture localization, (2) fracture morphology, (3) fracture fragmentation, and (3) healing status of the previous fracture. An alphanumeric code was included to identify each characteristic, allowing to describe up to 54 categories of PNFs, using a 3- to 4-digit code. The proposal of the consensus-based classification reporting the most relevant aspects for PNF treatment might be a useful tool to guide the orthopaedic surgeon in the appropriate management of these fractures.

1. Introduction

Fractures around nails are a huge challenge for the orthopaedic surgeon with a constantly rising incidence due to the increased frequency of hip fragility fractures worldwide [1, 2]. These fractures are commonly classified into two groups "intracapsular" and "extracapsular" (EF). Although considered as a unique entity, these two types differ largely in terms of pathoanatomy, clinics, epidemiology, and management [3]. In this regard, while intracapsular fractures are treated using hemiarthroplasty (HA) or total hip arthroplasty (THA), EF is generally fixed, most commonly, using trochanteric nails (TNs) [4]. However, TNs are associated with some complications, including perinail fractures (PNFs), whose incidence is expected to grow up in the next years [5]. The available evidence on PNFs concerning their clinical and treatment issues is poor and confusing, since these fractures are generally described along with those occurred around femoral plates, and both anterograde and retrograde interlocking nails (namely, peri-implant fractures) [5–7]. Moreover, the treatment of PNFs is often extrapolated by periprosthetic fracture (PPF) management [7, 8]. These latter fractures are generally treated using revision surgery or plate fixation, depending on fracture localization, prosthesis loosening, and bone stock, as defined by the Vancouver classification [9]. However, PNFs present several differences with respect to PPF, including treatment outcomes, particularly higher mortality rate in PNFs [10, 11]. Moreover, in our opinion, Vancouver classification use for PNFs is somewhat questionable and PNFs must be considered more appropriately a unique entity [7]. The growing interest in these fractures led some authors to propose other classifications of peri-implant fractures [5–7]. To the best of our knowledge, there is a gap in classifying PNFs and, consequently, guiding their treatment. This unmet need has driven us in a stepwise procedure aiming to propose a specific classification system and a practical guide for the treatment of PNFs.

2. Materials and Methods

The present study was the first of a three-step protocol based on (1) a consensus conference aimed to identify the fracture characteristics considered relevant for their classification and management; (2) retrospective multicentre observational study to apply the new classification system to our patients with PNFs; and (3) a position statement aimed to define the most appropriate PNFs treatment protocol. This kind of approach was recommended by Audigé et al. [12] and has been widely used for the proposal of new classifications [13].

In this first study, a steering committee, consisting of 7 members (5 orthopaedic surgeons with expertise in fragility fractures and 2 clinical researchers with expertise in performing systematic reviews), identified by the Italian group for the study of severe osteoporosis (*Gruppo Italiano per lo studio dell'osteoporosi severa, G. I. S. O. O. S.*) and the Association of Orthopaedics and Traumatologists of Campania (*Associazione Campana Ortopedici e Traumatologi Ospedalieri, A. C. O. T. O.*), conducted a comprehensive literature review in October 2018. The steering committee identified key evidence on the diagnosis and treatment of PNFs. The systematic research was conducted in MEDLINE and EMBASE, using different combinations of keywords (i.e., peri nail fractures AND diagnosis; peri implant fractures AND diagnosis; peri prosthetic fracture AND diagnosis; trochanteric nail AND fracture AND diagnosis; peri nail fractures AND treatment; peri implant fractures AND treatment; peri prosthetic fracture AND treatment; trochanteric nail AND fracture AND treatment) between January 2000 and November 2018.

All articles in English, Italian, and Spanish languages were included.

The committee selected the most relevant papers among those identified, based on the following inclusion criteria:

(1) Articles on femoral peri-implant fractures

(2) Articles on surgical techniques and related outcomes on periprosthetic Vancouver B1 and C fractures

(3) Articles on surgical techniques and related outcomes on interprosthetic and/or interimplant femoral fractures

(4) Articles on trochanteric nail complications (excluding those designed on specific complications like the cutout)

Articles on periprosthetic knee femoral fractures were also excluded.

After the literature research, the steering committee defined some questions concerning current unmet needs in the management of PNFs during their first meeting in January 2019.

The open issues identified by the steering committee were as follows:

(1) PNF definition

(2) PNF management

(3) PNF classification

These open issues were proposed to a panel of 18 orthopaedics with specific expertise in geriatric orthopaedics and trauma surgery, during two further meetings. The entire procedure through which the present study was conducted is summarized in Figure 1.

During the last meeting, the steering committee asked the panel of experts to give their consensus on the open questions and treatment statements on PNFs. During this meeting, the research group decided that all the characteristics of PNFs considered relevant for their treatment would be included in a specific classification system. A secret voting session was performed, and the relevant characteristics that got more than 65% of votes would have been included in the classification proposal. The classification categories were identified in hierarchical order according to the grade of consensus. Finally, the classification proposal was approved by both steering committee and panel members.

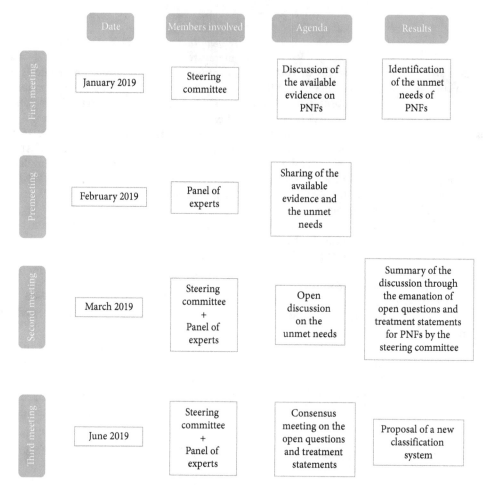

FIGURE 1: Summary of the entire procedure done to obtain the consensus for the classification system.

3. Results and Discussion

2919 articles were analysed after the first literature research. After title and abstract revision and duplicates removal, 2510 articles were excluded. Further 150 articles were excluded after full-text reading because it was considered inconclusive for the main objective of the study. Therefore, 259 articles were included and discussed by the steering committee during their first meeting (Figure 2).

The answers to each open question are summarized in Table 1, while the statements proposed for the management of PNFs are shown in Table 2.

According to the research group (namely, the steering committee and the panel of expert), the definition of PNF is "a fracture occurred around or next to a TN".

The research group included four PNF characteristics considered relevant for their treatment in the classification proposal in the following hierarchical order:

(1) Fracture localization (around the nail (namely, from the cephalic to the distal screw), around the distal screw, and distal from the tip of the nail), consensus 98%

(2) Fracture morphology (spiral, oblique, and transverse), as defined by AO [14], consensus 98%

(3) Fracture fragmentation (2, 3, or more than 3 fracture fragments), consensus 92%

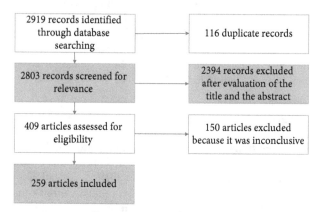

FIGURE 2: Research strategy.

(4) Healing status of the previous EF (healed or not healed), consensus 92%

The type of the implanted nail was not considered relevant, whereas no consensus was obtained regarding the nail length.

An alphanumeric code was proposed to identify each characteristic: (A) fracture around the nail; (B) fracture around the distal screw; (C) fracture distal from the tip of the nail; (S) spiral fracture; (O) oblique fracture; (T) transverse

TABLE 1: Open question answers and grade of consensus.

Question	Answer	Grade of consensus (%)
Is the definition of perinail fracture a fracture occurred around or next to an implanted nail?	Yes	100
Is fracture localization (around the nail (namely, from the cephalic to the distal screw), around the distal screw, distal from the tip of the nail) a pivotal factor for PNF management?	Yes	98
Is fracture morphology (spiral, oblique, and transverse), as defined by AO, a pivotal factor for PNF management?	Yes	98
Is the fracture fragmentation (number of fragments (2, 3, and more than 3 fragments)) a pivotal factor for PNF management?	Yes	92
Is the healing status of the previous EF (healed or not healed) a pivotal factor for PNF management?	Yes	92
Is the type of implanted TN (namely, biaxial or monoaxial) a pivotal factor for PNF management?	No	100
Is TN length (short or long using 300 mm as a threshold) a pivotal factor for PNF management?	Yes	50
Do you think that the currently available classification systems are useful for the management of PNFs?	No	100

TABLE 2: Statements on the management of PNFs.

Statement	Description
Statement #1	Fracture localization is a pivotal factor for PNF management. The fixation device used depends largely on the part of the femur involved by the fracture line and its relationship with the implanted nail.
Statement #2	Fracture morphology is a pivotal factor for PNF management, considering the fracture intrinsic stability. The description of fracture line orientation made by AO is appropriate for the definition of PNF morphology.
Statement #3	Fracture fragmentation is a pivotal factor for PNF management.
Statement #4	The healing status of the previous EF is a pivotal factor for PNF management as it can significantly reduce treatment options.
Statement #5	The type of implanted TN is not a pivotal factor for PNF management.
Statement #6	TN length may affect the fracture pattern, but it is unclear if it acts on PNF management.
Statement #7	The available classification systems are not useful for guiding the treatment decision making of PNFs

fracture; (2) two fracture fragments; (3) three fracture fragments; (3+) more than three fracture fragments; and (n) EF not healed. Therefore, a total of 54 potential categories were proposed in our classification and a single fracture would be described by 3 to 4 codes (see Figures 3–5).

Our study has the main purpose of covering a gap in the knowledge of PNF management, proposing, through a scientifically corroborated procedure, an algorithm for treating it. This gap concerns, above all, an appropriate classification of PNFs since those available were considered inadequate as treatment guide by our research group and led us to propose a new classification system from which some statements concerning specific management indications are derived.

PNFs (fractures occurred around or next to an implanted TN) have been a challenge for the orthopaedic surgeon. Some characteristics (fracture localization, fracture morphology, fracture fragmentation, and healing status of the previous fracture) were considered relevant for their management.

The relevance of PNFs was demonstrated by the growing literature around this topic [5–8, 15–17] and was justified by the expected increase in PNF incidence due to the rise of osteoporotic fractures [1, 2].

Osteoporosis is considered one of the main health problems in developed countries, considering the high morbidity and mortality of fragility fractures and the resulting economic burden [18]. The proximal femur is one of the most affected sites by fragility fractures [1].

Proximal femoral fractures are classified into intracapsular and EF depending on the anatomic localization of the fracture line. Although several studies reported that a clear difference did not exist between the plate and TNs for the treatment of EFs [19], these latter devices are the preferred fixation methods by the orthopaedic surgeons, probably because of their supposed easy-to-use and minimally invasive technique [4, 20]. In a recent epidemiological study on EF management in Sweden, over 6,000 nails were used to treat 10548 fractures [21]. However, some implant-related complications were frequently reported including cutting out, cut through, secondary fracture displacement, and PNFs [22].

These were an emerging complication of TN fixation with high mortality and morbidity [15], and their incidence was reported to be around 2% [16, 23].

Generally, PNFs were treated using the recommendation of PPF [7]. However, several differences could be seen in terms of both technical issues and patient outcomes comparing PNFs and PPF [10, 11]. For example, the former demonstrated a 1-year mortality rate higher than PPF (21% vs. 13%) [10, 11]. Moreover, factors that guide the treatment decision making of PPF (i.e., prosthesis stability and bone loss) could not be used for PNFs.

According to our classification, fracture localization, fracture morphology, fracture fragmentation, and healing status of the previous EF were the most relevant factors for the management of PNFs. The fracture localization was considered relevant because fixation devices are anatomically shaped (i.e., distal femur plates are specifically designed for the distal part of the femur) and the choice of a specific fixation device depends also on the relationship of the fracture line with the implanted TN. However, for 1 of the

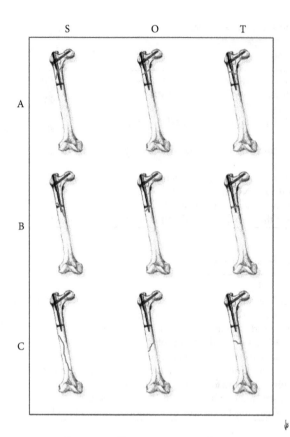

FIGURE 3: The main 9 types of PNFs.

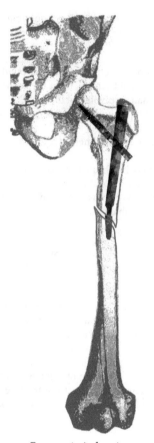

FIGURE 4: A drawing representing a BO2 fracture.

members of the panel, the definition of B type (around the distal screw) should be more appropriately as "parting from the distal screw"; nevertheless, during the discussion, the vast majority of the members agreed with the proposal of the steering committee, considered less confusing.

One of the members does not consider relevant fracture morphology because in his experience all fractures were oblique. Moreover, two other members of the research group questioned the relevance of fracture fragmentation because, in their personal experience, most of the PNFs were simple 2 fragment fractures. However, most of the members of the research group were in agreement that fracture morphology and fragmentation must be considered relevant because they affect primary fracture stability [24, 25] and guide the fixation technique (i.e., the choice between relative or absolute stability) [26]. For example, the intrinsic stability and the difficulty in obtaining nail-periosteum contact in femoral spiral fractures make mandatory the use of locked nails or plates [24]. However, the relevance of the afore-mentioned factors was generally known, considering that these were at the base of the AO classification of bone fractures since its first edition [27].

The healing status of the previous EF might complicate the fracture pattern, resembling an ipsilateral femoral neck and shaft fracture. These considerations were not accepted by two research members, especially regarding the choice of the fixation device, because several reports proposed the use of a single fixation device (namely the nail) for the treatment of ipsilateral femoral neck and shaft fractures [28, 29].

The aforementioned relevant factors were in line with some reported in the previously published classifications [6, 7]. In fact, while Skela-Rosenbaum et al. considered fracture localization (from proximal to distal) and mor-phology (spiral fractures) as a guide for the treatment de-cision making [6], the healing status of the previous fracture was considered relevant by Chan et al. [7].

Other proposed factors were not part of the classification proposal since the research group did not consider the type of implant (monoaxial and biaxial) a pivotal factor for the management of PNFs. The difference between a monoaxial and a biaxial TN depends on the number of pins, screws, or blades that cross the fracture line [16]. In fact, while the biaxial TN presents two screws, pins, or blades that cross the fracture line, the monoxial just one. Norris et al. demon-strated that biaxial TNs were associated with lower fracture risk compared with monoaxial ones [16]. This could be linked to the lower positioning of the lower screw of the biaxial TN that allows a reduction in the stress concentration on the proximal femur [16]. However, in our opinion, this supposed difference in the pathogenesis of PNFs did not affect the treatment decision making.

The relevance of nail length in determining PNFs is still a matter of debate [30–32]. Recently, Shannon et al. in their randomized controlled trial reported a similar rate of PNFs around both short and long nails (2.4% vs. 2.7%) [30]. Moreover, Daner et al. in their biomechanical study did not observe any difference in stiffness between long and short

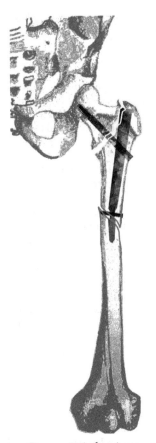

FIGURE 5: A drawing representing a BO2n fracture.

nails under rotational forces, thus making the fracture risk similar [17]. These inconclusive evidences on the role of nail length in determining PNFs and the observation that a clear definition of long nail did not exist (long nails are considered those longer than 240 mm, 300 mm, and 340 mm depending on the nail and the authors [32–35]) did not lead the research group to reach a consensus on the putative role played by nail length in their PNF management.

Our classification proposal was not the first on femoral peri-implant fractures [5–7]. Interestingly, all these classifications have been published in the last four years, underlying the relevance of the topic and the need for treatment guidance. However, in our opinion, none of the previously published classifications was able to accurately describe the PNF pattern and to guide treatment decision making (see Table 3 for further details).

The classification proposal by Videla-Cés et al. was performed by studying 143 peri-implant fractures. The classification extrapolated some concepts from the AO/OTA classification (i.e., the alphanumeric code). Their classification aimed to morphologically describe all peri-implant femoral fractures, giving information on fracture localization (from 1 to 3), the type of implant used (N for nails, P for plates, and D for retrograde implants), and fracture relationship with the implant (from A to E). In the classification proposed by Videla-Cés et al., fracture fragmentation or previous fracture healing (except for type E) was not considered. Although the comprehensive anatomical and morphological description was made by this classification,

the lack of some relevant factors (fracture fragmentation and healing status of the previous fracture) reduced its applicability for treatment purpose.

Chan et al., instead, classified peri-implant fractures according to the type of implant (N for nail and P for plate), fracture localization (at the tip of the implant or distal from the implant), and healing status of the previous fracture. Their classification proposal hereby authorised to classify peri-implant fractures regardless of the bone affected, but they performed an extreme simplification of the fracture characterization, excluding several types of fractures (i.e., fracture around the implant and comminuted fractures).

Skela-Rosenbaum et al., evaluating a series of 21 PNFs, proposed a simple classification system based on three types and two subtypes (IA trochanteric metaphyseal, IB proximal metadiaphyseal; IIA fracture at the tip of the nail, IIB fractures extending from the tip of the nail; and III fractures of the distal femur). The main factors evaluated in their classification were fracture localization and morphology. However, the classification is purely descriptive, and it was impossible to combine the factors included (i.e., it is not possible to classify a spiral fracture occurred around the nail). Moreover, in their classification proposal, the fragmentation and the healing status of the previous fracture were not evaluated. These factors represented a limit for an appropriate fracture characterization, reducing the applicability of their classification as a treatment guide only to some specific types of PNFs.

TABLE 3: Published peri-implant femoral fracture classifications.

Authors	Journal	Year of publication	Pros	Limitation	Main differences with the present classification
Skela-Rosenbaum et al.	Injury	2016	Treatment-oriented classification; classification included only PNFs; evaluated fracture occurred around a single type of nail	Not validated; did not consider the original fracture healing status; classified fracture occurred only around short nails	Original EF healing status considered; classification of fracture occurred around long nails; comprehensive morphological classification; evaluation of fracture fragmentation
Chan et al.	Arch Orthop Trauma Surg	2017	Treatment-oriented; evaluated the original EF healing state	Included also fractures occurred around plates; did not include fracture occurred in the proximal part of the nail; did not consider fracture fragmentation and morphology	Comprehensive morphological and anatomical classification; classification of fracture occurred only around TN; evaluation of fracture fragmentation
Videla-Cés et al.	Injury	2018	Large cohort, comprehensive anatomical and morphological classification	Not treatment-oriented; included also fractures around plates; not validated; did not consider the original fracture healing status; did not consider fracture fragmentation	Original EF healing status considered; fracture fragmentation considered; classification of fracture occurred only around TN

When proposing a classification system, it should be reliable, simple to use, and serve as the basis for treatment [36]. In these perspectives, we choose a simple alphanumerical code also exploiting some of the codes used in well-known classifications of the orthopaedic world. In fact, the use of the ABC code for the fracture localization was the same as the Vancouver classification of PPF [9]. Instead, we preferred the SOT code to describe the fracture morphology using the first letter of the words "spiroid", "oblique," and "transverse". In a similar way, the fragmentation was encoded using the number of fragments observed (2, 3, and +3). Lastly, the nonhealing status was coded adding an "n" at the end of the alphanumeric code. Therefore, a two-fragment oblique fracture occurred around the distal screw of a TN would be classified as B (around the distal screw) O (oblique fracture) 2 (see Figure 4). In case the previous EF was not healed yet, then the same fracture should be classified as BO2n (see Figure 5).

Our classification proposal, based on expert opinions, included 54 possible categories of PNFs, to characterize them considering fracture localization, morphology, and fragmentation and healing status of the previous fracture. These factors are all considered relevant for the management of PNFs; therefore, this new classification system fulfils the intended purpose of providing a simple tool for guiding treatment choice for PNFs. However, before its applicability, a cohort study is required.

4. Conclusions

The growing incidence of proximal femoral fractures and the large use of TN will lead to a constant increase of PNFs. However, their diagnosis is still underrated, considering that they are generally included along with fractures occurred around plates in a generic "peri-implant" fracture category.

However, PNFs are a separate entity with high patients' morbidity and mortality that needs specific strategies to be treated. The proposal of a simple classification based on the most relevant aspects for fracture treatment might be a useful tool to guide the orthopaedic surgeon. Moreover, the use of a specific classification system would be beneficial also to standardize the literature terminology to improve the evidence around PFNs. However, case-based studies are needed to validate the present classification before its widespread use.

Acknowledgments

The authors would like to thank Ms. Valentina Bocchino, for her consistent support with the artworks of the present study.

References

[1] C. Cooper, Z. A. Cole, C. R. Holroyd et al., "Secular trends in the incidence of hip and other osteoporotic fractures," Osteoporosis International, vol. 22, no. 5, pp. 1277–1288, 2011.

[2] U. Tarantino, G. Iolascon, L. Cianferotti et al., "Clinical guidelines for the prevention and treatment of osteoporosis: summary statements and recommendations from the Italian Society for Orthopaedics and Traumatology," Journal of Orthopaedics and Traumatology, vol. 18, no. S1, pp. 3–36, 2017.

[3] G. Toro, F. Lepore, S. D. Cicala et al., "ABO system is not associated with proximal femoral fracture pattern in Southern Italy," HIP International, vol. 28, no. 2, pp. 84–88, 2018.

[4] E. Niu, A. Yang, A. H. S. Harris, and J. Bishop, "Which fixation device is preferred for surgical treatment of intertrochanteric hip fractures in the United States? A survey of orthopaedic surgeons," Clinical Orthopaedics and Related Research, vol. 473, no. 11, pp. 3647–3655, 2015.

[5] M. Videla-Cés, J.-M. Sales-Pérez, R. Sánchez-Navés, E. Romero-Pijoan, and S. Videla, "Proposal for the classification of peri-implant femoral fractures: retrospective cohort study," *Injury*, vol. 50, no. 3, pp. 758–763, 2019.

[6] J. Skála-Rosenbaum, V. DžupaDžupa, R. BartoškaBartoška, P. DoušaDouša, P. Waldauf, and M. Krbec, "Distal locking in short hip nails: cause or prevention of peri-implant fractures?" *Injury*, vol. 47, no. 4, pp. 887–892, 2016.

[7] L. W. M. Chan, A. W. Gardner, A. W. Gardner, M. K. Wong, K. Chua, and E. B. K. Kwek, "Non-prosthetic peri-implant fractures: classification, management and outcomes," *Archives of Orthopaedic and Trauma Surgery*, vol. 138, no. 6, pp. 791–802, 2018.

[8] F. A. Liporace, R. S. Yoon, and C. A. Collinge, "Interprosthetic and peri-implant fractures," *Journal of Orthopaedic Trauma*, vol. 31, no. 5, pp. 287–292, 2017.

[9] B. A. Masri, R. M. D. Meek, and C. P. Duncan, "Periprosthetic fractures evaluation and treatment," *Clinical Orthopaedics and Related Research*, vol. 420, no. 420, pp. 80–95, 2004.

[10] J. M. Drew, W. L. Griffin, S. M. Odum, B. Van Doren, B. T. Weston, and L. S. Stryker, "Survivorship after periprosthetic femur fracture: factors affecting outcome," *The Journal of Arthroplasty*, vol. 31, no. 6, pp. 1283–1288, 2016.

[11] C. Kleweno, J. Morgan, J. Redshaw et al., "Short versus long cephalomedullary nails for the treatment of intertrochanteric hip fractures in patients older than 65 years," *Journal of Orthopaedic Trauma*, vol. 28, no. 7, pp. 391–397, 2014.

[12] L. Audig, M. Bhandari, B. Hanson, and J. Kellam, "A concept for the validation of fracture classifications," *Journal of Orthopaedic Trauma*, vol. 19, no. 6, pp. 404–409, 2005.

[13] M. Reinhold, L. Audigé, K. J. Schnake, C. Bellabarba, L.-Y. Dai, and F. C. Oner, "AO spine injury classification system: a revision proposal for the thoracic and lumbar spine," *European Spine Journal*, vol. 22, no. 10, pp. 2184–2201, 2013.

[14] E. Meinberg, J. Agel, C. Roberts, M. Karam, and J. Kellam, "Fracture and dislocation classification compendium-2018," *Journal of Orthopaedic Trauma*, vol. 32, no. 1, p. S1, 2018.

[15] F. Müller, M. Galler, M. Zellner, C. Bäuml, A. Marzouk, and B. Füchtmeier, "Peri-implant femoral fractures: the risk is more than three times higher within PFN compared with DHS," *Injury*, vol. 47, no. 10, pp. 2189–2194, 2016.

[16] R. Norris, D. Bhattacharjee, and M. J. Parker, "Occurrence of secondary fracture around intramedullary nails used for trochanteric hip fractures: a systematic review of 13,568 patients," *Injury*, vol. 43, no. 6, pp. 706–711, 2012.

[17] W. E. Daner, J. R. Owen, J. S. Wayne, R. B. Graves, and M. C. Willis, "Biomechanical evaluation of the risk of secondary fracture around short versus long cephalomedullary nails," *European Journal of Orthopaedic Surgery & Traumatology: Orthopedie Traumatologie*, vol. 27, no. 8, pp. 1103–1108, 2017.

[18] G. Iolascon, A. Moretti, G. Toro, F. Gimigliano, S. Liguori, and M. Paoletta, "Pharmacological therapy of osteoporosis: what's new?" *Clinical Interventions in Aging*, vol. 15, pp. 485–491, 2020.

[19] M. J. Parker, "Sliding hip screw versus intramedullary nail for trochanteric hip fractures; a randomised trial of 1000 patients with presentation of results related to fracture stability," *Injury*, vol. 48, no. 12, pp. 2762–2767, 2017.

[20] J. O. Anglen and J. N. Weinstein, "Nail or plate fixation of intertrochanteric hip fractures: changing pattern of practice," *The Journal of Bone and Joint Surgery-American Volume*, vol. 90, no. 4, pp. 700–707, 2008.

[21] L. Mattisson, A. Bojan, and A. Enocson, "Epidemiology, treatment and mortality of trochanteric and subtrochanteric hip fractures: data from the Swedish fracture register," *BMC Musculoskeletal Disorders*, vol. 19, no. 1, p. 369, 2018.

[22] B. Buecking, C. Bliemel, J. Struewer, D. Eschbach, S. Ruchholtz, and T. Müller, "Use of the gamma3 nail in a teaching hospital for trochanteric fractures: mechanical complications, functional outcomes, and quality of life," *BMC Research Notes*, vol. 5, no. 1, p. 651, 2012.

[23] M. J. Parker and H. H. Handoll, "Gamma and other cephalocondylic intramedullary nails versus extramedullary implants for extracapsular hip fractures in adults," *Cochrane Database of Systematic Reviews*, vol. 8, no. 9, Article ID CD000093, 2010.

[24] A. Herrera, J. Rosell, E. Ibarz et al., "Biomechanical analysis of the stability of anterograde reamed intramedullary nails in femoral spiral fractures," *Injury*, vol. 51, pp. S74–S79, 2020.

[25] S. Samsami, R. Pätzold, M. Winkler, S. Herrmann, and P. Augat, "The effect of coronal splits on the structural stability of bi-condylar tibial plateau fractures: a biomechanical investigation," *Archives of Orthopaedic and Trauma Surgery*, vol. 140, 2020, http://link.springer.com/10.1007/s00402-020-03412-8.

[26] K. E. Kojima and R. E. S. Pires, "Absolute and relative stabilities for fracture fixation: the concept revisited," *Injury*, vol. 48, p. S1, 2017.

[27] M. E. Müller, P. Koch, S. Nazarian, and J. Schatzker, "Principles of the classification of fractures," in *The Comprehensive Classification of Fractures of Long Bones [Internet]*, pp. 4–7, Springer Berlin Heidelberg, Berlin, Heidelberg, 1990, http://link.springer.com/10.1007/978-3-642-61261-9_2.

[28] K.-T. Wu, S.-J. Lin, Y.-C. Chou et al., "Ipsilateral femoral neck and shaft fractures fixation with proximal femoral nail antirotation II (PFNA II): technical note and cases series," *Journal of Orthopaedic Surgery and Research*, vol. 15, no. 1, p. 20, 2020.

[29] W.-Y. Wang, L. Liu, G.-L. Wang, Y. Fang, and T.-F. Yang, "Ipsilateral basicervical femoral neck and shaft fractures treated with long proximal femoral nail antirotation or various plate combinations: comparative study," *Journal of Orthopaedic Science*, vol. 15, no. 3, pp. 323–330, 2010.

[30] S. F. Shannon, B. J. Yuan, W. W. Cross et al., "Short versus long cephalomedullary nails for pertrochanteric hip fractures," *Journal of Orthopaedic Trauma*, vol. 33, no. 10, pp. 480–486, 2019.

[31] J. Vaughn, E. Cohen, B. G. Vopat, P. Kane, E. Abbood, and C. Born, "Complications of short versus long cephalomedullary nail for intertrochanteric femur fractures, minimum 1 year follow-up," *European Journal of Orthopaedic Surgery & Traumatology*, vol. 25, no. 4, pp. 665–670, 2015.

[32] D. S. Horwitz, A. Tawari, and M. Suk, "Nail length in the management of intertrochanteric fracture of the femur," *Journal of the American Academy of Orthopaedic Surgeons*, vol. 24, no. 6, pp. e50–e58, 2016.

[33] Gamma3 | Stryker, 2020, https://www.stryker.com/us/en/trauma-and-extremities/products/gamma3.html.

[34] Proximal Femoral Nail Antirotation, (PFNA), 2020, https://www.jnjmedicaldevices.com/en-EMEA/product/proximal-femoral-nail-antirotation-pfna.

[35] G. Okcu, N. Ozkayin, C. Okta, I. Topcu, and K. Aktuglu, "Which implant is better for treating reverse obliquity fractures of the proximal femur: a standard or long nail?" *Clinical Orthopaedics and Related Research*, vol. 471, no. 9, pp. 2768–2775, 2013.

[36] J. Bernstein, B. A. Monaghan, J. S. Silber, and W. G. DeLong, "Taxonomy and treatment - a classification of fracture classifications," *The Journal of Bone and Joint Surgery. British Volume*, vol. 79-B, no. 5, pp. 706-707, 1997.

9

Does Open Reduction in Intramedullary Nailing of Femur Shaft Fractures Adversely Affect the Outcome?

Syed Imran Ghouri, Abduljabbar Alhammoud ⓘD, and Mohammed Mubarak Alkhayarin ⓘD

Hamad Medical Corporation, Doha, Qatar

Correspondence should be addressed to Mohammed Mubarak Alkhayarin; Alkhayarin@hamad.qa

Academic Editor: Panagiotis Korovessis

Aim. This study aims to assess the results of open versus closed reduction in intramedullary nailing for femoral fractures and whether it delays union, predisposes to nonunion, or increases the rate of infection. *Materials and Methods*. A retrospective review of all adult patients with isolated femoral shaft fractures treated by intramedullary nailing was done. The primary outcome is union rate, and the secondary outcomes are operation time and the infection rate. *Results*. 110 isolated femoral shaft fractures, with 73 (66.4%) in the closed reduction group and 37 (33.6%) in the open reduction group, 90.4% males and 9.6% females, and the average age was 32.6 years. RTA is the most common cause of these injuries followed by the fall from height. The delayed union rate was 20% (22/110) with no difference between the two groups, *p* value 0.480, and the nonunion rate was 5.5% (6/110), and no statistical difference was observed between the two groups. The operation time was shorter in the closed groups, and no difference in the time to union was observed between two groups. No infection was found in the two groups. *Conclusions*. There is no statistical difference between the healing rates in closed and open reduction in femoral shaft fractures. In cases where closed reduction is difficult, it is better to open reduce the fracture if closed reduction cannot be achieved in 15 minutes, especially in polytrauma.

1. Introduction

Fractures of the femoral shaft are due to high energy trauma and therefore can be associated with life-threatening injuries and causes of permanent disability. Intramedullary nailing is the standard of care for the management of femoral shaft fractures in adults with union rates between 95 and 99% [1]. Though the complication such as nonunion and malunion is still a challenge in such fracture especially in subtrochantric, pediatrics age group, and floating knee, this technique can be done with either closed (without disruption of the fracture site with indirect reduction) or open reduction (through small incision over the fracture with direct reduction) [2]. Remarkable improvements in the operative treatment of these injuries in the last 15 years have dramatically lessened the morbidity and mortality associated with these fractures [3]. Closed locked intramedullary nailing is now the management of choice in femoral diaphyseal fractures. However, closed reduction may not always be achievable, and the only

option then is to open the fracture site to achieve an acceptable reduction. This is an additional trauma to the patient and alters the biology of the fracture.

The aim of this study to ascertain if open reduction during intramedullary nailing of femoral shaft fractures is detrimental to fracture healing, operating times, and infection rates comparing to the closed one.

2. Materials and Methods

A retrospective review of all adult patients with isolated femoral shaft fractures treated by intramedullary nailing at level one trauma center between 2011 and 2015 was done after obtaining the ethical approval from Medical Research Center.

Patients with isolated closed, diaphyseal femur shaft fracture were included, whereas those with fractures of the proximal or distal femur treated with other modalities, open fractures, head injury and polytrauma, inadequate data availability, and nonavailability of follow-up were excluded.

Data were collected for general demographic (age and gender), injury characteristic (mechanism of injury and fracture classification), and outcome finding (union rate, infection rate, secondary procedure, and operation time).

Delayed union was considered when no bridging callus was seen at 6 months after surgery as per standard FDA definition, whereas nonunion was established when no bridging callus was seen on radiographs at 12 months after surgery [4].

All patients were operated in the lateral decubitus position using statically locked AO Synthes femoral nails, and in cases with open reduction, an additional incision was made over the fracture site, and with one or two fingers, the reduction and rotation were checked.

Descriptive statistics were used to summarize demographic data and injury characteristics. We used a chi-squared test and a Fisher exact test to express the associations between two or more qualitative data points, whereas an unpaired t-test was used to compare the quantitative data between the two groups. Frequency (percentage) and mean ± SD or median and range were used for categorical and continuous values as appropriate. A p value of <0.05 was considered statistically significant. All statistical analyses were done using statistical packages SPSS 23.0 (SPSS Inc., Chicago, IL) and Epi InfoTM 2000 (Centers for Disease Control and Prevention, Atlanta, GA).

3. Results

110 adult patients with isolated femoral shaft fractures treated by intramedullary nailing were included in the study, and 73 (66.4%) underwent closed reduction and 37 (33.6%) required open reduction and subsequent insertion of a femoral nail.

3.1. Demographic. Out of a total of 110 patients, 90.4% were males and 9.1% were females with 62 males and 5 females in the closed reduction group and 32 males and 5 females in the open reduction group (Table 1 and Figure 1).

The mean age of the patients in the closed reduction group was 31.6 years and in the open reduction group was 33.08 years.

3.2. Injury Characteristic. Mechanism of injury in most of patients in our series was victims of road traffic accidents with head on or side impact injuries; others sustained falls, especially the laborers working on construction sites (Figure 1 and Table 1).

We adopted the Winquist and Hansen classification for this study for fracture classification. Eighty fractures were Winquist type 1 (53 in the closed reduction group and 27 in the open reduction group). Twenty-four were Winquist type 2 (16 in the closed reduction group and 8 in the open reduction group). Three fractures were Winquist type 3 (2 in the close group and one in the open group). Three fractures

TABLE 1: Demographic data.

	Total	Closed group	Open group	p value
Number	110	73 (66.4%)	37 (33.6%)	
Gender				
Male	94 (90.4%)	62 (92.5%)	32 (86.5%)	0.316
Female	10 (9.6%)	5 (7.5%)	5 (13.5%)	
Age (year)		31.16 + 11.04	33.08 + 14.62	0.453
Mechanism of injury				
RTA	80 (74.8%)	53 (75.7%)	27 (73.0%)	0.696
Fall	26 (24.3%)	16 (22.9%)	10 (27.0%)	
Others	1 (0.9%)	1 (0.9%)	0 (0%)	
Fracture classification:				
Type 1	80 (72.7%)	53 (72.6%)	27 (73.0%)	1.0
Type 2	24 (21.8%)	16 (21.9%)	8 (21.7%)	
Type 3	3 (2.7%)	2 (1.8%(	1 (0.9%)	
Type 4	3 (2.7%)	2 (1.8%)	1 (0.9%)	

were segmental (2 in the closed reduction group and 1 in the open reduction group) (Table 1).

3.3. Bone Healing Outcome. The union was delayed in 22 (20%) patients, comprising 16 cases in the closed reduction and 6 in the open reduction group, and no statistical difference in delay union between two groups was observed, p value (0.480).

Six patients had nonunion of the fracture with 4 nonunions in the closed reduction group (5.5%) and 2 in the open reduction group (5.4%). The p value again was not significant. All the nonunion patients were managed by secondary autogenous bone grafting, and union was achieved in all cases (Table 2 and Figure 2).

The mean time to union in the closed reduction group was 7.11 months with a standard deviation of 3.496. The mean time to union in the open reduction group was 7.35 months with a standard deviation of 4.673. The p value here again was not significant.

3.4. Other Outcomes. The mean operating time in the closed reduction group was 113.2 minutes with a standard deviation of 34.725. The mean operating time in the open group was 132 minutes with a standard deviation of 35.670. The p value was significant. However, we believe that the longer operating time in the open group was probably due to the complex nature of these fractures to start with. No patient in our series developed any superficial or deep infection.

4. Discussion

This study aims to find out whether open reduction with subsequent drainage of the fracture hematoma and the

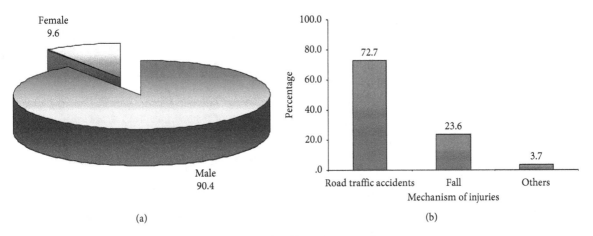

FIGURE 1: (a) Gender; (b) mechanism of injuries.

TABLE 2: Outcome data.

	Total	Closed group	Open group	p value
Delay union	22 (20%)	16 (21.9%)	6 (16.2%)	0.480
Nonunion	6 (5.5%)	4 (5.5%)	2 (5.4%)	0.987
Time to union (months)		7.111 + 3.4	7.3 + 4.6	0.802
Operation time (minutes)		113 + 34.7	132 + 35.6	0.010
Infection rate	0	0	0	

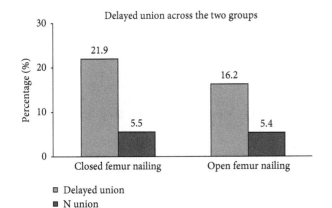

FIGURE 2: Delayed union and no union.

additional tissue trauma affects the union and rehabilitation with more complication rates in femoral shaft fractures when compared with the closed reduction technique which is the gold standard of management of these injuries [2, 3].

That being said, open intramedullary nailing of the femur does have certain advantages like using less expensive equipment than that required for closed nailing; no special fracture table is required; image intensifier is not (or briefly) required; or absolute anatomical reduction is easier to obtain than with closed means [5]. Direct observation of the bone may identify undisplaced and undetected comminution not noted radiographically which can be dealt with. Precise interdigitation of the fracture fragments improves rotational stability. In segmental fractures, the middle segment can be stabilized, preventing torquing and twisting associated with closed reduction and medullary reaming. In nonunions,

opening of the medullary canals of sclerotic bones is easier, and rotational malalignment is rare after open reduction.

Some disadvantages of the open technique have also been described which include the consideration of skin scars, loss of fracture hematoma which is important for fracture healing, and bone shavings obtained from reaming the canal are lost. Infection rates are increased, union rates are decreased, and image intensification may still be required if a locking nail is used [6].

Because it requires no special equipment and achieves quick reduction, some authors advocate open nailing in the polytrauma patients [5]. Open intramedullary nailing is invaluable in the first trimester pregnant polytrauma patient with least radiation exposure [7].

Grundnes et al. in their study on open versus closed femur nailing in rats concluded that the fractures did heal faster initially with closed nailing, but at 12 weeks, there was no significant difference in the mechanical characteristics [8]. Furthermore, some studies actually showed judicious use of open reduction techniques during intramedullary nailing of closed fractures which appeared to have a minimal risk of infection [7–9]. Our study has shown that the overall risk of nonunion or infection is unchanged in both types of reduction. Wolinsky et al. demonstrated a union rate of 93.6% after initial nailing and an overall union rate of 98.9% following an additional procedure [10]. Leighton et al. also showed 97% satisfactory results with open nailing as compared to 92% with closed nailing [11]. Closed reamed intramedullary nailing technique is still the preferred method and has a greater chance of healing and lower rate of complications [12–16]. However, there are still controversies in results of femoral shaft fractures treated by close versus open nailing [17–20]. This study also reveals the fact that a well-timed and proper open reduction of a femoral fracture during nailing does not impede the healing or eventual functional outcome of the fracture, and the incidence of infection is similar. We did not record intraoperative radiation exposure in both groups by dosimetry; this may be considered as a relative weak point of the study along with the relatively small sample size.

One important factor that may impact in the outcome of femur fracture is using the locking screws as using the locking screws leads to increase surgical time, blood loss, and radiation exposure without significant impact in the fracture healing.

Dealing with nonunion and malunion is challenging in femur fracture, and proper and systematic follow-up is a key to deal with any delay union which can be managed by dynamization which leads to optimal results in such fractures.

Retrograde nailing is considered a good option for antegrade nailing in treatment of femur fracture with almost similar results with regard to the functional and radiological outcomes.

Open reduction and intramedullary nailing of femoral shaft fractures did not significantly increase delayed union or nonunion rates or predispose to infection. It only resulted in a longer operative time which was probably due to the complexity of the injury itself and can be considered a safe alternative to closed reduction in situations where closed reduction cannot be obtained and or in polytrauma patients.

The operating surgeon ought to be prepared to open the fracture if a satisfactory closed reduction cannot be attained within a reasonable interval of operating time. The potential benefits for the patient outweigh the theoretical pitfalls of this additional procedure. This, in our study, did not increase the risk of reducing the functional result. A prospective study in this regard will perhaps shed more light on the topic.

Acknowledgments

The medical research center at Hamad medical corporations provided the financial support for publication of this study.

References

[1] P. Wolinsky, N. Tejwani, J. H. Richmond et al., "Controversies in intramedullary nailing of femoral shaft fractures instruction course lectures," *Journal of Bone and Joint Surgery*, vol. 51, pp. 291–303, 2002.

[2] J. D. Kingsey and J. C. Krieg, "Femoral malrotation following intramedullary nail fixation," *Journal of the American Academy of Orthopaedic Surgeons*, vol. 19, no. 1, 2011.

[3] R. W. Bucholz and A. Jones, "Fractures of the shaft of the femur," *Journal of Bone and Joint Surgery*, vol. 73, no. 10, 1991.

[4] J. C. Taylor, *Delayed Union and Nonunion of Fractures: Campbell's Operative Orthopaedics*pp. 1287–1345, Mosby, St. Louis, MO, USA, 8th edition, 1992.

[5] L. Davlin, E. Johnson, T. Thomas, and G. Lian, "Open versus closed nailing of femoral fractures in the polytrauma patient," *Contemporary Orthopaedics*, vol. 22, no. 5, pp. 557–563, 1991.

[6] S. Terry Canale and J. Beaty, *Campbell's Operative Orthopaedics*, Elsevier, Amsterdam, Netherlands, 11th edition, 2007.

[7] A. Ogbemudia, R. Enemudo, and E. Edomwonyi, "Closed interlocked nailing of a fractured femur without x-ray guide in first trimester pregnancy: a case report," *The Internet Journal of Third World Medicine*, vol. 5, no. 2, 2006.

[8] O. Grundnes and O. Reikeras, "Closed versus open medullary nailing of femoral fractures," *Acta Orthopaedica Scandinavica*, vol. 63, no. 5, pp. 492–496, 1992.

[9] J. Schatzker, "Open intramedullary nailing of the femur," *The Orthopedic Clinics of North America*, vol. 11, pp. 623–631, 1980.

[10] P. R. Wolinsky, E. McCarty, Y. Shyr, and K. Johnson, "Reamed intramedullary nailing of the femur," *The Journal of Trauma: Injury, Infection, and Critical Care*, vol. 46, no. 3, pp. 392–399, 1999.

[11] R. K. Leighton, J. P. Waddell, J. F. Kellam, and K. G. Orrell, "Open versus closed intramedullary nailing of femoral shaft fractures," *The Journal of Trauma: Injury, Infection, and Critical Care*, vol. 26, no. 10, pp. 923–926, 1986.

[12] K. F. King and J. Rush, "Closed intramedullary nailing of femoral shaft fractures. A review of one hundred and twelve cases treated by the küntscher technique," *The Journal of Bone & Joint Surgery*, vol. 63, no. 8, pp. 1319–1323, 1981.

[13] S. Aiyer, J. Jagiasi, H. Argekar, S. Sharan, and B. Dasgupta, "Closed antegrade interlocked nailing of femoral shaft fractures operated up to 2 weeks postinjury in the absence of a fracture table or c-arm," *The Journal of Trauma: Injury, Infection, and Critical Care*, vol. 61, no. 2, pp. 457–460, 2006.

[14] B. D. Crist and P. R. Wolinsky, "Reaming does not add significant time to intramedullary nailing of diaphyseal fractures of the tibia and femur," *The Journal of Trauma: Injury, Infection, and Critical Care*, vol. 67, no. 4, pp. 727–734, 2009.

[15] R. J. Brumback and W. W. Virkus, "Intramedullary nailing of the femur: reamed versus nonreamed," *Journal of the American Academy of Orthopaedic Surgeons*, vol. 8, no. 2, pp. 83–90, 2000.

[16] S. Debrauwer, K. Hendrix, and R. Verdonk, "Anterograde femoral nailing with a reamed interlocking titanium alloy nail," *Acta Orthopaedica Belgica*, vol. 66, no. 5, pp. 484–489, 2000.

[17] C.-C. Wu and Z.-L. Lee, "Treatment of femoral shaft aseptic nonunion associated with broken distal locked screws and shortening," *The Journal of Trauma: Injury, Infection, and Critical Care*, vol. 58, no. 4, pp. 837–840, 2005.

[18] L. A. Taitsman, J. R. Lynch, J. Agel, D. P. Barei, and S. E. Nork, "Risk factors for femoral nonunion after femoral shaft fracture," *The Journal of Trauma: Injury, Infection, and Critical Care*, vol. 67, no. 6, pp. 1389–1392, 2009.

[19] J. C. Liao, P. H. Hsieh, T. Y. Chuang, J. Y. Su, C. H. Chen, and Y. J. Chen, "Mini-open intramedullary nailing of acute femoral shaft fracture: reduction through a small incision without a fracture table," *Chang Gung Medical Journal*, vol. 26, no. 9, pp. 660–668, 2003.

[20] M. A. Tahririan and A. Andalib, "Is there a place for open intramedullary nailing in femoral shaft fractures?" *Advanced Biomedical Research*, vol. 31, no. 3, p. 157, 2014.

10

Predicting Fracture Risk in Patients with Metastatic Bone Disease of the Femur: A Pictorial Review Using Three Different Techniques

Shannon M. Kaupp ⓘ, Kenneth A. Mann ⓘ, Mark A. Miller ⓘ, and Timothy A. Damron ⓘ

SUNY Upstate Medical University, Department of Orthopedic Surgery, 750 East Adams Street, Syracuse, NY 13210, USA

Correspondence should be addressed to Timothy A. Damron; damront@upstate.edu

Academic Editor: Francesco Liuzza

One of the key roles of an orthopedic surgeon treating metastatic bone disease (MBD) is fracture risk prediction. Current widely used impending fracture risk tools such as Mirels scoring lack specificity. Two newer methods of fracture risk prediction, CT-based structural rigidity analysis (CTRA) and finite element analysis (FEA), have each been shown to be more accurate than Mirels. This case series illustrates comparative Mirels, CTRA, and FEA for 8 femurs in 7 subjects. These cases were selected from a much larger data set to portray examples of true positives, true negatives, false positives, and false negatives as defined by CTRA relative to the fracture outcome. Case illustrations demonstrate comparative Mirels and FEA. This series illustrates the use, efficacy, and limitations of these tools. As all current tools have limitations, further work is needed in refining and developing fracture risk prediction.

1. Introduction

Bone is the third most common site for cancer metastases after lung and liver [1]. Metastatic bone disease (MBD) has become an increasingly prevalent condition as the population of patients over forty increases and the longevity for patients with cancer continues to improve [2]. Patients with MBD often present with bone pain, impaired mobility, and impending or actual pathologic fracture [1, 3]. The challenge of impending fracture lies in determining which warrants prophylactic treatment, particularly operative stabilization. Early clinical and radiographic attempts to define impending pathologic fracture, including Mirels score [4], show poor specificity and variable sensitivity. Strict adherence to Mirels score and recommendations for prophylactic stabilization would lead to unnecessary surgeries [5]. Numerous other tools suffer the same limitations [6–8].

Two more recently utilized techniques, CT-based structural rigidity analysis (CTRA) and finite element analysis (FEA), have reported improved accuracy in

predicting fracture in long bones, particularly the proximal femur [5, 9–14]. Although not yet widely used as a clinical tool, CTRA accounts for changes in bone density and bone geometry due to the presence of MBD lesions. With CTRA analysis, the rigidity of the bone is calculated using CT data for the bone, and a predetermined loss of rigidity threshold is used to create a binary outcome of increased risk or not increased risk of fracture [13, 15]. CTRA has been shown to be superior to Mirels score in terms of predicting fracture risk in terms of sensitivity, specificity, positive predictive value, and negative predictive value [5]. With FEA, a computer model of the femur with the lesion is created from the CT scan with material properties of each element of the model assigned based on bone density. Force to failure can be calculated by applying loads to the model simulating daily activities including standing, walking, and stair ascent [9–11]. FEA has also been shown to be a superior method when compared to Mirels score and expert opinion [9, 16].

Although CTRA and FEA have been reported to be more accurate than Mirels score when assessing fracture risk, neither CTRA nor FEA has been clearly demonstrated to be the superior technique. The primary purpose of this pictorial essay is to demonstrate the comparative and complementary use of Mirels, CTRA, and FEA in the setting of MBD in cases where all three tests were performed. A secondary goal is to familiarize clinicians with these techniques. With CTRA as the reference test, cases of true positives, false positives, false negatives, and true negatives are illustrated. This is the first report of its kind for MBD.

2. Materials and Methods

This research was deemed exempt by the Institutional Review Board at SUNY Upstate Medical University (UMU). Cases were extracted from SUNY UMU patients enrolled in a prospective Musculoskeletal Tumor Society (MSTS) sponsored study. The MSTS multi-institutional study has enrolled MBD patients since July 2008 and has continued through 2021. The primary purpose was to establish the efficacy of fracture prediction using CTRA. Patients from the MSTS CTRA study at UMU have also been analyzed by FEA, and those patients from 2008 to 2012 have been previously reported [11].

Initial enrollment in the MSTS study included all long bones and involved assigning a Mirels score and obtaining X-ray imaging and a CT scan with phantom. The CT scans with phantom were used for initial CTRA and subsequent FEA. Patients who did not undergo prophylactic stabilization surgery were followed at approximately 4-month intervals to assess changes in their condition and radiographic lesional progression.

Enrollment criteria for the current report were patients enrolled at SUNY UMU with MBD lesions of the femur for which Mirels, CTRA, and FEA had been performed and with follow-up available to time of fracture or death or a minimum 12-month follow-up. Excluded criteria were patients who had nonfemoral lesions analyzed by CTRA, did not have all three prediction outcomes available, had undergone prophylactic stabilization, or had less than 12-month follow-up without fracture or death. Patients who died within 12 months were included if there was a minimum 4-month follow-up. For the cases with patients who went on to fracture, we eliminated any case thought to have potentially been caused by an osteoporosis. Additional reasons for exclusion included elective discontinuation from the study, lack of X-ray images, and incomplete medical records (Figure 1). From the final group, we selected the most illustrative true positive, false positive, false negative, and true negative cases using CTRA as the reference test.

Many of the subjects had bilateral femoral lesions at presentation. However, case presentations were selected based upon the criteria depicted in Figure 1. Hence, for the final selected cases, details and figures for the contralateral femur are only discussed briefly where applicable.

A Mirels score was assigned to each subject by a single orthopedic oncologist (TAD) using information from both the initial visit and imaging. Scoring was determined based on the X-ray imaging, not the CT scans. Mirels score consisted of four components (size, location, tumor type,

and pain level), with 1–3 points assigned to each component. A total score of up to 12 points was possible [4, 17].

Computed tomography (CT) scans were performed with a hydroxyapatite phantom (0, 500, 1,000 mg/cc HA or 0, 750, 1,500 mg/cc HA) in view to calibrate the mineral equivalent density of the patient's bone [11]. The phantom was used for both CTRA and FEA to correlate the degree of X-ray attenuation with an accurate bone mineral density (BMD) measurement. CTRA is a technique that estimates a bone's fracture threshold through loss of bone rigidity (in this case the femur). Of note, CTRA has traditionally been calculated using straight beam theory, but more recently a method of curved CTRA has been developed [13]. When referencing CTRA within this manuscript, all subjects were assessed using traditional straight beam theory. The likelihood of fracture is based on axial (EA), bending (EI), and torsional (GJ) bone rigidity at the weakest CT cross section through the lesion. Bone rigidity is an indirect measure of the bone's resistance to fracture when a force is applied. CTRA calculates the elastic modulus (stiffness, E or G) of each pixel in the bone cross section using the local bone mineral density. The product of the pixel modulus (E or G) and section properties (A, I, J) are then calculated. A more detailed description of this technique has been described in the literature previously [18]. CT scans obtained locally were electronically and securely transferred to Beth Israel Deaconess Biomechanics Laboratory, Harvard University, Boston, Massachusetts, for analysis. As a research tool in development, CTRA was not always available for clinical decision making.

FEA was not part of any clinical decision making but rather was performed at a later time and as a research tool only. The FEA data was not available concurrently with the patient evaluation and therefore played no role in a patient's treatment plan. For the analysis with FEA, Mimics software was used to create voxel-based finite element meshes based on the CT scan of the femur with lesion. Material properties were assigned to each finite element based on the mineral equivalent density using the CT scan gray scale. Femoral head and abductor loads were applied to the model consistently with axial load, level walking, and stair ascent [11]. The force needed to fracture the femur was calculated for each loading condition. The risk of fracture (ROF) was calculated as 3 times the body weight (3 BW) divided by the predicted fracture load. If the ROF was greater than 1, fracture was predicted. The loading conditions used in this study (femoral head load and abductor load) were sufficient to assess fracture risk for proximal and midshaft femoral lesions only but were not used sufficiently to assess cases with distal femoral lesions.

3. Case Summaries

Cases are grouped according to the category of fracture prediction using CTRA as the primary technique relative to the true fracture outcome (Table 1). Mirels and FEA results are also presented for comparison. In only one of the cases, where both CTRA and FEA were available, was there a discrepancy in the findings (Case 7, left femur).

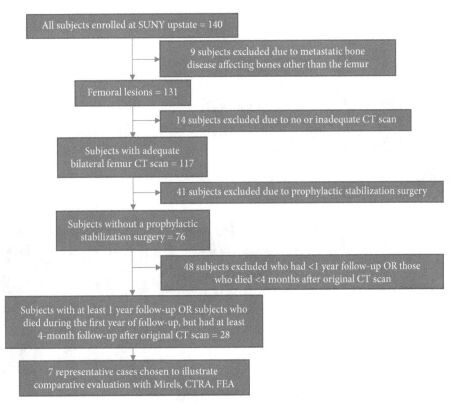

FIGURE 1: Subject exclusion flow chart.

TABLE 1: Case summary based upon CTRA statistical outcome.

Category (based on CTRA)	Case number	Fracture outcome	Mirels	CTRA	FEA
True positives	Case 1	Fracture	10	Increased risk	Increased risk
	Case 2	Fracture	11	Increased risk	Increased risk
False positives	Case 3	No fracture	7	Increased risk	Increased risk
	Case 4	No fracture	9	Increased risk	Increased risk
False negatives	Case 5	Fracture	9	Normal	N/A
True negatives	Case 6	No fracture	8	Normal	Normal
	Case 7 (left femur)	No fracture	8	Normal	Increased risk
	Case 7 (right femur)	No fracture	9	Normal	Normal

3.1. CTRA True Positive: Case #1 (Right Femur). A 68-year-old female presented with excruciating right thigh pain associated with a femoral metastatic lesion (Figure 2). She had a history of triple negative (ER-, PR-, Her2-) left breast infiltrating ductal carcinoma treated six years ago with bilateral mastectomies, radiation therapy, and multiple chemotherapeutic agents. Shortly following her office visit, while moving from the CT scanner, she fractured the proximal right femoral diaphysis. The following day, she underwent open biopsy followed by ORIF with an intramedullary reconstruction nail. Post-op EBRT was given. For the right femur, her Mirels score was 10, and both CTRA and FEA suggested that she was at increased fracture risk based on the prefracture CT. Due to the chronology, both the CTRA and FEA were calculated post hoc. Over the next year, new lesions were discovered in the left femur, but since the patient was asymptomatic, no surgical intervention occurred.

3.2. CTRA True Positive: Case #2 (Right Femur). A 77-year-old female with a history of renal cell carcinoma status following partial nephrectomy three years ago presented due to two years of progressive right thigh pain no longer responsive to oxycodone and causing difficulty with ambulation (Figure 3). A large right femoral diaphyseal lytic lesion was interpreted as an impending fracture. Mirels score was 11, and both CTRA and FEA suggested increased fracture risk.

She was directly admitted from the office due to poor health and need for additional malignancy staging and for interventional radiology biopsy prior to planned prophylactic stabilization. Additional metastatic lesions were noted on the chest wall and right humerus. Shortly after admission, she twisted her right lower extremity in bed resulting in increased right thigh pain, causing pathologic fracture through the lesion. Interventional radiology CT guided

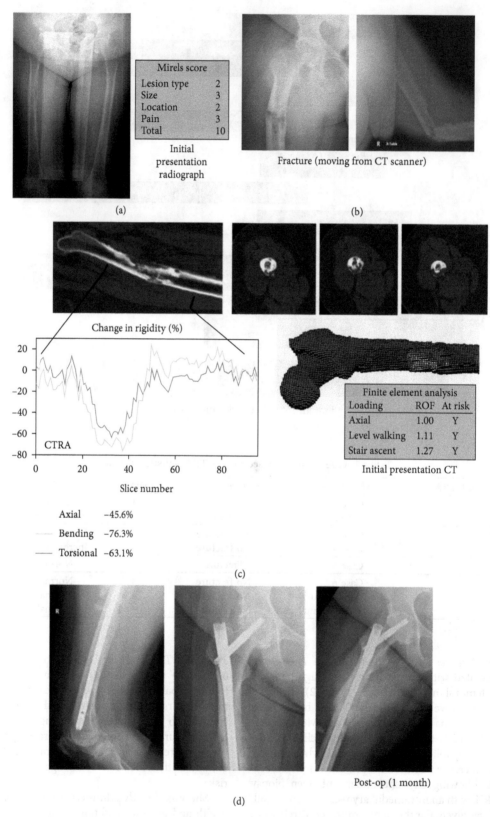

FIGURE 2: True positive (CTRA+/Fx+) (Case 1, R femur). (a) This is a 68-year-old female with metastatic breast cancer showing an osteolytic lesion in the right femoral diaphysis on X-ray imaging, (b) who, while moving from the CT scanner, fractured her right femur. (c) CTRA and FEA analysis both predicted fracture in this patient. (d) She was admitted and taken for surgical fixation of the right femur.

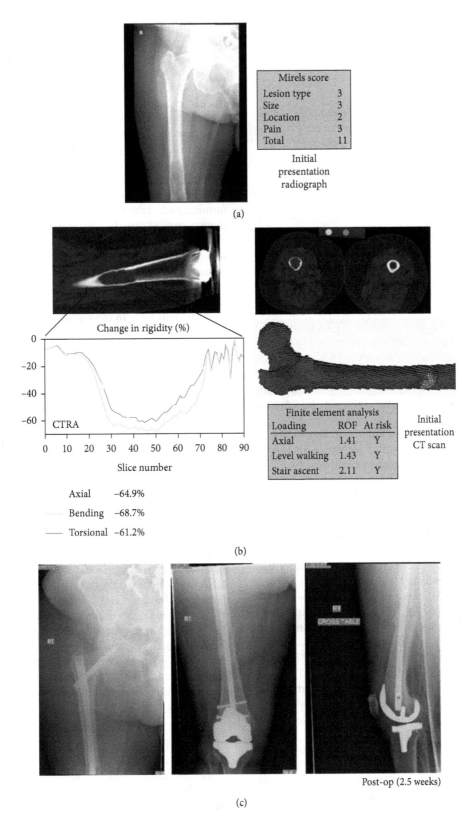

FIGURE 3: True positive (CTRA+/Fx+) (Case 2, R femur). (a) This is a 77-year-old female with metastatic renal cell carcinoma to the right femoral diaphysis. (b) CTRA and FEA both predicted fracture for this subject. (c) The patient was admitted to the hospital on the day of her initial appointment and twisted her leg in bed, likely causing a fracture. When taken to the OR for prophylactic stabilization, the patient was noted to have a fracture and thus was treated with ORIF.

biopsy confirmed metastatic renal cell carcinoma. Preoperative embolization the following day was followed by subsequent ORIF with a femoral reconstruction nail on the next day.

3.3. CTRA False Positive: Case #3 (Right Femur).

A 59-year-old female originally presented with persistent mild right hip pain (Figure 4). She had a history of breast cancer treated with lumpectomy, lymph node dissection, EBRT, and multiple chemotherapy agents 7 years ago. At presentation, she had known metastatic lesions in the sternum and L4 vertebrae. Imaging revealed a right greater trochanter lesion. Mirels score was 7, and prophylactic stabilization was not recommended. Instead, she underwent right proximal femoral EBRT.

Two years later, she returned with bilateral femoral metastatic lesions. The Mirels score for her right femur was unchanged at 7. However, both CTRA and FEA suggested increased fracture risk. Prophylactic right femoral stabilization was discussed due to the positive CTRA findings but ultimately was not recommended due to the low Mirels score and mild pain. Two years later, she returned with severe right hip pain associated with advanced osteoarthritis and a nondisplaced acetabular dome pathologic fracture through a periacetabular lytic lesion. However, there was no proximal femur fracture.

Images shown are for the right femur. Of note, for the left side, a Mirels score of 9 (2 for pain, 3 for size, 1 for lesional characteristics, and 3 for location) was followed by CTRA showing no increased risk of fracture. The left hip was treated with EBRT but no operative intervention.

3.4. CTRA False Positive: Case #4 (Right Femur).

A 68-year-old female presented to the ER with pathologic right humerus fracture and progressive right lower extremity pain rendering her nonambulatory (Figure 5). She had been diagnosed with metastatic neuroendocrine carcinoma one month ago. At that time, PET/CT scan showed metastatic lesions in the lymph nodes, liver, and multiple bones (right clavicle, right scapula, right humerus, left iliac crest, and bilateral femurs). For the right femoral midshaft diaphyseal lesion, Mirels score was 9, and both CTRA and FEA suggested increased fracture risk. The humerus was treated by ORIF. The right femoral lesion was treated nonoperatively with EBRT, and despite regaining an active lifestyle, she did not fracture over the subsequent year.

Images shown are for the right femur. Of note, the left femur demonstrated a distal metaphyseal lesion, for which Mirels was 9 and CTRA suggested no increased fracture risk. FEA was not run on the right femur because the model is not designed for distal femoral lesions. No fracture occurred over the year after EBRT.

3.5. CTRA False Negative: Case #5 (Left Femur).

A 63-year-old male presented with pain associated with a pathologic humeral fracture. Past medical history was significant for metastatic renal cell carcinoma to lung, lymph nodes, and bone (right ilium, right humerus, bilateral femurs). Due to the newly diagnosed bone metastases, he underwent dedicated X-ray and CT imaging of the bilateral femurs.

A lytic left distal femur lesion was identified (Figure 6). Mirels score was 9, and CTRA did not predict increased fracture risk. FEA was not run on the left femur because the model is not designed for distal femoral lesions. No specific treatment was recommended. Four months later, the patient fell and was found to have a closed pathological fracture of the left femoral shaft and underwent operative fixation with an intramedullary reconstruction nail. He went on to have a complicated hospital course with UTI, bilateral pleural effusions, and right-sided paralysis associated with hemorrhagic stroke due to metastatic brain lesions, leading ultimately to death. It is possible that prior prophylactic stabilization of the femur could have prevented this outcome. Pathologic fractures can be devastating complications of MBD, thus making accurate fracture prediction essential. However, prophylactic stabilization surgery comes with its own inherent risks to the patient, so weighing the risks and benefits for each patient is crucial.

All figures are for the left femur. For the right femur, CTRA was not run and a Mirels score was not assigned because a lesion was not recognized on X-ray imaging. It was only with CT imaging that the right side was noted to contain a metastatic lesion. Post hoc FEA was run for the right femur and predicted fracture. No prophylactic stabilization was recommended. Two months prior to the left femur fracture, he fell down some stairs and incurred both a right hip and right humeral fracture. He underwent hip hemiarthroplasty and ORIF humerus.

3.6. CTRA True Negative: Case #6 (Right Femur).

A 79-year-old male with a history of multiple myeloma diagnosed 12 years ago presented with a 9-month history of aching pain in his right pelvis that began suddenly while doing minor work in his yard (Figure 7). Both CT and X-ray showed right iliac pathologic fracture and numerous bilateral femoral lytic lesions. For his right femur, Mirels score was 8, and neither CTRA nor FEA suggested increased fracture risk. Biopsy of the iliac bone confirmed the lesions to be due to multiple myeloma. Treatment consisted of pelvic EBRT and systemic immunotherapy. At 4-year follow-up, no femoral fracture occurred. The patient had no left lower extremity pain, and therefore neither Mirels nor CTRA was assessed.

3.7. CTRA True Negative: Case #7 (Left and Right Femurs).

A 72-year-old female with a history of MBD due to breast cancer presented with a 7-month history of right upper extremity and left groin pain after a fall on ice. Multiple identified sites of MBD included bilateral femurs (Figures 8 and 9), bilateral humeri, anterior and posterior ribs, iliac bones, and sacrum, as well as diffuse spine and skull lesions.

The left proximal femoral diaphyseal lesion Mirels was 8, and CTRA did not suggest increased fracture risk. However, FEA suggested increased fracture risk. Prophylactic stabilization was not recommended. As she did not go on to

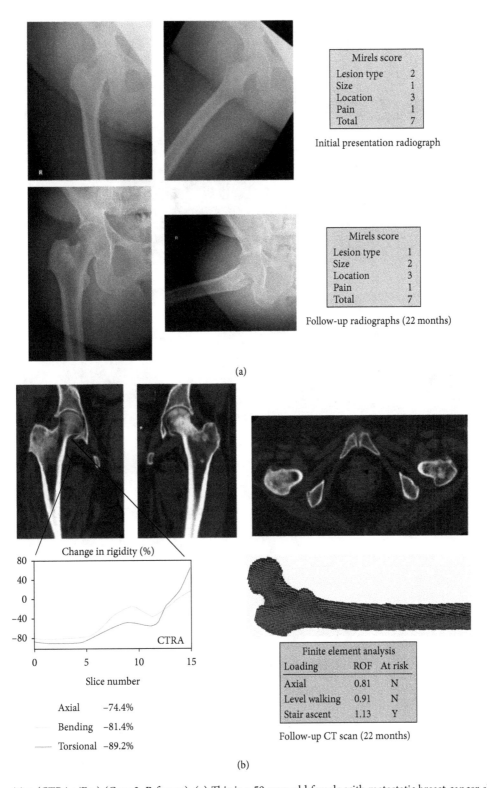

FIGURE 4: False positive (CTRA+/Fx-) (Case 3, R femur). (a) This is a 59-year-old female with metastatic breast cancer showing a mixed osteoblastic and osteolytic lesion in the right femoral neck. (b) Both CTRA and FEA predicted that the subject would fracture; however, due to a low Mirels' score and mild pain, she did not undergo prophylactic stabilization surgery.

fracture through 2-year follow-up, CTRA was a true negative while FEA was a false positive. This was the only case in our series where the findings for CTRA and FEA differed.

The right intertrochanteric femoral lesion Mirels was 9, and both CTRA and FEA did not suggest increased fracture risk. Prophylactic stabilization was not recommended. As

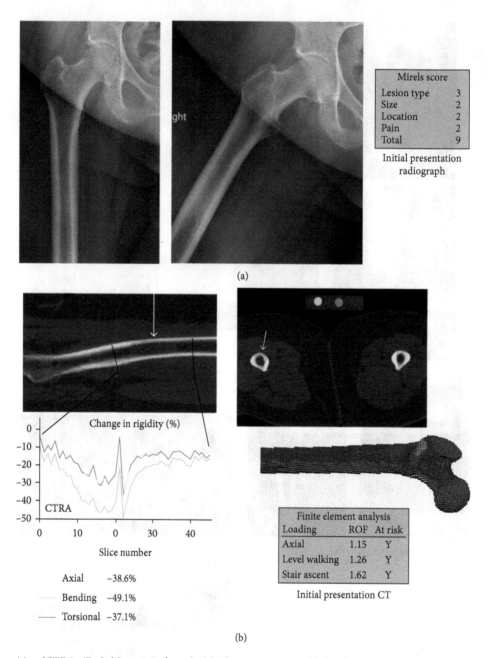

FIGURE 5: False positive (CTRA+/Fx-) (Case 4, R femur). (a) This is a 68-year-old female with metastatic neuroendocrine carcinoma demonstrating an osteolytic lesion in the right femoral diaphysis. (b) Both CTRA and FEA predicted that the patient would fracture; however, she was treated nonoperatively with EBRT and did not fracture over the course of her one-year follow-up.

noted above, no fracture occurred through 2-year follow-up.

4. Results

The above seven cases depict true positive, true negative, false positive, and false negative examples in respect of fracture outcome as predicted by CTRA. Since they were hand-selected for this case series, instead of randomly chosen, the results of the cases cannot be combined and instead are unique examples of CTRA prediction with outcome. Table 1 shows a summary of each of the cases. Case 5 is unique in that it is the only case out of the 140 we

analyzed where CTRA had not predicted fracture, but the patient indeed went on to fracture. As shown in Table 2, literature has reported CTRA sensitivity at 100%, so it is rare to find a false negative CTRA example. This is also why each category has two cases whereas there is only one case representing the false negative category.

5. Discussion

Fracture risk prediction in MBD is important to identify patients who will benefit from prophylactic stabilization by avoiding problems inherent to ORIF and separate them from those for whom operative intervention is unnecessary, poses

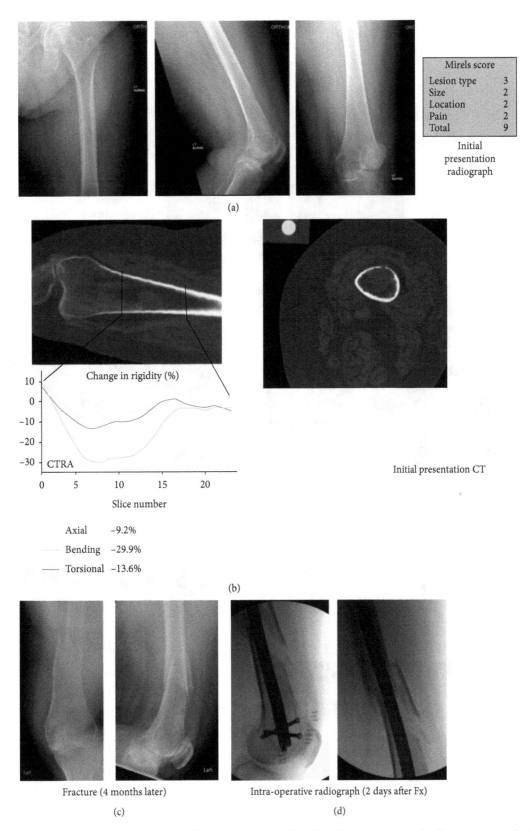

Mirels score	
Lesion type	3
Size	2
Location	2
Pain	2
Total	9

Initial presentation radiograph

(a)

Change in rigidity (%)

CTRA

Slice number

Axial   −9.2%
Bending   −29.9%
Torsional −13.6%

Initial presentation CT

(b)

Fracture (4 months later)   Intra-operative radiograph (2 days after Fx)

(c)   (d)

FIGURE 6: False negative (CTRA-/Fx+) (Case 5, L femur). (a) This is a 63-year-old male with metastatic renal cell carcinoma in the distal femoral diaphysis. (b) CTRA did not predict fracture in this patient, and FEA was not conducted due to the distal nature of this lesion. (c) The subject had a fall resulting in a fracture of the left femur and (d) underwent operative fixation.

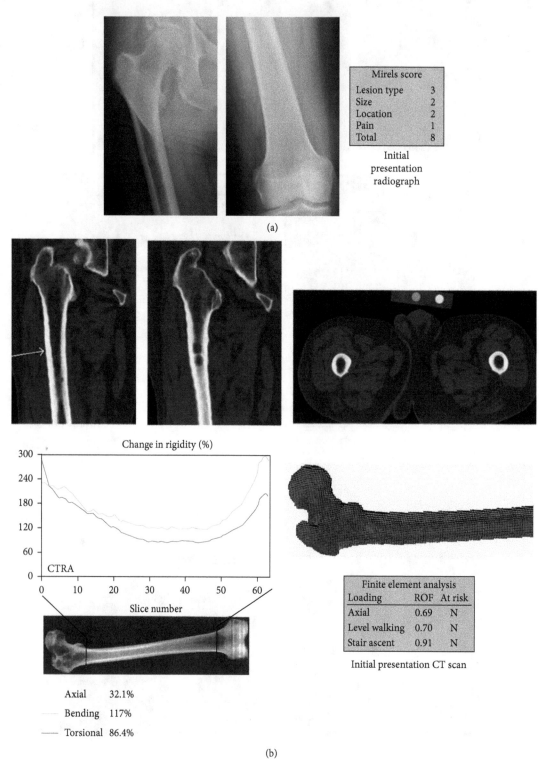

Mirels score	
Lesion type	3
Size	2
Location	2
Pain	1
Total	8

Initial
presentation
radiograph

(a)

Change in rigidity (%)

CTRA

Slice number

Axial   32.1%

Bending   117%

Torsional 86.4%

Finite element analysis		
Loading	ROF	At risk
Axial	0.69	N
Level walking	0.70	N
Stair ascent	0.91	N

Initial presentation CT scan

(b)

FIGURE 7: Continued.

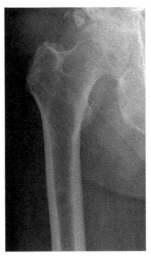

Follow-up radiograph (4 years)

(c)

FIGURE 7: True negative (CTRA-/Fx-) (Case 6, R femur). (a) This is a 79-year-old male with a 12-year history of multiple myeloma demonstrating osteolytic lesions within the right subtrochanteric femur. (b) CTRA and FEA were both run and did not predict fracture for this subject. (c) The patient was followed for several years, and follow-up imaging at four years demonstrates minimal change to the subtrochanteric lesion.

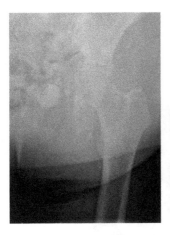 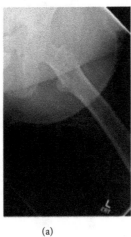

Mirels score	
Lesion type	2
Size	2
Location	3
Pain	1
Total	8

Initial presentation
radiograph

(a)

FIGURE 8: Continued.

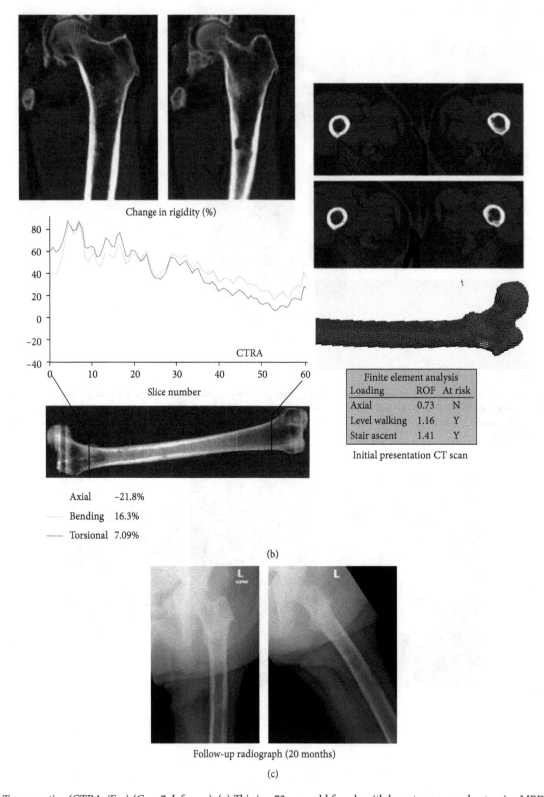

Change in rigidity (%)

CTRA

Axial	−21.8%
Bending	16.3%
Torsional	7.09%

Finite element analysis		
Loading	ROF	At risk
Axial	0.73	N
Level walking	1.16	Y
Stair ascent	1.41	Y

Initial presentation CT scan

(b)

Follow-up radiograph (20 months)

(c)

FIGURE 8: True negative (CTRA-/Fx-) (Case 7, L femur). (a) This is a 72-year-old female with breast cancer and extensive MBD showing a mixed osteoblastic and osteolytic lesion in the left femoral diaphysis. (b) While CTRA predicted that the subject would not fracture, FEA did predict fracture. (c) She was followed for two years without evidence of fracture. Imaging taken at 20 months demonstrates MBD without a fracture.

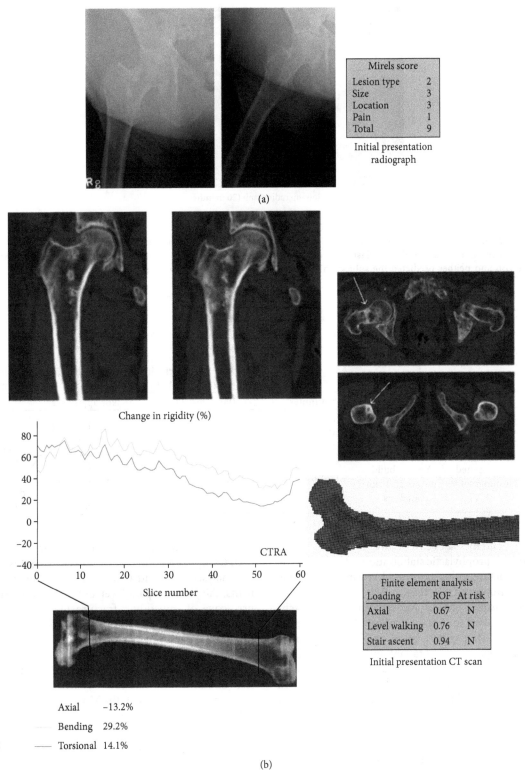

Figure 9: Continued.

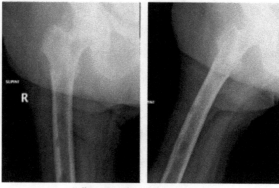

Follow-up radiograph (20 months)

(c)

FIGURE 9: True negative (CTRA-/Fx-) (Case 7, R femur). This figure is for the same subject in Figure 8 but now depicts the right femur. (a) Initial X-ray imaging shows a mixed osteoblastic and osteolytic lesion in the intertrochanteric region of the right femur. (b) Both CTRA and FEA were run and neither predicted the subject to fracture. (c) Imaging taken 20 months after her initial evaluation demonstrates progression of her MBD but without fracture.

TABLE 2: Comparison of Mirels, CTRA, and FEA technical considerations.

Prediction method	Imaging method	Specialized software	Analysis time	Reported sensitivity (%) [16]	Reported specificity (%) [16]	Types of loading	Anatomic/ modeling limitations
Mirels	Planar X-ray	No	<5 minutes	71–100	13–94	Not applicable	None
CTRA	Computed tomography (CT)	Yes, to calculate section rigidities	<15 minutes, with custom software	100	60–90	Axial, bending, torsion	Errors associated with the ends of long bones
FEA	Computed tomography (CT)	Yes, to build model and run analysis	2–8 hours, requiring engineering expertise	80–100	63–86	Functional loading (stance, gait, stair climb, etc.)	Models and loading for proximal femur different from distal femur

unneeded risks, and increases cost of care [19–24]. Although one of the goals of prophylactic stabilization is to prevent the morbidity of fracture, other purported advantages include pain relief and improved function.

Numerous historic clinical and radiologic based techniques have been used for fracture risk prediction in MBD [16, 25]. Mirels scoring system, based on plain radiographs and clinical findings, is widely taught and used, but newer CT-based techniques including CTRA and FEA have shown more accurate risk prediction [5, 9–13]. The cases presented in this pictorial review illustrate the nuances of utilization of all three (Mirels, CTRA, FEA) in individual cases.

5.1. Mirels Clinical Scoring. The Mirels score was originally developed and reported in 1989 [4]. Scoring ranges from four to twelve depending on the patient's reported pain level, the lesional characteristics (lytic/blastic/mixed), the size of the lesion, and the location of the bone lesion determined by X-ray imaging. Based upon the recommendation of Mirels, lesions deemed to have a total score of nine or more were considered to have an impending fracture, and prophylactic stabilization was recommended [4, 14]. Mirels found a sensitivity of 81% and specificity of 94% when doing a

retrospective analysis of 38 patients (78 lesions) on bones in both the upper and lower extremities using this criterion. In his analysis, he found that, among the four score components, the patient's pain level and lesion size were the most predictive of impending fracture [4]. However, it is important to note that Mirels developed the scoring system from a single training data set, with the goal of achieving the best combination of sensitivity and specificity. Ideally, this scoring system would have been applied to an independent test (or validation) data set.

Further application of the Mirels scoring system by other authors has not revealed results as promising as the original Mirels series, particularly with regard to specificity. Five more recent manuscripts have reported a sensitivity in the range of 67–100% but a specificity in the range of 13–50% [5, 11, 12, 26, 27] using Mirels scoring for femoral lesions, suggesting that the Mirels score may overpredict fracture risk among patients with MBD. This is an important consideration when using the Mirels scoring system clinically to identify patients who may need prophylactic stabilization surgery.

In the current pictorial review series, utilizing the suggested Mirels score of nine points or more as the criterion for prophylactic stabilization, there were three true positives, three true negatives, two false positives, and no false negatives relative to the actual clinical outcome (fracture vs no fracture). Although the purpose of this study was not to analyze the predictive capability of the Mirels scoring system given the small number of cases, these cases do illustrate the high sensitivity (100%) and modest specificity (60%) of Mirels scoring. The Mirels scoring system remains widely used by physicians, but, due to its low specificity and poor positive predictive value, relying purely on Mirels scoring could lead to many unnecessary prophylactic stabilization surgeries [14, 16, 28].

5.2. *Computed Tomography Rigidity Analysis (CTRA).* CTRA was developed in an effort to improve upon the Mirels scoring system through identification of bones that may be at an increased risk of fracture due to metastatic lesions. CTRA utilizes three-dimensional CT imaging sets of bone with metastatic lesions, in contrast to Mirels scoring which is based in part upon measures from two-dimensional radiographs. The geometry of the lesion is more fully characterized with CTRA, and the distribution of bone density is also determined. By incorporating the geometry of the bone and the density together, bone rigidity (axial, bending, and torsional) can be calculated. CT scan images are obtained for the bilateral femurs, and CTRA is performed on the involved femur as well as the contralateral femur, which serves as a control. If the femur rigidity has been reduced by 33% or more compared to the contralateral femur (without MBD), it is considered to be at a high risk of fracture [12, 16]. In cases where the contralateral femur cannot be used as a control, such as bilateral MBD, CTRA uses standardized age and sex matched femurs as the control. The use of the patient's contralateral femur is the preferred method and functions as a built-in control when calculating the loss of rigidity.

Several investigators have assessed the sensitivity and specificity of CTRA to determine its usefulness as a clinical tool [5, 10, 12, 18, 29–31]. CTRA has been applied to several different bony lesions including vertebral metastases [29], pediatric patients with benign skeletal lesions [30, 31], and femoral lesions [5, 12] demonstrating a higher specificity with CTRA analysis than what has been historically shown with Mirels for long bone lesions. Two manuscripts assessing fracture risk for femoral lesions directly compared CTRA and Mirels scoring. Nazarian et al. evaluated 104 patients with femur lesions and found the sensitivity of CTRA to be 100% and specificity to be 90%, while Mirels was found to be 71% sensitive and 50% specific [12]. Damron et al. analyzed 94 patients and found CTRA sensitivity and specificity to be 100% and 61%, respectively, while Mirels demonstrated 67% sensitivity and 48% specificity [5]. Interestingly, the same paper analyzed Mirels score cut-offs of 8, 9, and 10 and showed that CTRA was overall superior no matter which value was used as the cut-off. These manuscripts have shown that when using CTRA compared to Mirels scoring, sensitivity for identifying those at risk of fracture remains relatively high, but CTRA has improved specificity. Based on the high sensitivity and specificity of CTRA, this suggests

that clinical use of CTRA instead of Mirels scoring may better identify the patients at highest risk of fracture and who would benefit from prophylactic stabilization surgery, with less overtreatment of those who will not go on to fracture.

More recently, a curved beam CTRA approach has been developed to more accurately calculate rigidity for the ends of long bones, such as the femur, given the intrinsic curvature [32]. Traditional CTRA, which was used for the subjects in this study, uses straight beam theory and thus loses accuracy at the proximal and distal ends of long bones. The intertrochanteric region of the proximal femur has been shown to have significant intrinsic curvature and is also a common area for MBD [32]. The curved CTRA model is a promising improvement on the traditional straight CTRA predictions and has been reported as more accurate in predicting the magnitude of failure, as well as the location of failure [13]. These claims are based on a study using fresh frozen cadavers where one femur was used as a control while the other had a simulated lytic defect. While the results appear encouraging, further research is needed to assess the technique clinically.

5.3. *Finite Element Analysis (FEA).* FEA is the second CT-based tool used for fracture risk assessment in MBD examined in this study. Like CTRA, FEA uses both the 3D geometry and the density of the bone. However, FEA utilizes computer software to create a 3D femur model with lesions from the CT scan set. The model is discretized into small finite elements that are assigned bone strength and stiffness properties using the bone density information [33, 34]. Once the model is created, specific forces are applied to the femoral head and greater trochanter to simulate muscular and joint forces. The applied force is incrementally increased until the femur is predicted to fail [32, 33]. In the current series, the loading conditions included axial compression, level walking, and aggressive stair ascent as previously reported.

Direct comparison of FEA with Mirels illustrates the superiority of FEA. Goodheart et al. [11] compared FEA to the Mirels scoring system, showing a similarly high sensitivity for both tests, but in terms of specificity, FEA was found to be significantly higher. There is limited literature that assesses whether CTRA or FEA is superior in the ability to discriminate cases that fracture from those that do not. Anez-Bustillos et al. conducted a laboratory-based study in which femoral lesions were created in cadaver bones [10]. They found that the correlation between predicted and actual bone strength was not different for CTRA and FEA. Another laboratory-based study by Oftadeh et al. suggested that FEA is more accurate than straight beam CTRA [13], but curved beam analysis produced results that were similar to FEA in terms of predicted strength. In the series we report here, FEA was never used for clinical decision making, as all analyses were done post hoc. Among the cases reported, in only one case, did FEA differ from CTRA, and in that case, the FEA was a false positive.

One of the advantages of FEA over CTRA is that FEA accounts for true loading conditions, and this has been shown to be an important variable in fracture prediction. FEA is able to account for muscular attachment points and forces generated on the femur with both weight-bearing and muscular contraction [11, 32]. Despite the benefits and promising accuracy of FEA, using FEA as a fracture risk prediction tool remains cumbersome due to its complexity, time requirements, cost, and limited availability. FEA requires a trained expert to both build and run the models, and each model requires several hours of staff time to run. CTRA is much more computationally efficient compared to FEA but also requires custom software to generate the rigidity plots. In addition, neither FEA nor CTRA is currently available as plug-in to standard CT software.

Selection of these cases was based upon the CTRA results to illustrate each fracture prediction result (TP, TN, FP, FN) and obviates any conclusion regarding the accuracy of CTRA. However, examples of FP and FN CTRA results were few and far between within this much larger population of patients while TP and TN cases were the norm. This is consistent with the reported high rates of sensitivity and specificity for CTRA [5, 12, 30]. Use of CTRA is limited to only those institutions actively enrolling patients in the ongoing MSTS study and as a research tool is not always available in real time for clinical decision making.

As a pictorial review, this paper provides examples of fracture risk prediction in MBD focusing on CTRA with comparison to Mirels and FEA. Table 2 compares the utility and limitations of the three scoring systems (Mirels, CTRA, FEA) to summarize the technical considerations when using each of these tools. As seen within Table 2, all three scoring systems tend to have a high sensitivity; therefore, the differences in accurate detection lie in the different specificities of these scores. Reports of specificity for the different scoring systems have shown a wide range, but overall the trend is that Mirels has a poor specificity which has been improved with the use of CTRA or FEA. However, this is difficult to translate into practice since Mirels scoring can easily be used by the physician, whereas CTRA and FEA have much higher barriers to access. Mirels scoring can be done simply with an X-ray and some information from the patient. Both CTRA and FEA require CT scans, custom computer software, and people trained in the technique. Among these CT-based techniques, CTRA seems to be more accessible to physicians, whereas FEA is still a technique limited to the lab with minimal clinical utility at this point due to its limitations. No perfect system exists, and further refinement of these CT-based techniques in larger patient populations is needed.

Authors' Contributions

SMK contributed to data compilation and manuscript preparation and editing. KAM participated in finite element analysis, figure preparation, and manuscript editing. MAM performed finite element analysis and edited the manuscript. TAD helped with study conception, patient enrollment, and manuscript editing.

Acknowledgments

The authors would like to thank Brian Snyder, M.D., for CTRA development and validation and collaboration in CTRA study sponsored by Musculoskeletal Tumor Society; Ara Nazarian, Ph.D., for supervision of CTRA analysis; and Tina Craig, C.R.A., for assistance with IRB approval. This work was supported by Carol M. Baldwin Breast Cancer Research Fund (TAD, KAM), SUNY Upstate Research Foundation (TAD, KAM), David G. Murray Endowed Professorship (TAD), Musculoskeletal Tumor Society (TAD), and William Smythe Cancer Fund (TAD).

References

[1] F. Macedo, K. Ladeira, F. Pinho et al., "Bone metastases: an overview," *Oncology Reviews*, vol. 11, p. 321, 2017.

[2] United Nations, *World Population Ageing 2013*, E. S. Affairs, Ed., UN iLibrary, New York, NY, USA, 2013.

[3] D. A. Müller and R. Capanna, "The surgical treatment of pelvic bone metastases," *Advances in Orthopedics*, vol. 2015, Article ID 525363, 10 pages, 2015.

[4] H. Mirels, "Metastatic disease in long bones A proposed scoring system for diagnosing impending pathologic fractures," *Clinical Orthopaedics and Related Research*, vol. 249, pp. 256–264, 1989.

[5] T. A. Damron, A. Nazarian, V. Entezari et al., "CT-based structural rigidity analysis is more accurate than Mirels scoring for fracture prediction in metastatic femoral lesions," *Clinical Orthopaedics & Related Research*, vol. 474, no. 3, pp. 643–651, 2016.

[6] P. Carnesale, *Campbell's Operative Orthopaedics*, Elsevier, Amsterdam, Netherlands, 10th edition, 2003.

[7] J. J. Willeumier, Y. M. van der Linden, M. A. J. van de Sande, and P. D. S. Dijkstra, "Treatment of pathological fractures of the long bones," *EFORT Open Reviews*, vol. 1, no. 5, pp. 136–145, 2016.

[8] Y. M. van der Linden, H. M. Kroon, S. P. D. S. Dijkstra et al., "Simple radiographic parameter predicts fracturing in metastatic femoral bone lesions: results from a randomised trial," *Radiotherapy and Oncology*, vol. 69, no. 1, pp. 21–31, 2003.

[9] L. C. Derikx, J. B. van Aken, D. Janssen et al., "The assessment of the risk of fracture in femora with metastatic lesions," *The Journal of Bone and Joint Surgery. British Volume*, vol. 94, no. 8, pp. 1135–1142, 2012.

[10] L. Anez-Bustillos, L. C. Derikx, N. Verdonschot et al., "Finite element analysis and CT-based structural rigidity analysis to assess failure load in bones with simulated lytic defects," *Bone*, vol. 58, pp. 160–167, 2014.

[11] J. R. Goodheart, R. J. Cleary, T. A. Damron, and K. A. Mann, "Simulating activities of daily living with finite element analysis improves fracture prediction for patients with metastatic femoral lesions," *Journal of Orthopaedic Research*, vol. 33, no. 8, pp. 1226–1234, 2015.

[12] A. Nazarian, V. Entezari, D. Zurakowski et al., "Treatment planning and fracture prediction in patients with skeletal metastasis with CT-based rigidity analysis," *Clinical Cancer Research*, vol. 21, no. 11, pp. 2514–2519, 2015.

[13] R. Oftadeh, Z. Karimi, J. Villa-Camacho et al., "Curved beam computed tomography based structural rigidity analysis of bones with simulated lytic defect: a comparative study with finite element analysis," *Scientific Reports*, vol. 6, no. 1, p. 32397, 2016.

[14] E. L. Howard, K. L. Shepherd, G. Cribb, and P. Cool, "The validity of the Mirels score for predicting impending pathological fractures of the lower limb," *The Bone & Joint Journal*, vol. 100, no. 8, pp. 1100–1105, 2018.

[15] A. Nazarian, V. Entezari, J. C. Villa-Camacho et al., "Does CT-based rigidity analysis influence clinical decision-making in simulations of metastatic bone disease?" *Clinical Orthopaedics & Related Research*, vol. 474, no. 3, pp. 652–659, 2016.

[16] T. A. Damron and K. A. Mann, "Fracture risk assessment and clinical decision making for patients with metastatic bone disease," *Journal of Orthopaedic Research*, vol. 38, no. 6, pp. 1175–1190, 2020.

[17] M. U. Jawad and S. P. Scully, "In brief: classifications in brief," *Clinical Orthopaedics & Related Research*, vol. 468, no. 10, pp. 2825–2827, 2010.

[18] J. C. Villa-Camacho, O. Iyoha-Bello, S. Behrouzi, B. D. Snyder, and A. Nazarian, "Computed tomography-based rigidity analysis: a review of the approach in preclinical and clinical studies," *BoneKEy Reports*, vol. 3, p. 587, 2014.

[19] N. K. Behnke, D. K. Baker, S. Xu, T. E. Niemeier, S. L. Watson, and B. A. Ponce, "Risk factors for same-admission mortality after pathologic fracture secondary to metastatic cancer," *Supportive Care in Cancer*, vol. 25, no. 2, pp. 513–521, 2017.

[20] C. Arvinius, J. L. C. Parra, L. S. Mateo, R. G. Maroto, A. F. Borrego, and L. L.-D. Stern, "Benefits of early intramedullary nailing in femoral metastases," *International Orthopaedics*, vol. 38, no. 1, pp. 129–132, 2014.

[21] A. Nooh, K. Goulding, M. H. Isler et al., "Early improvement in pain and functional outcome but not quality of life after surgery for metastatic long bone disease," *Clinical Orthopaedics & Related Research*, vol. 476, no. 3, pp. 535–545, 2018.

[22] A. T. Blank, D. M. Lerman, N. M. Patel, and T. B. Rapp, "Is prophylactic intervention more cost-effective than the treatment of pathologic fractures in metastatic bone disease?" *Clinical Orthopaedics & Related Research*, vol. 474, no. 7, pp. 1563–1570, 2016.

[23] T. A. Damron, "CORR insights: is there an association between prophylactic femur stabilization and survival in patients with metastatic bone disease?" *Clinical Orthopaedics & Related Research*, vol. 478, no. 3, pp. 547–549, 2020.

[24] R. N. Kotian, V. Puvanesarajah, S. Rao, J. M. El Abiad, C. D. Morris, and A. S. Levin, "Predictors of survival after intramedullary nail fixation of completed or impending pathologic femur fractures from metastatic disease," *Surgical Oncology*, vol. 27, no. 3, pp. 462–467, 2018.

[25] M. S. Spinelli, A. Ziranu, A. Piccioli, and G. Maccauro, "Surgical treatment of acetabular metastasis," *European Review for Medical and Pharmacological Sciences*, vol. 20, pp. 3005–3010, 2016.

[26] Y. M. Van der Linden, P. D. S. Dijkstra, H. M. Kroon et al., "Comparative analysis of risk factors for pathological fracture with femoral metastases," *The Journal of Bone and Joint Surgery. British Volume*, vol. 86, no. 4, pp. 566–573, 2004.

[27] T. A. Damron, H. Morgan, D. Prakash, W. Grant, J. Aronowitz, and J. Heiner, "Critical evaluation of Mirels, rating system for impending pathologic fractures," *Clinical Orthopaedics and Related Research*, vol. 415, pp. S201–S207, 2003.

[28] D. C. Ramsey, P. W. Lam, J. Hayden, Y. C. Doung, and K. R. Gundle, "Mirels scores in patients undergoing prophylactic stabilization for femoral metastatic bone disease in the veterans administration healthcare system," *Journal of the American Academy of Orthopaedic Surgeons. Global Research & Reviews*, vol. 4, Article ID e2000141, 2020.

[29] B. D. Snyder, M. A. Cordio, A. Nazarian et al., "Noninvasive prediction of fracture risk in patients with metastatic cancer to the spine," *Clinical Cancer Research*, vol. 15, no. 24, pp. 7676–7683, 2009.

[30] B. D. Snyder, D. A. Hauser-Kara, J. A. Hipp, D. Zurakowski, A. C. Hecht, and M. C. Gebhardt, "Predicting fracture through benign skeletal lesions with quantitative computed tomography," *The Journal of Bone and Joint Surgery-American Volume*, vol. 88, no. 1, pp. 55–70, 2006.

[31] N. L. Leong, M. E. Anderson, M. C. Gebhardt, and B. D. Snyder, "Computed tomography-based structural analysis for predicting fracture risk in children with benign skeletal neoplasms," *Journal of Bone and Joint Surgery*, vol. 92, no. 9, pp. 1827–1833, 2010.

[32] A. Sas, E. Tanck, A. Sermon, and G. H. van Lenthe, "Finite element models for fracture prevention in patients with metastatic bone disease. A literature review," *Bone Reports*, vol. 12, p. 100286, 2020.

[33] J. Mizrahi, M. J. Silva, and W. C. Hayes, "Finite element stress analysis of simulated metastatic lesions in the lumbar vertebral body," *Journal of Biomedical Engineering*, vol. 14, no. 6, pp. 467–475, 1992.

[34] E. J. Cheal, J. A. Hipp, and W. C. Hayes, "Evaluation of finite element analysis for prediction of the strength reduction due to metastatic lesions in the femoral neck," *Journal of Biomechanics*, vol. 26, no. 3, pp. 251–264, 1993.

11

Instrumentation Removal following Minimally Invasive Posterior Percutaneous Pedicle Screw-Rod Stabilization (PercStab) of Thoracolumbar Fractures Is Not Always Required

Neil Manson [ID],[1,2,3] Dana El-Mughayyar [ID],[1] Erin Bigney [ID],[1] Eden Richardson [ID],[1] and Edward Abraham [ID][1,2,3]

[1]Canada East Spine Centre, Saint John Regional Hospital, 400 University Ave, PO Box 2100, Saint John, New Brunswick E2L 4L4, Canada
[2]Saint John Regional Hospital, Horizon Health Network, 400 University Ave, PO Box 2100, Saint John, New Brunswick E2L 4L4, Canada
[3]Department of Surgery, Dalhousie University, 100 Tucker Park Rd, Saint John, New Brunswick E2K 5E2, Canada

Correspondence should be addressed to Dana El-Mughayyar; dana.el-mughayyar@horizonnb.ca

Academic Editor: Panagiotis Korovessis

Study Design. Clinical case series. *Background.* Percutaneous stabilization for spinal trauma confers less blood loss, reduces postoperative pain, and is less invasive than open stabilization and fusion. The current standard of care includes instrumentation removal. *Objective.* 1. Reporting patient outcomes following minimally invasive posterior percutaneous pedicle screw-rod stabilization (PercStab). 2. Evaluating the results of instrumentation retention. *Methods.* A prospective observational study of 32 consecutive patients receiving PercStab without direct decompression or fusion. Baseline data demographics were collected. Operative outcomes of interest were operative room (OR) time, blood loss, and length of hospital stay. Follow-up variables of interest included patient satisfaction, Numeric Rating Scales for Back and Leg (NRS-B/L) pain, Oswestry Disability Index (ODI), and return to work. Clinical outcome data (ODI and NRS-B/L) were collected at 3, 12, 24 months and continued at a 24-month interval up to a maximum of 8 years postoperatively. *Results.* 81.25% of patients ($n = 26$) retained their instrumentation and reported minimal disability, mild pain, and satisfaction with their surgery and returned to work (mean = 6 months). Six patients required instrumentation removal due to prominence of the instrumentation or screw loosening, causing discomfort/pain. Instrumentation removal patients reported moderate back and leg pain until removal occurred; after removal, they reported minimal disability and mild pain. Neither instrumentation removal nor retention resulted in complications or further surgical intervention. *Conclusions.* PercStab without instrumentation removal provided high patient satisfaction, mild pain, and minimal disability and relieved the patient from the burden of finances and resources allocation of a second surgery.

1. Introduction

Spine fractures compromise approximately 6% of all fractures worldwide [1, 2]. Surgical treatments are proposed to patients with unstable traumatic pathologies, with or without neurological deficit [3]. While traditional open surgical treatments are commonly used, they may result in considerable blood loss, complications, extended hospital stays, and delayed functional recovery [4–7]. Minimally invasive surgical (MIS) techniques are intended to minimize

approach morbidity and associated complications of open surgeries [5]. Posterior percutaneous pedicle screw fixation can provide spinal stabilization with placement through small incisions using specific MIS technologies, in an effort to minimize complications [8–11].

As this is a nonfusion technique, the current standard of care following minimally invasive posterior percutaneous pedicle screw-rod stabilization (PercStab) includes instrumentation removal [12]. There is no consensus on timing of hardware removal but it is considered once tissue healing occurs and stability is restored to prevent instrumentation failure, loosening at the bone-screw interface, or other instrument related complications [13, 14]. Vanek et al. showed that instrumentation was removed from the part of the lumbar spine (below L-2) between 12 and 18 months postoperatively [15, 16]. Yang et al. reported that seven patients of 64 opted out of having their instrumentation removed postoperatively as they reported feeling satisfied with their function and wished to avoid having a second procedure [11]. Satisfaction without any disruptions can eliminate a second procedure in patients.

The objectives of this study were (1) reporting patient outcomes following minimally invasive posterior percutaneous pedicle screw-rod stabilization to treat spine trauma and (2) evaluating the results of instrumentation retention.

2. Methods

A prospective observational study monitored 32 consecutive spine trauma patients meeting inclusion criteria: age of 18 years or older with unstable spinal trauma for which PercStab was the course of treatment. Baseline data collection included patient age, sex, body mass index (BMI), comorbidities, mechanism of injury (MOI), Injury Severity Score (ISS), AOSpine Classification system, numeric pain rating scale, and admission diagnosis. Operative variables of interest included operative room (OR) time, instrumentation type, blood loss, length of hospital stay, levels operated on and surgical morbidity/mortality. Outcome variables of interest are the Numeric Rating Scales for Back and Leg (NRS-B/L) pain, Oswestry Disability Index (ODI), patient satisfaction, and time to return to work. Clinical outcome data (ODI and NRS-B/L) were collected at 3, 12, 24 months and continued at a 24-month interval up to a maximum of 8 years postoperatively. Patient satisfaction was collected at the patient's final follow-up. When applicable, timing of instrumentation removal and reasoning was reported.

The AOSpine Classification system has been shown to have reasonable reliability and accuracy for clinical validation of a unified system to effectively communicate case-specific details of patient injuries [17, 18]. The ISS assesses severity of trauma and correlates with mortality and morbidity [19]. Patient satisfaction was measured through a 5-point Likert scale (1 = extremely dissatisfied, 2 = somewhat dissatisfied, 3 = neither satisfied nor dissatisfied, 4 = somewhat satisfied, and 5 = extremely satisfied) asking "Are you satisfied with the results of your surgery?". The NRS-B/L and ODI questionnaire were used to quantify disability related to leg and back pain [20]. ODI has been shown to have excellent test-retest reliability [21]. Leg and back pain intensity (NRS-B/L) were measured through an 11-point numeric pain rating scale. Pain ratings represented the typical pain experienced over the preceding 24 hours, with potential scores ranging from 0 ("no pain") to 10 ("worst pain imaginable"). Ratings are categorized as "mild" (0–3), "moderate" (4–6), or "severe" (7–10). The numeric pain rating scale has excellent test-retest reliability and responsiveness [22–24].

Instrumentation removal was not applied as a standard. Instrumentation removal was provided based on clinical complaint, physical exam findings, and imaging findings at the discretion of the surgeon and in shared decision-making with the patient. Without specific justification, instrumentation was not removed.

3. Surgical Technique

All patients received PercStab under general anesthesia. The patient was positioned prone on the OSI spine table with chest, hip, and leg bolsters placed to optimize alignment at the fracture site. Standard antiseptic skin preparation and draping was completed, and preoperative antibiotics were provided. Two C-arm fluoroscopy units provided simultaneous anteroposterior (AP) and lateral imaging capabilities. AP fluoroscopy guided placement of 1.5 cm stab incisions overlying each pedicle to be instrumented. The Pedicle Access Kit cannulated trochar (Medtronic Sofamor Danek) was tamped through the pedicle assuring that the tip of the trochar remained lateral to the medial pedicle wall at all times until the tip of the trochar passed into the vertebral body. Trochar position was confirmed on AP and lateral C-arm imaging. Guidewire was passed through the trochar followed by trochar removal. Guidewires were placed at each pedicle to be instrumented. The pedicles were then tapped, and cannulated screws were placed by hand.

The pedicle screw-rod construct was placed utilizing the Longitude or Sextant II systems (Medtronic Sofamor Danek; Legacy 5.5 titanium). The Sextant II system was utilized if the construct spanned one or two motion levels. The Longitude system was utilized if the construct was greater than two motion levels. Screws of 6.5 mm diameter were most commonly utilized. Screws were positioned to optimize construct stability and fracture alignment. If the spine and traumatic pathology permitted, screws were placed at the level of pathology as well. Bilateral titanium rods, 5.5 mm in diameter were measured, contoured, and passed in a subfascial plane through the pedicle screw extenders. Construct and fracture alignment were optimized with compression and distraction maneuvers, and final tightening of the set screws was completed. Insertion tools were removed. Final AP and lateral C-arm imaging were used to confirm the appropriate instrumentation placement and spinal alignment. Incisions were closed in layers and dressing was applied.

4. Results

The sample includes thirty-two consecutive trauma patients (24 males and 8 females; mean age 38.3 years; see Table 1 for demographics). The MOI for 75% of patients was motor vehicle crash (MVC) and the remaining 25% was caused by a fall. Of the sample, 40.62% had polytrauma with an ISS mean score of 9.5 showing moderate injury. Burst fractures account for 68.75% of the diagnoses; patient fracture diagnosis was classified using the AOSpine Classification System (Table 2). Within the sample, the presence of comorbidities was low with 15.62% of the sample impacted (see Table 1).

TABLE 1: Demographics.

	Sample (N = 32)		NRG (n = 26)		IRG (n = 6)	
	Mean	Range	Mean	Range	Mean	Range
Age	38.3	(18–61)	40.7	(18–61)	27.6	(19–36)
Gender						
Male	24		19		5	
Females	8		7		1	
BMI	22.1	(17.3–34.3)	23.7	(18.8–34.4)	20.8	(17.3–29.5)
Injury Severity Score	9.5	(8–41)	9	(8–34)	9.5	(9–27)
Numeric pain rating scale	7	(3–10)	7	(3–10)	7	(5–9)
	%		%		%	
Comorbidities						
Diabetic	6.2		7.7		0	
Smoker	6.2		7.7		0	
Morbidly obese	3.1		3.8		0	
Mechanism of injury						
MVC	75		73		67	
Fall	25		27		33	
Polytrauma	40.62		34.61		66.67	

TABLE 2: Diagnosis details.

Patient	Injury	AO classification	Instrumentation
1	L2 burst fracture	L2:A4, N0	Medtronic Sextant II
2	L1 chance fracture	L1:B1, N0	Medtronic Sextant II
3	T12-L1 chance fracture, L1 burst fracture	T12-L1:B2 (L1:A4), N2	Medtronic Longitude CD Horizon
4*	T12-L1 chance fracture, L1 burst fracture, T11 compression	T12-L1:B2 (L1:A4, T11:A1), N2	Medtronic Sextant II
5	T12 burst fracture, scoliosis	T12:A4 (M2), N0	Medtronic Longitude
6	T12-L1 chance fracture	T12-L1:C, N0	Medtronic Longitude
7	T12 burst fracture, L1 burst fracture	T12:A4, L1:A4, N1	Medtronic Longitude
8	L1 burst fracture and burst fracture	L1:B1 (L1:A4), N0	Medtronic Longitude
9*	L2 burst fracture	L2:A4, N3	Medtronic Longitude
10	T10-11 instability, T6 extension	T10-11:c, T6:B3, N0	Medtronic Legacy
11	L1 burst fracture	L1:A4, N3	Medtronic Sextant
12	T3-4 chance fracture, T4 burst fracture	T3-4:B2 (T4:A4), N3	Medtronic Longitude CD Horizon
13	T10 extension	T10:B3 (M2), N0	Medtronic Longitude
14	T11-12 chance Fracture, T12 burst fracture	T11-12:B2 (T12:A4), N0	Medtronic Sextant II
15	L1 burst fracture	L1:A4, N0	Medtronic Longitude
16	T3 chance fracture, T4 compression	T3:B1 (T3:A4), T4:A1, N0	Medtronic CD Horizon Legacy
17	T11-12 PLC, T12 burst fracture	T11-12:B2 (T12:A4), N0	Medtronic Sextant
18	T2 and T3 chance fracture, T4 compression	T2:B1, T3:B1, T4:A1, N0	Medtronic Sextant
19*	T12 chance fracture	T12:B1, N0	Medtronic Horizon Sextant
20*	T10 chance fracture	T10:B2, N0	Medtronic Sextant
21	L4 burst fracture	L4:A4, N0	Medtronic Sextant
22*	T4-5 PLC, T5 chance fracture, T6 burst fracture	T4-5:c (T4:A4), T6:A4, N0	Medtronic Sextant
23	L1 burst fracture, chance fracture	L1:B1 (L1:A4), N0	Medtronic Sextant
24*	T12 burst fracture, L1 chance fracture	L1:B1, T12:A4, N0	Medtronic Longitude
25	T10-11 PLC, T8, 11, 12 compression	T10-11:c (T11:A1), T8:A1, T12:A1, N0	Medtronic Sextant II
26	T6-7 instability	T6-7:c (T6:A4, T7:A4), N0	Medtronic Sextant
27	L1 burst fracture and PLC	T12-L1:B2 (L1:A4), N0	Medtronic Longitude CD Horizon
28	T12 burst fracture	T12:A4, N0	Medtronic Horizon Sextant
29	L5 burst fracture	L5:A4, N0	Medtronic Sextant II
30	L1 burst fracture	L1:A4, N0	Medtronic Longitude
31	T12 burst fracture and PLC	T12-L1:B2 (T12:A2), N0	Medtronic Longitude
32	L1 burst fracture, L2 compression	L1:A4, L2:A1, N0	Medtronic Sextant II

*Patients who later require removal. PLC = posterior ligamentous complex injuries.

TABLE 3: Operative details.

OR time*	Sample ($N = 32$)		NRG ($n = 26$)		IRG ($n = 6$)	
	Mean	Range	Mean	Range	Mean	Range
	3 h 00 min	(38 min–7 h 15 m)	2 h 51 min	(38 m–7 h 15 m)	2 h 8 min	(50 m–4 h 50 m)
Blood loss (ml)	179.6	(50–600)	188.5	(50–600)	141.6	(50–250)
Length of hospital stay (days) (median)	5	1–37	4.5	1–37	6.5	1–15
Number of levels (median)	2	1–6	2	1–6	3.5	2–5

*OR time was inclusive of preparation time, induction, incision, closure, and patient being transferred onto the floor.

Most patients received PercStab to treat spinal instability over a mean of 2 levels (range 1–6 levels).

PercStab as a surgical option resulted in no surgical induced morbidity/mortality but injury related morbidity preoperatively was seen in 21.87% of the sample which included superventricular tachycardia, blood abnormalities, urinary retention, low hemoglobin, sepsis, compromised respiratory function, and exacerbation of injuries due to poor compliance. Operative room morbidity was seen in 6.2% of the sample which included coagulation abnormalities and respiratory decline during intubation. Postoperative morbidity was seen in 35.9% of the sample which included poor pain control, hypervolemia, oxygen saturation fluctuations, low oxygen, *E. coli* in septum, staph epidemia in blood, fluid collection, ileus, staph aureus, and vomiting. The majority of patients were followed up for 48 months (time of final follow-up ranged from 4 to 8 years).

The majority of patients in this case series, 26 of 32 (19 males and 7 females; mean age of 40.7 years; see Table 1), did not require instrumentation to be removed; these patients will be referred to as the nonremoval group (NRG). Only 6 of 32 patients required instrumentation removal. The instrumentation removal group (IRG; 5 males and 1 female; mean age of 27.6 years; see Table 1) required removal due to radiologically confirmed screw loosening causing back pain or discomfort (4) or due to screw prominence causing discomfort with direct pressure (2). Time of removal ranged from 16 to 45 months. Patients who required removal completed a follow-up prior to their second surgery and were followed up for 24 months after removal. Operative details for both the NRG and IRG can be seen in Table 3.

Overall pain at baseline averaged 7 points. All patients show clinically meaningful reduction in pain from baseline to final follow-up from severe to mild. Patients who did not require removal on average reported moderate back and leg pain at 3 months postsurgery then mild back and leg pain at 12, 24, and 48 months (see Table 4). Patient presented with L1 burst fracture injury after a snowmobile accident (see Figure 1) is shown to have instrumentation retention at 12-month follow-up and back to rigorous activities (see Figure 2). Patients who required removal reported moderate back pain at all follow-up points until instrumental removal; after removal, reported back and leg pain dropped to mild (see Table 4). Reported ODI for both the NRG and IRG was within the lower range of moderate disability for 3, 12, and 24 months. At 48 months after surgery, the NRG reported minimal disability and 24 months after removal (48 months

TABLE 4: Pain and disability scores.

	NRG			IRG		
	NRS-B	NRS-L	ODI	NRS-B	NRS-L	ODI
3 months	4	4.5	26	6	5	23
12 months	3	2	23	4	4	21
24 months*	2	1	21	5	5	27
48 months**	2	1	16	3	3	14

*24-month follow-up ranged for the IRG cohort from 16 to 24 months depending on time of instrumentation removal. **This is an average of final follow-up periods which ranged from 4 to 8 years depending on time of surgery.

after surgery), the IRG reported minimal disability (see Table 4).

The median time to return to work following surgery reported by patients in the NRG was 6 months and 7 months for the IRG with all patients returning to full-time work by 12 months, aside from 5 patients who retired. All patients reported being somewhat satisfied to extremely satisfied with their surgery (NRG mean = 4.8, range = 4-5; IRG mean = 4.8, range = 4-5).

5. Discussion

Our case series supports the previous literature demonstrating favorable outcomes following MIS management of spinal trauma independent of removal or retention [11, 15, 25]. All patients showed positive outcomes following surgery, reporting minimal disability, mild pain, and high satisfaction with their surgery. PercStab is a reliable and accurate treatment for thoracic and lumbar spine fractures [26]. This case series demonstrated PercStab offers minimal surgical morbidity and blood loss similar to previous studies [27]. Minimally invasive percutaneous pedicle screw fixation without fusion for thoracolumbar fractures did not result in instrumentation failure or surgery-related complications [28] and resulted in patient satisfaction [29].

Previous research investigating PercStab as a treatment for thoracic and lumbar spine fractures followed a criteria of instrumentation removal as the standard of care; however, Yang et al. (2011) reported a small subset of their samples (10.94%) declined the second operation as the patients reported high satisfaction with their results [11]. The current case series was conducted to see how patients would fare if the standard was to retain the instrumentation, avoiding the patient burden, costs, and resource allocation that a second

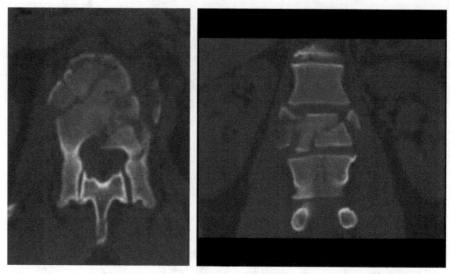

FIGURE 1: Axial and coronal CT scan of L1 burst fracture after a snowmobile accident.

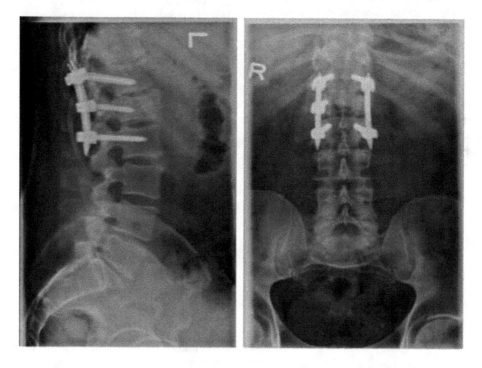

FIGURE 2: Lateral and AP X-ray of percutaneous stabilization of L1 burst fracture treated percutaneously at T12–L2 at 12-month follow-up.

surgery requires. In the current case series, 81.25% of the sample retained their instrumentation and reported long-term minimal disability, mild pain, and satisfaction with their surgery.

Removal is usually done to avoid an instrumentation failure, loosening at the bone-screw interface, or other instrument related complications [25]. In the current case series, this occurred but in only 18.75% of the sample, suggesting that instrumentation removal could be decided based on clinical indications (loosening of screws, reported pain) instead of being the standard of treatment for all cases. In the current study, the primary indicator for instrumentation

removal was patient-reported pain. Patients who required removal report moderate back and leg pain until removal. When follow-up occurred after removal, patients reported mild back and leg pain. The largest difference is seen at the 24-month follow-up; patients who needed removal reported more pain than those patients who did not require removal (difference score of 3 points for back pain and 4 points for leg pain).

Patients who retained their instrumentation were also older on average, had a lower incidence of polytrauma at admission, shorter average hospital stay, and fewer levels operated on. Comorbidities did not appear to influence removal though the low rate of reported comorbidities in the current sample (15.62% of the sample) could be responsible for this finding. None of these patients required removal.

Limitations of the presented study include the fact that it is a case series so no cause and effect conclusions can be drawn. The current case study had a variable final follow-up time with the majority having final follow-up at 4 years (range 4–8). It would be beneficial to extend the follow-up to ensure facet arthrosis and possible instrument failure do not occur at a later time. However, sustaining follow-up rates becomes more problematic as the time extends. The current study has a reasonably small sample and the proportion of patients needing removal could change with a larger population. Despite the limitations mentioned given the patient outcomes reported, we would suggest that compulsory instrumentation removal is not always required following minimally invasive percutaneous screw-rod stabilization for thoracolumbar pathology. Instrumentation removal can be safely guided by clinical complaints. Average follow-up of 4 years would suggest that no risk is posed to these patients by instrumentation retention. In fact, minimal pain and disability with good work capacity can be realized despite instrumentation retention. Thus, the elimination of a second surgery for instrumentation removal as a treatment standard could be considered.

6. Conclusions

Minimally invasive percutaneous screw-rod stabilization for thoracolumbar pathology resulted in high levels of patient satisfaction, minimal disability, mild pain, and high return to work with low perioperative risk. These findings were sustained despite eliminating the second surgery for instrumentation removal usually performed following this nonfusion procedure. While instrumentation removal may be provided for specific indications, removal in all cases may be unnecessary.

Acknowledgments

The authors thank Saint John Regional Hospital, Dalhousie University, and Canada East Spine Centre for supporting them.

References

[1] RL DeWald, "Burst fractures of the thoracic and lumbar spine," Clinical Orthopaedics and Related Research, vol. 189, pp. 150–161, 1984.

[2] C. P. Oboynick, M. F. Kurd, B. V. Darden, A. R. Vaccaro, and M. G. Fehlings, "Timing of surgery in thoracolumbar trauma: is early intervention safe?" Neurosurgical Focus, vol. 37, no. 1, 2014.

[3] A. Patel and A. Joaquim, "Thoracolumbar spine trauma: evaluation and surgical decision-making," Journal of Craniovertebral Junction and Spine, vol. 4, no. 1, pp. 3–9, 2013.

[4] S. H. Han, S.-H. Kang, Y.-J. Cho, and T. G. Cho, "Single incision percutaneous pedicle screw fixation for transforaminal lumbar interbody fusion," Korean Journal of Spine, vol. 9, no. 2, p. 92, 2012.

[5] W. W. G. Ee, W. L. J. Lau, W. Yeo, Y. Von Bing, and W. M. Yue, "Does minimally invasive surgery have a lower risk of surgical site infections compared with open spinal surgery?" Clinical Orthopaedics and Related Research, vol. 472, pp. 1718–1724, 2014.

[6] P. Huang, Y. Wang, J. Xu et al., "Minimally invasive unilateral pedicle screws and a translaminar facet screw fixation and interbody fusion for treatment of single-segment lower lumbar vertebral disease: surgical technique and preliminary clinical results," Journal of Orthopaedic Surgery and Research, vol. 12, no. 1, Article ID 117, 2017.

[7] B. Skovrlj, J. Gilligan, H. S. Cutler, and S. A. Qureshi, "Minimally invasive procedures on the lumbar spine," World Journal of Clinical Cases, vol. 3, no. 1, pp. 1–9, 2015.

[8] E. Kast, K. Mohr, H.-P. Richter, and W. Börm, "Complications of transpedicular screw fixation in the cervical spine," European Spine Journal, vol. 15, no. 3, pp. 327–334, 2005.

[9] Y. R. Rampersaud, N. Annand, and M. B. Dekutoski, "Use of minimally invasive surgical techniques in the management of thoracolumbar trauma: current concepts," Spine, vol. 31, no. 11S, pp. S96–S102, 2006.

[10] J. S. Smith, A. T. Ogden, and R. G. Fessler, "Minimally invasive posterior thoracic fusion," Neurosurgical Focus, vol. 25, no. 2, p. E9, 2008.

[11] H. Yang, J.-h. Shi, M. Ebraheim et al., "Outcome of thoracolumbar burst fractures treated with indirect reduction and fixation without fusion," European Spine Journal, vol. 20, no. 3, pp. 380–386, 2011.

[12] S. S. Sadrameli, R. Jafrani, B. N. Staub, M. Radaideh, and P. J. Holman, "Minimally invasive, stereotactic, wireless, percutaneous pedicle screw placement in the lumbar spine: accuracy rates with 182 consecutive screws," International Journal of Spine Surgery, vol. 12, no. 6, pp. 650–658, 2018.

[13] H. W. Alpert, F. A. Farley, M. S. Caird, R. N. Hensinger, Y. Li, and K. L. Vanderhave, "Outcomes following removal of instrumentation after posterior spinal fusion," Journal of Pediatric Orthopaedics, vol. 36, no. 6, pp. 612–617, 2014.

[14] M. Zotti, T. Fisher, W. W. Yoon et al., "The outcome of pedicle screw instrumentation removal for chronic low back pain," Global Spine Journal, vol. 5, no. 1_suppl, pp. s-0035, 2015.

[15] P. Vanek, O. Bradac, R. Konopkova, P. de Lacy, J. Lacman, and V. Benes, "Treatment of thoracolumbar trauma by short-segment percutaneous transpedicular screw instrumentation: prospective comparative study with a minimum 2-year follow-up," Journal of Neurosurgery: Spine, vol. 20, no. 2, pp. 150–156, 2014.

[16] A. Malhotra, V. B. Kalra, X. Wu, R. Grant, R. A. Bronen, and K. M. Abbed, "Imaging of lumbar spinal surgery complications," Insights Into Imaging, vol. 6, no. 6, pp. 579–590, 2015.

[17] S. N. Divi, G. D. Schroeder, F. C. Oner et al., "AOSpine-spine trauma classification system: the value of modifiers: a narrative review with commentary on evolving descriptive principles," Global Spine Journal, vol. 9, no. 1_suppl, pp. 77S–88S, 2019.

[18] Spinal fractures classification system," https://aosla.com.br/fractures/classification.pdf.

[19] S. P. Baker and B. O'Neill, "The injury severity score," The Journal of Trauma: Injury, Infection, and Critical Care, vol. 16, no. 11, pp. 882–885, 1976.

[20] R. W. J. G. Ostelo, R. A. Deyo, P. Stratford et al., "Interpreting change scores for pain and functional status in low back pain," Spine, vol. 33, no. 1, pp. 90–94, 2008.

[21] J. M. Fritz and J. J. Irrgang, "A comparison of a modified

Oswestry low back pain disability questionnaire and the quebec back pain disability scale," *Physical Therapy*, vol. 81, no. 2, pp. 776–788, 2001.

[22] E. E. Krebs, T. S. Carey, and M. Weinberger, "Accuracy of the pain numeric rating scale as a screening test in primary care," *Journal of General Internal Medicine*, vol. 22, no. 10, pp. 1453–1458, 2007.

[23] D. C. Zelman, E. Dukes, N. Brandenburg, A. Bostrom, and M. Gore, "Identification of cut-points for mild, moderate and severe pain due to diabetic peripheral neuropathy," *Pain*, vol. 115, no. 1, pp. 29–36, 2005.

[24] J. D. Childs, S. R. Piva, and J. M. Fritz, "Responsiveness of the numeric pain rating scale in patients with low back pain," *Spine*, vol. 30, no. 11, pp. 1331–1334, 2005.

[25] A. J. Smits, L. D. Ouden, A. Jonkergouw, J. Deunk, and F. W. Bloemers, "Posterior implant removal in patients with thoracolumbar spine fractures: long-term results," *European Spine Journal*, vol. 26, no. 5, pp. 1525–1534, 2016.

[26] F. Tian, L.-Y. Tu, W.-F. Gu et al., "Percutaneous versus open pedicle screw instrumentation in treatment of thoracic and lumbar spine fractures," *Medicine*, vol. 97, no. 41, Article ID e12535, 2018.

[27] M. H. Wild, M. Glees, C. Plieschnegger, and K. Wenda, "Five-year follow-up examination after purely minimally invasive posterior stabilization of thoracolumbar fractures: a comparison of minimally invasive percutaneously and conventionally open treated patients," *Archives of Orthopaedic and Trauma Surgery*, vol. 127, no. 5, pp. 335–343, 2007.

[28] M. Takami, H. Yamada, K. Nohda, and M. Yoshida, "A minimally invasive surgery combining temporary percutaneous pedicle screw fixation without fusion and vertebroplasty with transpedicular intracorporeal hydroxyapatite blocks grafting for fresh thoracolumbar burst fractures: prospective study," *European Journal of Orthopaedic Surgery & Traumatology*, vol. 24, no. S1, pp. 159–165, 2013.

[29] S.-T. Wang, H.-L. Ma, C.-L. Liu, W.-K. Yu, M.-C. Chang, and T.-H. Chen, "Is fusion necessary for surgically treated burst fractures of the thoracolumbar and lumbar spine?" *Spine*, vol. 31, no. 23, pp. 2646–2652, 2006.

12

The Necessity of CT Hip Scans in the Investigation of Occult Hip Fractures and Their Effect on Patient Management

Thomas Gatt⊕, **Daniel Cutajar, Lara Borg, and Ryan Giordmaina**

Department of Orthopaedics and Trauma, Mater Dei Hospital, Msida MSD2090, Malta

Correspondence should be addressed to Thomas Gatt; thomas.p.gatt@gmail.com

Academic Editor: Panagiotis Korovessis

The diagnostic challenge of negative plain radiography in the context of a previously ambulatory patient is increasing with the rise in geriatric trauma. These patients are often diagnosed with small undisplaced fractures of the pelvis and femur which may not alter management. This study aims to assess the frequency at which computed tomography (CT) hip scans altered patient management and whether two X-ray projections of the hip affected fracture detection rate. All CT hip scans performed over a three-year period were identified retrospectively. Only CT hips pertaining to the identification of occult fractures were included in the study. A total of 447 (63.6%) CT hips were performed to exclude an occult fracture, which was only detected in 108 (24.1%) of the scans requested. The majority were subcapital ($n = 58$, 53.7%) or intertrochanteric ($n = 39$, 36.1%). There was no significant difference between fracture detection rates when comparing one and two views of the pelvis. 82.4% ($n = 89$) of occult hip fractures were managed operatively. CT imaging led to a change in patient management in 20% of cases. The frequency at which CT scan detects and alters management in occult hip fractures confirms the justification for its use. Increasing the number of X-ray projection views does not decrease the reliance on CT. Pelvic ring fractures are common in nonambulatory patients following trauma, and if confirmed on initial imaging, subsequent imaging to exclude a concurrent occult hip is unnecessary. The focus of further research should be towards the development of investigation algorithms which decrease the reliance on CT and defining the optimal surgical criteria for occult hip fractures.

1. Introduction

Occult hip fractures are defined as fractures which are not visible on initial two-view conventional radiography of the hip. The incidence is reported to be as high as 10% on initial imaging [1]. Delayed diagnosis may lead to complications such as fracture displacement, delayed surgery, nonunion, and increased morbidity [2]. While magnetic resonance imaging (MRI) is the recognised gold standard for diagnosis, this is not always an easily accessible or cost-effective option in many centres. For this reason, there has been a move towards the use of computed tomography (CT) as first-line imaging for occult hip fractures, in view of its high sensitivity and specificity rates [3].

However, CT scanning is not without its own disadvantages. Even when using a lower dose protocol, CT is costly and leads to more radiation exposure than conventional radiography. Additionally, patients are subject to longer waiting times in the emergency department when subsequent imaging is requested following normal or inconclusive imaging. With respect to hip pathology in the acute setting, patients are often subjected to a single anteroposterior (AP) view of the pelvis, with some literature claiming that this is sufficient for fracture detection [4]. The diagnostic challenge of negative plain radiography in the context of a previously ambulatory patient is increasing with the rise in geriatric trauma. Often these patients are subsequently diagnosed with small undisplaced fractures of the pelvis and femur which might not alter management. This raises the question whether or not better initial imaging of the pelvis and hips can detect more subtle pathology, explaining the patient's symptomatology and decreasing reliance on CT.

This study aims to assess the frequency at which CT scans of the hip were deemed to change patient management. The secondary aims were to assess whether two projections of the hip had any effect on fracture detection rate and to obtain a better understanding of injury patterns in this patient cohort.

2. Method

All CT hip scans performed at Mater Dei Hospital, Malta, over a three-year period from January 1, 2018, to December 31, 2020, were identified retrospectively through the Centricity™ Universal Viewer Zero Footprint software. All CT hips pertaining to the identification of occult fractures were included in the study. Scans performed for chronic pain, preoperative planning, or postoperative complications were excluded. In our hospital, while there is currently no formal algorithm pathway for suspected occult hip fractures, CT is the commonly accepted imaging modality. Indications for CT imaging despite negative radiography included inability to weight bear, acute limb shortening following trauma, and severe pain on passive movement. Any patient who showed one of these indications formed part of the inclusion criteria to scan. Exclusion criteria were confirmed or suspected pregnancy and patient refusal. The decision to perform a CT hip is normally a joint decision between the emergency physician and the orthopaedic specialist on call, after reviewing the initial X-rays. On occasion, it may also be a recommendation in the X-ray report issued by the radiologist. Requests for CT scans need to be vetted by the CT radiologist on call.

For each scan performed, data on patient demographics, mechanism of injury, indication, time from injury, X-ray number of projections, X-ray findings, fracture types detected, and management outcomes were collected. Only the official imaging reports as issued by the medical imaging department were considered.

SPSS Statistics software was used to collect and analyse the data. Chi square testing was used to assess the relationship between categorical variables. A p value of <0.05 was deemed statistically significant.

3. Results

A total of 702 CT hip scans were performed over the study period. The majority of these were to exclude occult hip fractures ($n = 447$, 63.6%), with the rest performed for preoperative planning ($n = 53$, 7.5%), postoperative assessment ($n = 71$, 10.1%), and chronic conditions ($n = 131$, 18.7%) (Table 1).

Of the 447 suspected occult hip fractures analysed further, the majority were females ($n = 256$, 57.3%) with a mean age of 75.6 years (SD = 14.4). A fracture was detected in 251 cases (56.1%); however, an occult fracture of the proximal hip was only detected in 108 (24.1%) of the CTs requested. The other fractures were primarily isolated pubic ramus fractures ($n = 51$, 20.3%), isolated greater trochanter fracture ($n = 31$, 12.4%), isolated acetabulum fractures ($n = 18$, 7.2%), or a combination of pelvic ring fractures

Table 1: Indications for CT hip scans.

	N (%)
Total CT hip scans performed	702 (100)
Suspected occult hip fracture	447 (63.7)
Preoperative planning	53 (7.5)
Postoperative assessment	71 (10.1)
Chronic pathology	131 (18.7)
Longstanding hip pain	96 (13.7)
Malignancy	14 (2)
Infection	9 (1.3)
Postreduction	7 (1)
Miscellaneous	5 (0.7)

($n = 33$, 13.1%). Of the 108 occult hip fractures identified, the majority were subcapital ($n = 58$, 53.7%) or intertrochanteric ($n = 39$, 36.1%) (Table 2).

An X-ray was taken prior to CT in the majority of cases ($n = 432$, 96.6%). X-rays performed were either a single AP view of the pelvis including both hips ($n = 112$, 25.9%), a single AP of the affected hip ($n = 84$, 19.4%), or an AP of the pelvis with a lateral view of the affected hip ($n = 236$, 54.6%). There was no significant difference between the proximal femur fracture detection rate when comparing AP view of the whole pelvis and AP view of only the affected hip ($p = 0.65$). There was also no significant difference in fracture detection rate when comparing one-view and two-view radiography ($p = 0.22$).

Of the 108 occult hip fractures, 82.4% ($n = 89$) were managed operatively. Operative fixation was performed most frequently by dynamic hip screw ($n = 34$, 31.5%), hemiarthroplasty ($n = 28$, 25.9%), or cannulated screws ($n = 15$, 13.9%) (Table 3).

CT imaging for suspected occult hip fractures led to a change in patient management in 20% of cases. Repeat X-ray imaging within 6 months, despite negative CT findings, was performed in 6 cases. In one instance, an old subcapital fracture was picked up, which was not visible on CT imaging. This patient underwent a total hip replacement, with good recovery.

4. Discussion

Previously, mobile patients who are unable to ambulate following trauma are a diagnostic challenge. The complications of overinvestigation must be balanced against the high morbidity of missing a hip fracture [5]. CT imaging is typically reserved for patients with a clinical suspicion of a hip fracture despite initial negative or inconclusive imaging. This includes, for instance, patients complaining of pain out of proportion to X-ray findings, pain on axial compression of the limb, or being unable to mobilize adequately following trauma. Unfortunately, these presentations are very common in frail individuals, and clinical signs cannot be relied upon to exclude an occult fracture [6]. While some authors have tried to describe tests to aid clinical diagnosis, such as the patellar percussion test, these are no replacement for imaging [7]. CT imaging has emerged as a cost-effective imaging alternative with very high sensitivity and specificity

TABLE 2: Fracture patterns for positive CT hip results.

	N (%)
Fracture detected	
Yes	251 (56.2)
No	196 (43.8)
Fracture types	
Occult proximal femur	108 (43)
Pubic ramus	51 (20.3)
Greater trochanter	31 (12.4)
Acetabulum	18 (7.2)
Iliac crest	4 (1.6)
Sacrum	1 (0.4)
Combination*	33 (13.1)
Others#	5 (2)
Occult proximal femur types	
Subcapital	58 (53.4)
Intertrochanteric	39 (36.1)
Basicervical	4 (3.7)
Transcervical	4 (3.7)
Pertrochanteric	1 (0.9)
Subtrochanteric	2 (1.9)

*Combination patterns include any two or more of the following: ramus, sacrum, acetabulum, ilium, and ischium. #Other fracture patterns include distal femur (1), femoral head (2), femoral shaft (1), and lesser trochanter (1).

TABLE 3: Outcomes of confirmed occult hip fractures.

	N (%)
Conservative	19 (17.6)
Dynamic hip screw	34 (31.5)
Hemiarthroplasty	28 (25.9)
Cannulated screws	15 (13.9)
Total hip arthroplasty	6 (5.5)
Proximal femoral nail	5 (4.6)
Open reduction internal fixation	1 (0.9)

rates [1, 2, 8, 9]. The concern is that this may be used excessively and pick up clinically irrelevant pathology in this patient cohort, ultimately not altering the management or patient disposition significantly.

Our study confirmed similar findings from previous literature that the lateral view of the hip contributes little to detecting occult fractures and decreasing the subsequent need of CT imaging [4, 10]. However, the authors' experience is that it is still relevant in the detection of nonoccult hip fractures and planning surgical techniques. We therefore still recommend both AP and lateral radiographs of the hip as the initial imaging. Some studies have looked at performing novel Bristol views of the hip, which involves a 30-degree angulation film instead of a conventional lateral. If needed, it is found to be more comfortable for the patient, and initial studies show that it is superior to lateral views, despite not having been assessed in large cohorts yet [11].

A significant portion of the patients were found to have some degree of pelvic ring injury, either isolated or in combination. Our study confirmed that pelvic ring injuries and occult hip fractures tend not to occur

simultaneously [12]. This also confirms that an established pelvic ring fracture does not always warrant further investigation for occult hip fractures [13]. Only 3 patients sustaining pelvic ring fractures required surgical fixation, and this was typically reserved for younger patients. Older patients are typically treated with a period of rest, gradual weight-bearing, and physiotherapy. Therefore, the CT scan did little to alter the management in these cases once a pelvic ring fracture was already identified [14].

In this study, the CT detection rate for occult fractures of 24.2% was similar to other studies, ranging from 13 to 39% [1, 2, 15, 16]. Greater trochanter (GT) fractures were mostly isolated, and only a minority extended to the capsule. This was in keeping with the findings of some reports [1]; however, it is in contrast to the findings from other studies which found that up to 90% are extending into the intertrochanteric region [16, 17]. In fact, Kim et al. recommend MRI for all isolated GT fractures, in view of it leading to significant fixation rates [18]. Operative fixation in our study was 82.4% and was significantly higher for occult hip fractures when compared to the meta-analysis performed by Haj-Mirzaian et al. [16] Conservative management for these fractures is generally reserved for older, medically unfit patients with incomplete fracture extending to less than 50% [19]. This discrepancy is probably due to variations in local practice; however, further study focusing on this discrepancy in fixation rates is warranted.

The fact that CT imaging changed the management in 20% of patients in this study shows that low-dose CT remains a relevant investigation for occult hip fractures. This would also be true if we were to have followed a more conservative fixation rate than this study recorded. It may also be argued that the remaining 80% of scans were needed to achieve a diagnosis and reassure patients. Some authors have attempted to devise an algorithm to guide management on initial presentation of this patient cohort. Such algorithms would ensure more stringent criteria to decrease unnecessary imaging. Gangopadhyay et al. proposed sending home ambulatory patients to undergo repeat X-ray in one week, or admitting nonambulatory patients to scan the following day if symptoms persist [20]. This may lead to reducing unnecessary CT scans in these patients. The development of such algorithms coupled with cost-effectiveness studies for these approaches should serve as the focus for further studies on the topic.

4.1. Limitations. This study is limited by its retrospective nature. Data were collected from the official X-ray and CT reports issued online by the radiology department. The medical grade of the person reporting is not documented, and this in itself may affect the data. It may well be that a more experienced radiologist may have picked up the more subtle signs, reducing the need for a CT scan, giving rise to a degree of sampling bias. Furthermore, the patient outcomes following the management of these occult fractures were unable to be obtained.

5. Conclusion

The frequency at which CT scan detects and alters management in occult hip fractures confirms the justification for its use. Increasing the number of X-ray projection views does little to increase detection rate and decrease reliance on CT. However, we still advocate a minimum of two views for the benefit of nonoccult hip fractures. Pelvic ring fractures are very common in nonambulatory patients following trauma, and if confirmed to be stable on initial imaging, subsequent imaging to exclude a concurrent occult hip is unnecessary. The focus of further research should be towards the development of investigation algorithms which decrease the need for CT and defining the optimal surgical criteria for occult hip fractures.

References

[1] R. W. Thomas, H. L. Williams, E. C. Carpenter, and K. Lyons, "The validity of investigating occult hip fractures using multidetector CT," *British Journal of Radiology*, vol. 89, no. 1060, Article ID 20150250, 2016.

[2] S. K. Gill, J. Smith, R. Fox, and T. J. Chesser, "Investigation of occult hip fractures: the use of CT and MRI," *The Scientific World Journal*, vol. 2013, Article ID 830319, 4 pages, 2013.

[3] H. Rehman, R. G. Clement, F. Perks, and T. O. White, "Imaging of occult hip fractures: CT or MRI?" *Injury*, vol. 47, no. 6, pp. 1297–1301, 2016.

[4] B. Almazedi, C. D. Smith, D. Morgan, G. Thomas, and G. Pereira, "Another fractured neck of femur: do we need a lateral X-ray?" *British Journal of Radiology*, vol. 84, no. 1001, pp. 413–417, 2011.

[5] S. Je, H. Kim, S. Ryu et al., "The consequence of delayed diagnosis of an occult hip fracture," *Journal of Trauma and Injury*, vol. 28, no. 3, pp. 91–97, 2015.

[6] M. Hossain, C. Barwick, A. K. Sinha, and J. G. Andrew, "Is magnetic resonance imaging (MRI) necessary to exclude occult hip fracture?" *Injury*, vol. 38, no. 10, pp. 1204–1208, 2007.

[7] S. J. M. Smeets, W. Vening, M. B. Winkes, G. P. Kuijt, G. D. Slooter, and P. V. van Eerten, "The patellar pubic percussion test: a simple bedside tool for suspected occult hip fractures," *International Orthopaedics*, vol. 42, no. 11, pp. 2521–2524, 2018.

[8] S. Heikal, P. Riou, and L. Jones, "The use of computed tomography in identifying radiologically occult hip fractures in the elderly," *Annals of the Royal College of Surgeons of England*, vol. 96, no. 3, pp. 234–237, 2014.

[9] T. T. Kellock, B. Khurana, and J. C. Mandell, "Diagnostic performance of CT for occult proximal femoral fractures: a systematic review and meta-analysis," *American Journal of Roentgenology*, vol. 213, no. 6, pp. 1324–1330, 2019.

[10] D. S. Kumar, S. D. Gubbi, B. Abdul, and M. Bisalahalli, "Lateral radiograph of the hip in fracture neck of femur: is it a ritual?" *European Journal of Trauma and Emergency Surgery*, vol. 34, no. 5, pp. 504–507, 2008.

[11] J. Harding, T. J. Chesser, and M. Bradley, "The Bristol hip view: its role in the diagnosis and surgical planning and occult fracture diagnosis for proximal femoral fractures," *The Scientific World Journal*, vol. 2013, Article ID 703783, 4 pages, 2013.

[12] T. Ohishi, T. Ito, D. Suzuki, T. Banno, and Y. Honda, "Occult hip and pelvic fractures and accompanying muscle injuries around the hip," *Archives of Orthopaedic and Trauma Surgery*, vol. 132, no. 1, pp. 105–112, 2012.

[13] P. Lakshmanan, A. Sharma, K. Lyons, and J. P. Peehal, "Are occult fractures of the hip and pelvic ring mutually exclusive?" *Journal of Bone and Joint Surgery*, vol. 89, no. 10, pp. 1344–1346, 2007.

[14] M. Oka and J. U. Monu, "Prevalence and patterns of occult hip fractures and mimics revealed by MRI," *American Journal of Roentgenology*, vol. 182, no. 2, pp. 283–288, 2004.

[15] J. Williams, F. Allen, M. Kedrzycki, Y. Shenava, and R. Gupta, "Use of multislice CT for investigation of occult geriatric hip fractures and impact on timing of surgery," *Geriatric Orthopaedic Surgery & Rehabilitation*, vol. 10, 2019.

[16] A. Haj-Mirzaian, J. Eng, R. Khorasani et al., "Use of advanced imaging for radiographically occult hip fracture in elderly patients: a systematic review and meta-analysis," *Radiology*, vol. 296, no. 3, pp. 521–531, 2020.

[17] J. Noh, K. H. Lee, S. Jung, and S. Hwang, "The frequency of occult intertrochanteric fractures among individuals with isolated greater trochanteric fractures," *Hip & Pelvis*, vol. 31, no. 1, pp. 23–32, 2019.

[18] S. J. Kim, J. Ahn, H. K. Kim, and J. H. Kim, "Is magnetic resonance imaging necessary in isolated greater trochanter fracture? A systemic review and pooled analysis," *BMC Musculoskeletal Disorders*, vol. 16, p. 395, 2015.

[19] G. Rubin, I. Malka, and N. Rozen, "Should we operate on occult hip fractures?" *The Israel Medical Association Journal*, vol. 12, no. 5, pp. 316-317, 2010.

[20] S. Gangopadhyay, G. A. Akra, and A. M. Nanu, "Occult hip fractures in the elderly: a protocol for management," *European Journal of Orthopaedic Surgery and Traumatology*, vol. 17, no. 2, pp. 153–156, 2007.

13

Delayed Presentation of Patients with Hip Fractures during the COVID-19 "Stay-at-Home" Order in the Southmost Region of the United States

Michael Serra-Torres(ID),[1,2] **Raul Barreda**(ID),[2,3] **David Weaver**(ID),[2] and **Annelyn Torres-Reveron**(ID)[2]

[1]DHR Health Orthopedic Institute, Edinburg, TX 78539, USA
[2]DHR Health Institute for Research and Development, Edinburg, TX 78539, USA
[3]DHR Health Surgery Institute, McAllen, TX 78504, USA

Correspondence should be addressed to Michael Serra-Torres; m.serra@dhr-rgv.com

Academic Editor: Francesco Liuzza

To evaluate the effects of COVID-19 and stay-at-home orders in traumatic hip fractures presentation, we conducted a retrospective chart review cohort study from March 13 to June 13 in 2020 compared to 2019 from a single-hospital Trauma Level 2 Center. Males and females, 18 years of age and older presenting with a diagnosis of displaced or nondisplaced, intracapsular, or extracapsular hip fracture, underwent standard of care—comparative analysis of the patient's characteristics and clinical outcomes. The primary study outcomes included age, sex, ethnicity, and body mass index, the onset of injury, date of arrival, payer, the primary type of injury and comorbidities, mechanism of injury, treatment received, postoperative complications, days in an intensive care unit (ICU), discharge disposition, pre- and postinjury functional status, and COVID-19 test. Age, sex, ethnicity, and body mass index were similar in the patients in 2019 compared to 2020. The patients' average age was 76 years old, 80% reported Hispanic ethnicity, and 63% of the patients were females. Most injuries (90%) occurred due to falls. On average, patients in 2020 presented 4.8 days after the injury onset as compared to 0.7 days in 2019 ($p < 0.05$). There was an increase in displaced fractures in 2019 compared to 2020 and an increase in patients' disposition into rehabilitation facilities compared to skilled nursing facilities. Despite the delay in presentation, length of stay, days in the ICU, or functional outcomes of the patients were not affected. Although the patients showed a delayed presentation after hip fracture, this does not appear to significantly interfere with the short-term or the 6-month mortality outcomes of the patients, suggesting the possibility of guided delayed care during times of national emergency and increased strain in hospital resources.

1. Introduction

The COVID-19 pandemic has introduced many challenges to healthcare systems around the world, presenting added changes, pressures, and strains at all levels of the system, including but not limited to doctor–patient relationships and health organization resources [1, 2]. The pandemic has, in turn, produced several changes in the patient's behavior and clinical outcomes. Nevertheless, these changes have provided us the opportunity to examine variations in clinical presentations that would not have been possible under normal circumstances. On March 13, 2020, the State of Texas declared a state of emergency, shortly followed (March 22) by an order for the postponement of elective surgical procedures anticipating an increase in COVID-19-infected patients requiring usage of hospital resources. On April 2, the State entered into a stay-at-home order that extended until April 30. On May 1, the State started a phase one reopening, as recommended by the Department of State Health Services [3]. On May 18, Texas expanded to a phase two reopening plan, allowing for most of the economy to resume operations with some restrictions on their capacity.

The sum of all these orders created a decrease in the mobility of the general public, resulting in a reduction of all traumatic injuries presenting at our hospital emergency service, including hip fractures. Changes in population behavior during the COVID-19 restrictions have given us an inside perspective on the impact of states of emergency in traumatic hip fractures.

Most hip fractures occur in the elderly population, with 90% occurring after the age of 50 years and 52% occurring after the age of 80 years [4]. Ninety percent of hip fractures occur due to falls from a standing height or less [5, 6]. Women experience 75% of all hip fractures, mainly due to the increased frequency of osteoporosis [7]. The State of Texas has the highest number across the United States for older adults who fall, reported at 33.9% [8]. Injuries due to falls represent a cost of 1.6 billion in Medicare expenses for Texas [9] and 29 billion for the United States annually [10].

Hip fractures can be categorized using multiple classifications. In this study, we classified fractures by displacement (displaced versus nondisplaced) and anatomic sites (femoral neck, intertrochanteric/subtrochanteric) since this classification guides the surgical options. Clinical guidelines recommend immediately surgical repair of hip fractures within 24 hours, preferably, or as soon as medically stable, but avoiding a delay in surgery beyond 72 hours [11–13]. However, there is still controversy in the literature regarding the definition of a delayed intervention in hip fracture repairs [14]. Mortality appears to decrease when patients are intervened within the 72 hours following the injury [15]. On the other hand, two large studies that adjusted for demographic characteristics and comorbidities reported that mortality rates are not affected by a delay in the surgical intervention of more than 120 hours [11–13]. Based on previous findings, we are defining a delayed presentation of hip fracture as any presentation for more than four days (96 hours).

The purpose of this study was to evaluate the effects of COVID-19 and stay-at-home orders in traumatic hip fractures presenting at a functioning Level 1 Trauma center in Texas. It was hypothesized that the behavior of patients seeking care during the COVID-19 pandemic has been altered by the governmental regulations with possible changes to the mechanism of injury, time of presentation, and outcomes of treatment. While other hospitals in the region entered into the diversion of patients, our hospital system continued to receive all types of patients. We were the only center able to allocate 200 beds for patients arriving with COVID-19 symptoms. Therefore, our orthopedic department continued uninterruptedly caring for all patients, including those being transferred from other hospitals into our hospital, regardless of their COVID-19 status. In light of this, the hospital implemented treatment algorithms designed to deliver timely treatment to patients while protecting the medical personnel in the emergency room and the operating rooms. Understanding how government-imposed restrictions affect clinical outcomes may provide a working framework for optimal healthcare delivery during state and national emergencies.

2. Methods

2.1. Study Design and Setting. This is a retrospective chart review cohort study of patients from a single hospital, Level 2 Trauma Center in South Texas. The Institutional Review Board approved this study, and it conformed to the Declaration of Helsinki and the US Federal Policy for the Protection of Humans Subjects. A full waiver of authorization under the Health Insurance Portability and Accountability Act (HIPAA, 1996) was submitted by the study team and approved by the Institutional Review Board to conduct this retrospective study. The retrospective period of chart review was set from March 13, 2020, to June 13, 2020. We used March 13, 2020, as the start because on that day, the state government issued the emergency order and up to three months after. This period includes data for the four weeks following phase two reopening of the State, allowing for a possible return to normal behavior and mobility in the population. To compare, we used the data extracted from the same period in 2019.

2.2. Subjects. Male and female subjects 18 years and older with a diagnosis of the displaced or nondisplaced femoral neck and intertrochanteric/subtrochanteric fractures with all its modifiers (ICD10: S72.0, S72.1, and S72.2) were eligible for the study. The patients were excluded from the study if they presented with a fracture already treated at another institution (referred to a rehabilitation hospital), if the onset of the injury or presentation was outside the study period, for the repair of nonunion fractures, or lack of documentation for the onset of the injury.

2.3. Variables. The demographic variables included were age, sex, ethnicity, body mass index, date of injury arrival (presentation), date of arrival, presentation site, health insurance, or self-pay. From the medical record, we obtained the onset of the injury, the primary diagnosis and secondary diagnosis, the mechanism of injury, treatment received and date, postoperative complications (i.e., respiratory failure, hypotension, anemia, infection, deep vein thrombosis, and hemorrhage), intensive care unit (ICU) usage, comorbidities and discharge disposition, pre- and postinjury functional level, and the COVID-19 test results, for patients who received it in 2020. The delay in the presentation was calculated from the date reported by the patient, when the injury occurred, to the date of arrival to the hospital (emergency room or clinic). The delay in surgery was calculated from the date of arrival to the date of surgery, as reported in the medical record. If surgical treatment was delayed due to medical optimization needed (i.e., coagulation), it was also noted during the data collection process.

To determine whether the delay in presentation represented a difference in functionality for the patients, we quantified the presurgical and postsurgical functionality level of patients into three main categories: walking with aid (walker, crutches, and rollator), bed-bound (nonambulating, including those that use a wheelchair for transportation or stand for transfer only), and walking independently. The functional level received a categorical score of zero (0) for bed-bound, one (1) for walking with aid, and two (2) for walking independently. To calculate the change in functionality, we subtracted the value on the level of functionality at discharge from that of the admission. A zero indicates no change in function from preinjury to postinjury, a minus 1 (−1) indicates a decrease in function (e.g., from walking independently to walking with aid), and a minus two (−2) indicates a decrease in functionality of two levels (e.g., from walking independently to bed-bound).

2.4. Data Source/Measurements. The hospital system maintains a trauma databank as part of the trauma quality improvement program from the American College of Surgeons. The trauma databank is populated by trained nurses for this task. Patients' meeting inclusion criteria from 2019 were identified via an electronic report from the hospital trauma databank. For 2020, we requested a report from the business intelligence department in the hospital for the three months' period under review, using the ICD-10 codes reported above. Once the list of patients and the corresponding medical record number were obtained, the same variables for all patients were extracted. All the presented information was part of the subject's standard of care, as documented in their medical record or the trauma data bank, and there was no intervention or variable collected directly from the patient. To maintain quality and consistency in the data extraction process, the same trauma data analyst extracted patient's additional information not present in the trauma databank "record from 2019" and 2020. Inclusion and exclusion criteria were verified by the orthopedic trauma surgeon before the patient was included in the analysis. After six months of the event, the patient's mortality was verified by their recorded attendance to follow-up visits or by notes from our hospital call center in charge of following up patient's status via phone calls.

2.5. Statistical Methods. Descriptive statistics were used for the entire study population and subdivided by year. Frequencies and column percentages were used to summarize categorical variables. The normal distribution of continuous variables was measured using the Shapiro–Wilk goodness-of-fit test. Nonnormally distributed variables were analyzed using the Wilcoxon test, and normally distributed variables were analyzed using the Student *t*-test for independent samples. Chi-square or Fisher's exact test was used for categorical variables. Multinomial regression analyses were used to explore the changes in function across injury types. The statistical analyses were two-sided and conducted using JMP 15.0 (SAS Institute, Inc., Carry, NC, USA). The significance was set at $p < 0.05$.

3. Results

3.1. Participants. From March 13, 2020, to June 13, 2020, 41 patients met the inclusion criteria. Six patients were excluded for the following reasons: (1) a visit related to a nonunion treatment, (2) a visit associated with the removal of the implant, (3) patient unable to report the onset of injury due to a history of multiple falls, (4) patient left against medical advice from the emergency room, (5) patient requested a transfer to a different institution, and (6) patient with rule-out treatment, with negative results. Data from 2019 was extracted from the trauma databank at our institution, and all encounters have already been reviewed and verified by qualified trauma data analysis. During the same period for 2019, 45 records were reported to the trauma databank. Four patients' records were eliminated because these were transferred to our institution with fractures already treated; forty-one records met the inclusion criteria in 2019.

3.2. Demographic Characteristics. Table 1 presents the demographic characteristics of patients per year. There was a female's predominance in the cohort of patients for both years with no difference in the gender distribution between years. The majority of the patients in both years (>80%) self-reported Hispanic ethnicity, which represents the demographic distribution of our region. The average age for the patient's cohort was 76.4 ± 14.9 years, and the mean age for both years was very similar. The body mass index was also similar between the 2019 and 2020 cohorts. There was no statistical difference in the demographic characteristics of patients between years (all $p > 0.05$).

3.3. Outcome Data. Table 2 presents the categorical clinical characteristics of the patients. The modes of injury for the hip fractures were in the majority (>90%) due to falls of less than a meter height (e.g., transferring from bed to commode) for both years ($X^2 = 1.7$, d.f. = 2, $p > 0.05$). Similarly, 90% of the patients presented directly to the emergency room, with an average of 9% of patients going directly to clinics ($X^2 = 0.674$, d.f. = 1, $p > 0.05$). The types of injuries that the patients presented upon arrival were different across years ($X^2 = 18.76$, d.f. = 3, $p < 0.01$), with displaced fractures more frequently presented in 2019 than in 2020. Displaced intertrochanteric hip fractures were more frequent in 2019 than in 2020 compared to nondisplaced intertrochanteric, OR = 22.28 (95% CI, 2.12 to 233.85). Similarly, displaced femoral neck hip fractures were also more frequent in 2019 than in 2020 compared to the nondisplaced femoral neck, OR = 15.37 (95% CI, 2.37 to 99.56). The majority of the patients (>70%) had Medicare as the principal payer, which was predicted from the cohort's age range. We observed a significant difference in the payer between years ($X^2 = 8.69$, d.f. = 3, $p < 0.05$). There was an increased odds ratio for the patients having Medicare instead of private/other insurance as a payer in 2019 compared to 2020: OR = 3.48 (95% CI, 0.5 to 24.06). The disposition of patients varied between 2019 and 2020 ($X^2 = 12.61$, d.f. = 4, $p < 0.05$). While more than half of the patients were discharged to rehabilitation facilities during both years, an increased proportion of patients were discharged to skilled nursing facilities in 2019 compared to 2020 (OR: 8.88 (95% CI, 1.42 to 55.45). Only one patient died in 2020 (cardiopulmonary arrest in a 92-year-old male) and none in 2019. The proportion of patients with postsurgical

TABLE 1: Demographic characteristics of patients.

Variable	All	2019	2020	P-value
Gender, n (column %)				
Males	28 (36.8)	15 (36.6)	13 (37.1)	0.967
Females	48 (63.2)	26 (63.4)	22 (62.9)	
Ethnicity, n (row %)				
Hispanic	61 (80.3)	33 (80.5)	28 (80.0)	0.942
Non-Hispanic	15 (19.7)	8 (19.5)	7 (20.0)	
Age, mean (SD)	76.4 (14.9)	76.3 (15.6)	76.5 (14.3)	0.907
BMI, mean (SD)	25.4 (4.9)	25.2 (5.3)	25.5 (4.5)	0.751

BMI: body mass index.

complications was not different between years ($X^2 = 2.819$, d.f. = 5, $p > 0.05$). The mortality of the patients at 6 months after the presentation was evaluated. Four patients were lost at follow-up: two in 2019 and two in 2020. There was a nonsignificant increase in mortality for 2020 at 17.1% as compared to 2019 at 9.8% ($X^2 = 0.969$, d.f. = 1, $p > 0.05$). Despite the lack of significant difference, the odds of mortality at 6 months in 2020 compared to 2019 were moderately higher: OR = 1.94 (95% CI, 0.542 to 6.53). When only the patients with a delayed presentation were considered, only one patient from the 2020 cohort died and none from 2019.

3.4. Main Results. Table 3 presents the quantitative variables related to their inpatient period. The average time from injury onset to presentation in 2020 was 7.5 times higher compared to 2019 (0.7 days in 2019 vs. 4.8 days in 2020). Patients in 2020 presented to the hospital on average, four days later than in 2019. The delay in the presentation was significantly different between years ($Z = 2.13$, $p < 0.01$). The average among only those patients with the delayed presentation was 8.33 (range: 7 to 11) days in 2019 compared to 20.87 (range: 4 to 55) days in 2020. In 2019, only three (7.31%) patients showed up to the hospital with a delay larger than four days in 2019; in 2020, eight (22.85%) patients had a delayed presentation. Despite the significant delay in presentation between years, the time to surgical care was similar ($Z = 1.41$, $p > 0.05$). There was no difference between years regarding the total hospital length of stay ($Z = 1.09$, $p > 0.05$), the number of days spent in the ICU ($Z = 1.43$, $p > 0.05$), and the number and type of comorbidities ($Z = -0.59$, $p > 0.05$). The most frequently observed comorbidities were type 2 diabetes and hypertension.

We explored the change in functionality within each type of fracture and presentation delay. Neither the type of fracture nor the delay in presentation affected the change in functionality across the years (Figure 1(a)). The categorical decrease function is maintained across both years and is not affected by the delay in presentation (Figure 1(b)). The percentage of patients that maintained the same level of function (zero category) was 45% and 41% in nondelayed compared to delayed presentation, respectively. Similarly, 45% and 49% of patients decreased one level of functionality (−1 category) in 2019 and 2020, respectively. Less than 10%

of the patients decreased two levels of functionality (−2 category) regardless of delayed presentation.

In 2020, 8 patients had a delayed presentation to our institution. Qualitative analysis of the reasons for the delay in seeking care in 2020, as documented in the chart, revealed that two patients did not seek immediate care because they were afraid of COVID-19 contagion; one patient had an injury out of the country. One patient tried avoiding the emergency room due to COVID-19 and visited their primary care physician (PCP). Two patients had delayed diagnosis (X-ray) before the final diagnosis by advanced imaging (MRI and CT), and both were nondisplaced femoral neck fractures. Finally, two patients were bed-bound prior to the injury, and their respective families brought them to the hospital only after symptoms did not resolve for more than a week. On the other hand, in 2019, three patients had delayed presentation: one patient had a missed diagnosis of the fracture, one had a delay in workup at PCP, and for the third one, the reason for the delay could not be found in the chart.

3.5. COVID-19 Testing. From the 35 patients included in 2020, twenty patients had the COVID-19 test done. From May 28, 2020, to June 15, 2020, all patients received a COVID-19 test (13 patients). Before that, the test was done only upon the request of the orthopedic surgeon and depending on the test kit availability. All tested patients were negative for SARS-CoV-2. At the 6-month follow-up, one patient from the 2020 cohort resulted positive for COVID-19 shortly after the hip fracture and died due to the virus. This patient was not a delayed presentation.

4. Discussion

A delay in the presentation following hip fractures in the elderly population of South Texas during the COVID-19 pandemic did not significantly impact the length of stay, postsurgical complications, or functional outcomes compared to a similar demographic population with hip fractures during the same period of the last year. The delay in the presentation was significantly influenced by the absence or presence of displaced fractures. A lower number of displaced fractures were observed in 2020 compared to 2019. Displaced fractures are prone to increased complications and decreased patients' quality of life compared to nondisplaced

TABLE 2: Categorical clinical characteristics of patients.

Variable n (column %)	All	2019	2020	P-value
Mode of injury				
Fall	71 (93.4)	38 (92.7)	33 (94.3)	
MVC	3 (4.0)	2 (4.9)	1 (2.9)	0.419
Other	2 (2.6)	1 (2.4)	1 (2.9)	
Type of injury				
D-femoral neck	15 (19.7)	10 (24.4)	5 (14.3)	
D-Inter.	22 (28.9)	18 (43.9)	5 (11.4)	<0.001*
ND-femoral neck	12 (15.8)	4 (9.8)	8 (22.9)	
ND-Inter.	27 (35.5)	9 (21.9)	18 (51.4)	
Arrived at				
ER	69 (90.8)	38 (88.6)	31 (90.8)	0.412
Clinic	7 (9.2)	3 (7.3)	4 (11.4)	
Payer				
Medicare	56 (73.7)	32 (78.1)	24 (68.6)	
Medicaid	4 (5.3)	3 (7.3)	1 (2.9)	0.0336*
Private/other	13 (17.1)	5 (12.2)	8 (22.8)	
Self-paid	3 (3.9)	1 (2.4)	2 (5.7)	
Disposition				
Rehabilitation	43 (56.6)	19 (46.3)	24 (68.6)	
Skilled nursing	16 (21.1)	12 (29.3)	4 (11.4)	0.013*
Home/self-care	15 (19.7)	9 (21.9)	6 (17.1)	
Other	1 (1.3)	1 (2.4)	0 (0)	
Died	1 (1.3)	0 (0)	1 (2.9)	
Postsurgical complications*				
None noted	63 (82.9)	34 (83.0)	28 (80.0)	
Respiratory complications	5 (6.6)	3 (7.3)	2 (5.7)	
Cardiac complications	3 (3.9)	1 (2.4)	2 (5.7)	0.728
Anemia	3 (3.9)	1 (2.4)	2 (5.7)	
Stroke	1 (1.3)	1 (2.4)	0	
UTI	1 (1.3)	1 (2.4)	0	
Mortality at 6 months				
Died	6 (7.9)	4 (9.8)	6 (17.1)	0.332
Unknown status	4 (5.2)	2 (4.9)	2 (5.7)	

fractures [16]. This could, in part, explain the incidence of nondisplaced fractures with a late presentation. Avoidance behavior, such as going to the PCP instead of the emergency room or family members expecting symptoms resolution, was observed. Our results align with a previous study using data from the American College of Surgeons, indicating that a surgical delay for pathological hip fractures was not associated with increased complications [17].

Delaying medical care, or otherwise known as medical care avoidance, is a multifactorial process. The three main categories that explain this behavior are (1) unfavorable evaluations, (2) low perceived needs, and (3) barriers to medical care, such as high cost and time constraints [18]. Unfavorable assessments are influenced by affective behavior as presented by Taber et al.; fear of bad news and unspecified fear, in general, were two of the factors documented in her work. While medical insurance was not a factor in the current study that statistically explained the delay, the lower perceived need, fear of bad news, a saturated medical system, and fear of COVID-19 contagion seem to have played a role in explaining patient's presentation. Additional studies in our hospital and other facilities across the nation are needed to understand the behavioral patterns in light of the pandemic and how it affects outcomes.

The current pandemic presents a significant strain on hospital resources and a possible increased risk of contagion for patients. With future emergencies leading to an overloaded system, it might become necessary to stratify care by weighing the risks and benefits of early/delayed intervention versus exposure. Our study appears to suggest that a possible delay, specifically in the treatment of nondisplaced hip fractures of an average of three weeks, does not result in an adverse effect on early outcomes. Furthermore, during emergencies, when the medical system is saturated, such as during the COVID-19 pandemic, the patient could be triaged at other clinical care facilities and brought into the hospital with decreased urgency (guided delayed treatment) to reduce exposure to external risk factors such as high contagious infectious diseases with increased mortality. We strongly believe that the clinical guidelines for surgical repair within the shortest time frame should always be followed. However, the possibility of guided delay during emergencies will require further research to measure feasibility and acceptability by patients and health care providers.

We observed an increase in rehabilitation disposition as compared to skilled nursing facilities in 2020. The most reasonable explanation for this observation results from the increased risks of COVID-19 infections and mortality in nursing homes that have been observed across the nation [19]. Thus, in times of emergency, the patient's postsurgical disposition might need to be weighed by both the benefit to the patient functionality and preventive measures to preserve optimal health. Discharge disposition could also explain the marginal increase in the length of stay in 2020 since some patients had to wait for placement at the rehabilitation hospital.

Cultural differences are well known to influence the type of care that is given to the elderly. The majority of the patients in this study were of Mexican-American descent due to the close proximity that our hospital has with the northern border of Mexico. When faced with a hip fracture diagnosis, Mexican-Americans prefer informal caregivers (family members or friends), rather than formal care in comparison to non-Latino whites [20]. Yet, Mexican-American elders are more functionally impaired than their non-Latino whites' counterparts [21]. Crist and Speaks [22] have documented that within the Mexican-American cultural norm, familism is strong: the care of the elderly is the responsibility of the family. During the stay-at-home order to reduce COVID-19 spread, there was an increased number of family members available to care for the elderly in the family nucleus. We presume that this availability resulted in increased supervising and assistance with activities of daily living to the senior members. An increased number of helping hands within the family structure may lead to a reduction in the risk factors for falls [23] or in the severity of the falls that occurred. This factor may partially explain the general decrease in the presentation of trauma arriving at

TABLE 3: Quantitative clinical characteristics of patients.

Variables, n (SD)	All	2019	2020	P-value[+]
Delay in presentation (days)	2.6 (8.2)	0.7 (2.3)	4.8 (11.5)	**0.033**[*]
Hours from arrival to surgery	40.5 (29.0)	40.2 (29.0)	40.9 (28.9)	0.920
Hospital LOS in days	5.9 (3.2)	5.4 (2.5)	6.5 (3.7)	0.275
Number of days in ICU	0.4 (1.7)	0.1 (0.4)	0.8 (2.4)	0.152
Number of comorbidities	2.7 (1.6)	2.7 (1.6)	2.5 (1.6)	0.550

+: nonparametric test.

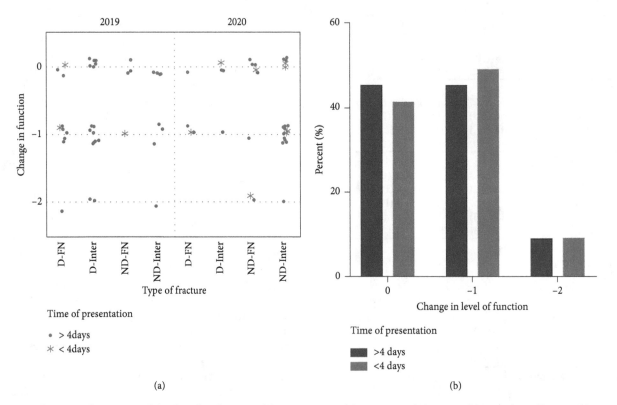

(a) (b)

FIGURE 1: Changes in function resulting from hip fractures. (a) Comparison of the categorical change in function for each type of fractures. Change in function was assigned a value based on the mobility capacity before fracture and after fracture. A zero indicates no change from pre- to postfracture; negative one indicates a one-level decrease in function (i.e., from previously walking to using aid to walk); and negative two indicates a two-level decrease in function (i.e., from previously walking to being bedridden). No significant differences in functionality were observed between years. (b) The percent of patients within each categorical change in functionality was not affected by the delay in presentation (data collapsed across years). D = displaced, ND = nondisplaced, FN = femoral neck, and Inter. = intertrochanteric.

our emergency room due to the reduction of exposure and potential severity of the fall.

In other parts of the world, significantly impacted by the COVID-19 pandemic, orthopedic surgeries have continued due to the essential nature of this service. Orthopedic surgeons and other surgeons in charge of trauma services have the imminent urgency to take care of the patients, with the increased susceptibility to contagious diseases of any type [24]. For example, in China, 26 orthopedic surgeons tested positive for COVID-19, with 80% of these exposures in the wards [25]. On the other hand, patients' undergoing surgical interventions due to traumatic injuries have poorer outcomes if they have active COVID-19 infections. This is confirmed by independent reports from New York [24], United Kingdom [26], France [27], and China [28]. While we only had one patient who resulted positive for COVID-19

shortly after surgery, the delay in surgical intervention in light of poorer outcomes in patients with active COVID-19 deserves additional attention at the national and multinational levels.

4.1. Study Limitations. One of the limitations of our study is the lack of long-term outcomes for the patients. The best indicator of outcome for hip fractures is mortality within a year [29]. However, the assessment of mortality at 6 months did not show a significant difference between 2019 and 2020. It still needs to be determined if the same outcome remains true at one year after fracture. We did not assess whether the delay in the presentation of care resulted in increased medical costs, family burden, or psychological stress. These are areas that could be explored in light of the multiple changes that have been implemented at hospitals in response to the pandemic. The sample size of the study was limited by the number of presentations within the selected time frame. As with any retrospective study, there was the confounding factor of information bias. A rigorous protocol for data extraction was uniformly followed for both years and verified by the orthopedic surgeon. As mentioned before, the majority of the patient population in this study was of Hispanic ethnicity. When extrapolating the current results to other populations, demographic and contextual variables within the population of interest should be considered. While we explored access to healthcare, some other social determinants of health remained unexplored. Future studies might consider marital status/family living environment, income, education level, and access to healthcare facilities that might serve as factors to explain presentation delays following hip fracture.

5. Conclusions

Major emergencies present challenges for patients seeking healthcare. Although patients have been showing delayed presentation after hip fracture, it does not appear to interfere with the patients' short-term outcomes. The stay-at-home orders likely lead to an increase in familism in Mexican-American families, impacting the incidence and severity of fractures in seniors. A decrease in the severity of the hip fractures may explain the higher tolerance to delays in the presentation. The observed changes in delayed presentation for hip fractures may be unique to this pandemic; thus, permanent changes in patients' behavioral patterns need to be confirmed with longer exposure times and subsequent studies. Although we propose the possibility of guided delayed treatment in future emergency events, additional studies are necessary to determine the criteria, feasibility, and sequelae of treatment delay.

Disclosure

The research work presented in this manuscript did not receive funding and was of the original conception of the authors.

References

[1] D. De Mauro, G. Rovere, A. Smimmo et al., "COVID-19 pandemic: management of patients affected by SARS-CoV-2 in Rome COVID Hospital 2 Trauma Centre and safety of our surgical team," *International Orthopaedics*, vol. 44, no. 12, pp. 2487–2491, 2020.

[2] B. C. Service, A. P. Collins, A. Crespo et al., "Medically necessary orthopaedic surgery during the COVID-19 pandemic," *Journal of Bone and Joint Surgery*, vol. 102, no. 14, p. e76, 2020.

[3] Texas Department of State Health Services, *Coronavirus Disease 2019 (COVID-19)*, Texas Department of State Health Services, Austin, TX, USA, 2020, https://www.dshs.texas.gov/coronavirus/.

[4] C. Cooper, G. Campion, and L. J. Melton, "Hip fractures in the elderly: a world-wide projection," *Osteoporosis International*, vol. 2, no. 6, pp. 285–289, 1992.

[5] A. V. Schwartz, J. L. Kelsey, S. Maggi et al., "International variation in the incidence of hip fractures: cross-national project on osteoporosis for the World Health Organization Program for Research on Aging," *Osteoporosis International*, vol. 9, no. 3, pp. 242–253, 1999.

[6] D. Dhanwal, E. Dennison, N. Harvey, and C. Cooper, "Epidemiology of hip fracture: worldwide geographic variation," *Indian Journal of Orthopaedics*, vol. 45, no. 1, pp. 15–22, 2011.

[7] Centers for Disease Control and Prevention, *Older Adults Falls. In: CDC Features [Internet]*, Centers for Disease Control and Prevention, Atlanta, GA, USA, 2018, https://www.cdc.gov/features/falls-older-adults/index.html.

[8] Centers for Disease Control and Prevention National Center for Injury Prevention and Control, *Leading Causes of Death Reports, 1981 - 2017*, WISQARS, Atlanta, GA, USA, 2019, https://webappa.cdc.gov/sasweb/ncipc/leadcause.html.

[9] C. S. Florence, G. Bergen, A. Atherly, E. Burns, J. Stevens, and C. Drake, "Medical costs of fatal and nonfatal falls in older adults," *Journal of the American Geriatrics Society*, vol. 66, no. 4, pp. 693–698, 2018.

[10] Y. K. Haddad, G. Bergen, and C. S. Florence, "Estimating the economic burden related to older adult falls by state," *Journal of Public Health Management and Practice*, vol. 25, no. 2, pp. E17–E24, 2019.

[11] J. P. Grimes, P. M. Gregory, H. Noveck, M. S. Butler, and J. L. Carson, "The effects of time-to-surgery on mortality and morbidity in patients following hip fracture," *The American Journal of Medicine*, vol. 112, no. 9, pp. 702–709, 2002.

[12] G. M. Orosz, J. Magaziner, E. L. Hannan et al., "Association of timing of surgery for hip fracture and patient outcomes," *JAMA*, vol. 291, no. 14, pp. 1738–1743, 2004.

[13] M. T. Vidán, E. Sánchez, Y. Gracia, E. Marañón, J. Vaquero, and J. A. Serra, "Causes and effects of surgical delay in patients with hip fracture: a cohort study," *Annals of Internal Medicine*, vol. 155, no. 4, pp. 226–233, 2011.

[14] T. Klestil, C. Röder, C. Stotter et al., "Impact of timing of surgery in elderly hip fracture patients: a systematic review and meta-analysis," *Scientific Reports*, vol. 8, no. 1, p. 13933, 2018.

[15] N. Simunovic, P. J. Devereaux, S. Sprague et al., "Effect of early surgery after hip fracture on mortality and complications: systematic review and meta-analysis," *Canadian Medical Association Journal*, vol. 182, no. 15, pp. 1609–1616, 2010.

[16] J. Tidermark, "Quality of life and femoral neck fractures," *Acta Orthopaedica Scandinavica*, vol. 74, no. 2, pp. 1–62, 2003.

[17] N. H. Varady, B. T. Ameen, and A. F. Chen, "Is delayed time to surgery associated with increased short-term complications in patients with pathologic hip fractures?" *Clinical Orthopaedics & Related Research*, vol. 478, no. 3, pp. 607–615, 2020.

[18] J. M. Taber, B. Leyva, and A. Persoskie, "Why do people avoid medical care? A qualitative study using national data," *Journal of General Internal Medicine*, vol. 30, no. 3, pp. 290–297, 2015.

[19] M. L. Barnett, L. Hu, T. Martin, and D. C. Grabowski, "Mortality, admissions, and patient census at SNFs in 3 US cities during the COVID-19 pandemic," *JAMA*, vol. 324, no. 5, pp. 507–509, 2020.

[20] J. W. Min and C. Barrio, "Cultural values and caregiver preference for Mexican-American and non-Latino White elders," *Journal of Cross-Cultural Gerontology*, vol. 24, no. 3, pp. 225–239, 2009.

[21] C. Torres, "Elderly Latinos along the Texas-Mexico border: a healthcare challenge for the 21st century," *Board Health Journal*, vol. 1, pp. 28–36, 2001.

[22] J. D. Crist and P. Speaks, "Keeping it in the family," *Home Healthcare Nurse: The Journal for the Home Care and Hospice Professional*, vol. 29, no. 5, pp. 282–290, 2011.

[23] G. F. Fuller, "Falls in the elderly," *American Family Physician*, vol. 61, no. 7, pp. 2159–2168, 2000.

[24] K. A. Egol, S. R. Konda, M. L. Bird et al., "Increased mortality and major complications in hip fracture care during the COVID-19 pandemic," *Journal of Orthopaedic Trauma*, vol. 34, no. 8, pp. 395–402, 2020.

[25] G. Guo, L. Ye, K. Pan et al., "New insights of emerging SARS-CoV-2: epidemiology, etiology, clinical features, clinical treatment, and prevention," *Frontiers in Cell and Developmental Biology*, vol. 8, p. 410, 2020.

[26] H. Hope, V. Gulli, D. Hay et al., "Outcomes of orthopaedic trauma patients undergoing surgery during the peak period of COVID-19 infection at a UK major trauma centre," *The Surgeon: Journal of the Royal Colllege of Surgeons of Edinburgh and Ireland*, vol. 1479-666X, no. 20, pp. 30182–30187, 2020.

[27] M. Rizkallah, E. Melhem, M. Sadeqi, J. Meyblum, P. Jouffroy, and G. Riouallon, "Letter to the editor on the outcomes in fracture patients infected with COVID-19," *Injury*, vol. 51, no. 10, pp. 2333-2334, 2020.

[28] B. Mi, L. Chen, Y. Xiong, H. Xue, W. Zhou, and G. Liu, "Characteristics and early prognosis of COVID-19 infection in fracture patients," *Journal of Bone and Joint Surgery*, vol. 102, no. 9, pp. 750–758, 2020.

[29] R. Cornwall, M. S. Gilbert, K. J. Koval, E. Strauss, and A. L. Siu, "Functional outcomes and mortality vary among different types of hip fractures," *Clinical Orthopaedics and Related Research*, vol. 425, pp. 64–71, 2004.

14

The Role of Additional K-Wires on AO Type C Distal Radius Fracture Treatment with External Fixator in Young Population

Ivan Micic,[1] Erica Kholinne ⓘ,[2,3] Yucheng Sun,[3,4] Jae-Man Kwak,[3] and In-Ho Jeon ⓘ[3]

[1]Clinic for Orthopaedic Surgery and Traumatology, Clinical Center Nis, Nis, Serbia
[2]Department of Orthopedic Surgery, St. Carolus Hospital, Jakarta, Indonesia
[3]Department of Orthopedic Surgery, Asan Medical Center, University of Ulsan College of Medicine, Seoul, Republic of Korea
[4]Department of Hand Surgery, Affiliated Hospital of Nantong University, Nantong, Nantong University, Jiangsu, China

Correspondence should be addressed to In-Ho Jeon; jeonchoi@gmail.com

Academic Editor: Allen L. Carl

Objectives. Several methods have been proposed to treat AO type C distal radius fracture. External fixator has gained popularity for its simple procedure and rapid recovery. Some surgeons suggested that additional K-wires may play a critical role in the outcome. The purpose of study is to evaluate the role of additional K wires in treating distal radial fracture with external fixator regarding its outcome. *Material and Methods*. From January 2006 to January 2010, 40 patients with AO type C distal radius fracture were treated with external fixator, with (EF) or without additional K wires (EFK). Radiologic outcome parameters include radial inclination, volar tilt, radial length, and the presence of radiocarpal arthritis according to Knirk and Jupiter. Clinical outcomes include New York Orthopedic Hospital (NYOH) wrist scoring scale. *Results*. Radiographic outcome showed significant difference in regard of articular congruency at the final follow-up with the EFK group showing the advantage in maintaining the articular incongruity. NYOH wrist scoring scale showed no significant difference between both groups at final follow-up. The amount of articular step-off was less in EFK group with significant statistical finding on the final follow up. *Conclusion*. Both EF and EFK technique were able to provide satisfactory result in treating AO type C distal radius fractures. We observed that EFK is superior in reducing the number of radiocarpal arthritic changes compared to EF group due to its superiority in reducing articular step-off.

1. Background

The extra-articular distal radius fractures occur frequently in osteoporotic geriatric group, while the intra-articular type is more frequent in young adult patients with high-energy trauma [1]. The high energy injury pathomechanism involved axial load transfer from hand to the articular surface of distal radius. This causes shearing force which leads to impacted fracture and marked displacement [2]. Most of this high energy fracture is unstable and classified as AO type C fracture. Several studies have reported the comparison between external and internal fixation and concluded that volar locking plate (VLP) is superior to the external fixator (EF) [1, 3–5]. Nevertheless, EF showed its distinctive advantages with nondemanding surgical procedures and unnecessity for hardware removal surgery for intra-articular distal radius fracture [3, 6, 7].

External fixation for distal radius fracture is applied after ligamentotaxis achieved following fracture reduction [8]. Unfortunately, comminuted fracture type is often difficult to reduce and maintain. Hence, additional K-wires are needed as a reduction tool and later provide additional stability to fracture site. To date, not many studies focus on the role of additional K-wires in external fixator. Therefore, the aim of our study is to define whether additional K-wires in external fixator will influence the outcome of distal radius fracture in young population.

2. Materials and Method

This retrospective cohort study enrolled forty patients from January 2006 to 2010. Institutional review board approval was obtained prior to study. The power of study was estimated at 0.8 with 10% of type 1 error and the above sample size. The inclusion criteria were patients aged between 18 and 50 years, AO type C distal radius fractures, dorsal comminution, > 10 degrees' dorsal tilt, > 3mm radial shortening, and >1 mm intra-articular step-off after manipulative reduction. Patients with medical contraindications, open fractures, bilateral fractures, concomitant injuries, previous wrist injuries and diseases, and AO type A/B fractures were excluded. Preoperative radiographic assessment was obtained for all patients. All patients were treated with closed reduction under fluoroscopic guide and followed by external fixation (EF group) (Figures 1(a) and 1(b)) or with additional K-wires fixation (EFK group) (Figures 2(a) and 2(b)).

2.1. Surgical Technique. All patients were treated with closed manipulation and splinting prior to surgical intervention. Patients whose radiographs following closed manipulation demonstrated unacceptable reduction of the metaphyseal-diaphyseal junction were scheduled for surgical intervention. Procedure was performed under general anesthesia with patient in supine position on radiolucent table. A 250mmHg tourniquet was applied proximally. Stab incisions were made on the dorsal-radial side superior from the extensor pollicis longus tendon and on the lateral side of the second metacarpal. Two 4-mm pins were inserted proximally and two were inserted distally in a different trajectory angle. Pins were then connected to the bar with clamps. Traction was applied, respectively, under fluoroscopic control after satisfactory radiologic parameters (radial inclination, volar tilt, and radial length) were achieved.

In EFK group, the articular fragment was reduced percutaneously using pointed reduction forceps followed by percutaneous 0.45-in K-wire insertion under fluoroscopy guidance through either the radial styloid and/or the intermediate column of the wrist. External fixator was applied accordingly. All patients were treated by single orthopedic surgeon.

2.2. Postoperative Management. Active and passive range-of-motion exercise of the digits and the elbow were initiated on the second day after operation under the supervision of a hand physical therapist. Wound dressing was carried out once daily. The K-wires were removed at six weeks after operation and two weeks later external fixators were removed subsequently. Range-of-motion exercise of the wrist and hand exercises was encouraged afterwards.

2.3. Evaluation. Patients were followed up for at least 1 year with the interval at 3, 6, and 12 months. The mean of final follow-up is 33 months (range: 26 to 55 months). Demographic data included age, sex, hand dominance, and fracture type. Serial postoperative outcome follow-up assessment was done by orthopedic surgeon with NYOH wrist scoring scale. Postoperative radiographic evaluation was carried out by radiologist for radial inclination, volar tilt, radial length, articular congruency status, amount of articular step-off, and the presence of radiocarpal arthritis according to Knirk and Jupiter (Figures 1(c) and 2(c)). Pre- and postoperative radiographic evaluations were compared.

2.4. Statistical Analysis. The *t*-test was used to compare the ages, sex, hand dominance, fracture type, NYOH wrist

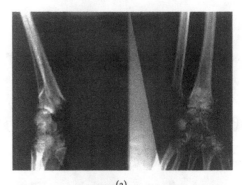

(a)

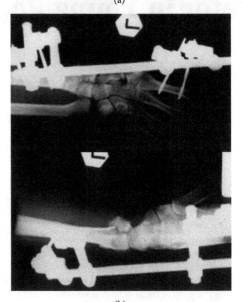

(b)

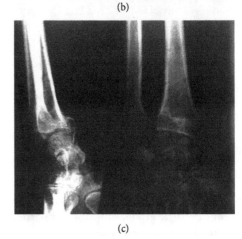

(c)

FIGURE 1: Preoperative (a), postoperative (b), and final follow-up radiographs of EF group (c).

scoring scale (pain, function, movement, grip strength, and presence of arthrosis), and radiographic parameters (radioulnar angle, volar angle, radial length, and articular congruency). Chi-square test was used to compare the articular step-off in both EF and EFK group. The relationship between articular step-off to the presence of radiocarpal arthritis, mobility, and pain was analyzed with Pearson correlation test. A *p* value ≤ 0.05 was considered to be statistically significant.

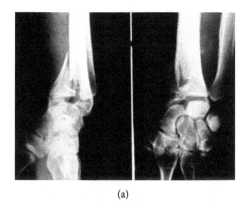

(a)

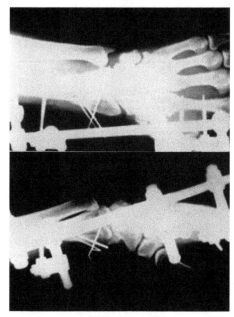

(b)

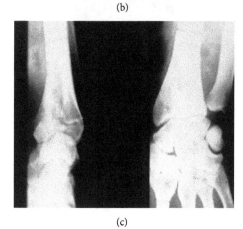

(c)

FIGURE 2: Preoperative (a), postoperative (b), and final follow-up radiographs of EFK group (c).

3. Results

The mechanism of injury was fall on an outstretched hand for twenty-four patients and motor-vehicle accident for sixteen patients. Patients' demographics are shown in Table 1. All fractures healed accordingly without any additional

intervention. No distal radioulnar instability was found at the final follow-up. Superficial pins-track infection developed in four (10%) patients. Oral antibiotic and daily dressing care around the pins was performed accordingly. Deep bone infection was not observed at final follow-up. There was no refracture or tendon rupture observed. No patients reported digital stiffness or reflex sympathetic dystrophy at the end of follow-up.

We found a significant difference of patients' demographics in terms of sex ratio between two groups ($p= 0.048$). Functional outcome according to NYOH wrist scoring scale showed no significant difference between both groups at final follow-up (Table 1). Radiographic outcome showed significant difference in regard of articular congruency at the final follow-up with the EFK group showing the advantage in maintaining the articular incongruity ($P<0.001$) (Table 2). The amount of articular step-off was less in EFK group with significant statistical finding at the final follow-up (Table 3).

The relationship between articular step-off and the presence of radiocarpal arthritis showed a significant negative linear correlation for EFK group ($p < 0.001$). Articular step-off also showed a negative linear correlation with pain but nonstatistically significant. The relationship between articular step-off and mobility showed a positive linear correlation with no statistical significance for both groups (Table 4).

At the final follow-up, 6 patients in EF group and 4 patients in EFK group presented with articular incongruence with radiocarpal arthritic changes in their radiographic examination. Only one patient in EFK group showed radiocarpal arthritic changes despite congruent articular surface of the wrist. Overall, the total incidence of arthritis in EF and EFK group is 30% and 20%, respectively.

4. Discussion

AO type C distal radius fractures are mostly hard to reduce and stabilize due to their multifragmentary and unstable characteristics. The aim of treatment is to achieve congruent articular surface and correct axial malalignment while maintaining good reduction to preserve function. Inability to achieve congruent articular surface has been shown to cause posttraumatic arthritic changes in the wrist joint.[9]

Many strategies have been widely studied in terms of distal radius fracture fixation type. VLP has gained its popularity for the treatment of distal radius comminuted fracture. Direct visualization allows us to achieve stable rigid fixation with direct manipulation to the fracture fragments. Thus, early mobilization will result in good wrist function. Studies had been done to compare external fixation with percutaneous pin and open reduction with plate fixation for distal radius fracture [1, 3–5]. Wright et al. and Rizzo et al. reported better recovery in open reduction and internal fixation (ORIF) compared with EF group in ulnar variance and volar tilt [10, 11]. Williksen et al. and Roh et al. found that ORIF group showed advantage in ulnar variance compared with EF group [4, 12]. Kreder et al. and Jeudy et al. found that articular step-off status in ORIF group is superiorly maintained [13, 14]. Most of the results are in favor of

TABLE 1: Patients' demographics and NYOH wrist scoring scale assessment.

Variable	EF	EFK	P-value
Age (years)	41(6)	39(10)	0.504
Range	27-49	18-48	
Sex			0.048*
Male	9	16	
Female	11	4	
Hand dominance affected			0.191
Yes	15	10	
No	5	10	
AO type of fracture			0.939
C 1.	4	4	
C 2.	7	8	
C 3.	9	8	
Pain(points)	17.8 (2.4)	18.6 (2.0)	0.258
Function(points)	26.8 (3.4)	27.8 (3.0)	0.328
Movement(points)	12.9 (1.7)	13.3 (1.8)	0.430
Grip(points)	12.7 (2.1)	12.9 (1.9)	0.752
Arthrosis			0.545
No	14	16	
Minimal	4	4	
Moderate	1	0	
Severe	1	0	
NYOH Total points	86.7 (11.8)	91.3 (10.0)	0.195
Results			0.806
Excellent	10	12	
Fair	1	1	
Good	9	7	

EF: external fixation group; EFK: external fixation adjuvant K-wires group. NYOH: New York Orthopaedic Hospital wrist scoring scale consists of pain, function, movement, and grip.
*Statistically significant (p<0.05).

TABLE 2: Radiographic assessment.

		EF	EFK	P value
Radial inclination (degree)	Preoperation	2,9 (1,1)	4,2 (1,2)	0,415
	Postoperation	20,4 (0,4)	20,1 (0,3)	0,574
	Final follow-up	19,5 (0,4)	19,3 (0,5)	0,775
Volar tilt (degree)	Preoperation	-6,1 (1,8)	-6,7 (1,2)	0,355
	Postoperation	9,6 (0,3)	9,2 (0,3)	0,289
	Final follow-up	7,7 (0,5)	8,2 (0,7)	0,201
Radial length (mm)	Preoperation	-0,4 (1,2)	1,0 (0,8)	0,513
	Postoperation	11,2 (0,3)	10,4 (0,4)	0,123
	Final follow-up	10,7 (0,4)	10,1 (0,4)	0,278
Articular incongruity (mm)	Preoperation	2,5 (0,3)	2,5 (0,3)	0,910
	Postoperation	0,4 (0,1)	0,1 (0,1)	0,103
	Final follow-up	1,0 (0,2)	0,1 (0,1)	≤0,001*

*Statistically significant (p<0.05).

volar locking plate, for its radiological and clinical outcome [1, 3, 4].

To date, there is still no cogent conclusion to favor VLP fixation over external fixation or vice versa. External fixation relies solely on ligamentotaxis to correct and maintain fracture alignment until healing is achieved [15]. Being less invasive and hence with less surgical trauma and moreover low technically demanding tools to apply, external fixator is favorable for some surgeons. Lin et al. reported that external fixation is widely used to treat these fractures for its minimally

TABLE 3: Articular step-off assessment.

		EF	EFK	P value
Articular step-off ≥ 2mm	Preoperation	15	13	0.490
	Postoperation	2	0	0.487
	Final follow-up	6	0	0.020*

*Statistically significant (p<0.05).

TABLE 4: Correlation of articular step-off to radiocarpal arthritic changes, mobility, and pain.

Pearson correlation test	EF	EFK
Articular step-off ≥ 2mm – radiocarpal arthritic changes	r = (-) 0.306 p = 0.189	r = (-) 0.793 p ≤ 0.001*
Articular step-off ≥ 2mm – mobility	r = (+) 0.120 p = 0.614	r = (+) 0.111 p = 0.641
Articular step-off ≥ 2mm – pain	r = (-) 0.112 p = 0.638	r = (-) 0.250 p = 0.288

*Statistically significant (p<0.05).

invasive technique [16]. External fixation application did not cause any trauma to soft tissue adjacent to fracture site and thus prevented devascularization of the fracture site [17, 18]. The unnecessity for further implant removal surgery is considered to be a favorable factor in some developing countries. Therefore, health care cost would be reduced. EF is also able to prevent further complications that could arise from secondary surgery (implant removal) since EF removal is feasible to be done in office setting under local anesthesia manner [3]. In a multicenter randomized control trial, Kreder et al. noted that indirect reduction and percutaneous fixation were associated with a rapid recovery and better functional outcome in comparison with open reduction and internal fixation [14]. In a prospective randomized control trial, Williksen et al. found that EF surgery was simpler and needed less time compared with VLP surgery, though their result was still in favor of the VLP fixation [5].

Our study showed homogenous demographic data for age, hand dominance, and fracture type in our sample. Male predominance was seen in EFK group due to the possibility of having higher trauma energy pathomechanism. NYOH wrist scoring scale showed better outcome in EFK group especially in clinical parameters (pain, function, ROM, and grip strength) without statistical significance. Radiological parameter (arthrosis) only showed slightly higher score in EFK group without statistical significance. The mainstay of having an additional K wire in EF is to maintain articular surface reduction and provide additional stability. Hence, we postulated that this could reduce and minimize the incidence of secondary radiocarpal arthritis. All radiographic parameters were corrected at immediate postoperative radiographic evaluation. Our study showed that radial inclination, volar tilt, and radial length correction were not statistically significant for both groups in immediate postoperative and final follow-up time frame. We found that only articular step-off parameter showed significant correction in the final follow-up in both groups. Moreover, our study showed that there is strong statistical correlation for the presence of

radiocarpal arthritic changes in regard of coexistent articular step-off. EF was able to maintain all radiographic parameters except for articular congruency. In our study, the additional K-wires were removed at six weeks postoperatively. At this time fracture has consolidated and allowed radiological parameters to be maintained. This explains why EFK group have better articular congruence because the additional K-wires maintain articular reduction until consolidation is achieved.

According to Knirk and Jupiter scale [19], there were 4 patients in EFK group and 6 patients in EF group who showed radiocarpal arthritis. All patients in EFK groups presented with minimal arthritic changes while 6 patients in EF group presented with 4 minimal, 1 mild, and 1 severe arthritic change. The arthritis incidence of our study is 33.3%, which is low compared to study by Knirk and Jupiter with 65% prevalence with a mean of 6.7 years' follow-up [19]. Another study by Arora et al. reported that 44% of elderly patients treated with VLP fixation presented with radiocarpal arthritis and 62% of them who received conservative treatment also had arthritis changes in the end [20]. Forward and colleagues reported that 68% of patients with intra-articular fractures developed radiographic evidence of arthritis at a mean follow-up of 38 years [7]. Our short-term follow-up explained the reason of having lower number of arthritic changes. Some authors suggested that patients should be counseled on the long-term risk of developing radiographic arthritic changes following distal radius fixation. On the other hand, the age of patients in our study is relatively young (range from 18 to 50 years); hence the incidence of arthritis is lower. The positive correlation between patient's age and arthritic changes has been studied well [21].

Our study has several limitations. The current study was a retrospective, nonrandomized, comparative trial with small sample size and short follow-up term with a single outcome assessment tool (NYOH wrist scoring scale). We suggested that a future randomized clinical trial will provide cogent conclusion towards this issue.

5. Conclusion

Both EF and EFK techniques were able to provide satisfactory result in treating AO type C distal radius fractures. We observed that EFK is superior in reducing the number of radiocarpal arthritic changes compared to EF group due to its superiority in reducing articular step-off.

Acknowledgments

This study was supported by the Global Frontier R&D Program on Human-centered Interaction for Coexistence and funded by the National Research Foundation of Korea via the Korean Government (MSIP) (grant no. 2017-0522).

References

[1] F. Leung, Y. Tu, W. Y. Chew, and S. Chow, "Comparison of External and Percutaneous Pin Fixation with Plate Fixation for Intra-articular Distal Radial Fractures," *The Journal of Bone and Joint Surgery-American Volume*, vol. 90, no. 1, pp. 16–22, 2008.

[2] T. E. Trumble, R. W. Culp, D. P. Hanel, W. B. Geissler, and R. A. Berger, "Intra-articular fractures of the distal aspect of the radius," in *Instructional course lectures*, vol. 48, pp. 465–480, 1999.

[3] Y. H. Roh, B. K. Lee, J. R. Baek, J. H. Noh, H. S. Gong, and G. H. Baek, "A randomized comparison of volar plate and external fixation for intra-articular distal radius fractures," *Journal of Hand Surgery*, vol. 40, no. 1, pp. 34–41, 2015.

[4] J. H. Williksen, F. Frihagen, J. C. Hellund, H. D. Kvernmo, and T. Husby, "Volar locking plates versus external fixation and adjuvant pin fixation in unstable distal radius fractures: A randomized, controlled study," *Journal of Hand Surgery*, vol. 38, no. 8, pp. 1469–1476, 2013.

[5] J. H. Williksen, T. Husby, J. C. Hellund, H. D. Kvernmo, C. Rosales, and F. Frihagen, "External fixation and adjuvant pins versus volar locking plate fixation in unstable distal radius fractures: A randomized, controlled study with a 5-year follow-up," *Journal of Hand Surgery*, vol. 40, no. 7, pp. 1333–1340, 2015.

[6] N. D. Downing and A. Karantana, "A revolution in the management of fractures of the distal radius?" *The Journal of Bone and Joint Surgery—British Volume*, vol. 90, no. 10, pp. 1271–1275, 2008.

[7] D. P. Forward, T. R. C. Davis, and J. S. Sithole, "Do young patients with malunited fractures of the distal radius inevitably develop symptomatic post-traumatic osteoarthritis?" *The Journal of Bone & Joint Surgery*, vol. 90, no. 5, pp. 629–637, 2008.

[8] J. M. Agee, "Application of multiplanar ligamentotaxis to external fixation of distal radius fractures.," *The Iowa Orthopaedic Journal*, vol. 14, pp. 31–37, 1994.

[9] T. E. Trumble, S. R. Schmitt, and N. B. Vedder, "Factors affecting functional outcome of displaced intra-articular distal radius fractures," *Journal of Hand Surgery*, vol. 19, no. 2, pp. 325–340, 1994.

[10] M. Rizzo, B. A. Katt, and J. T. Carothers, "Comparison of Locked Volar Plating Versus Pinning and External Fixation in the Treatment of Unstable Intraarticular Distal Radius Fractures," *HAND*, vol. 3, no. 2, pp. 111–117, 2008.

[11] T. W. Wright, M. Horodyski, and D. W. Smith, "Functional outcome of unstable distal radius fractures: ORIF with a volar fixed-angle tine plate versus external fixation," *Journal of Hand Surgery*, vol. 30, no. 2, pp. 289–299, 2005.

[12] Y. H. Roh, B. K. Yang, J. H. Noh, G. H. Baek, C. H. Song, and H. S. Gong, "Cross-cultural adaptation and validation of the Korean version of the Michigan hand questionnaire," *Journal of Hand Surgery*, vol. 36, no. 9, pp. 1497–1503, 2011.

[13] J. Jeudy, V. Steiger, P. Boyer, P. Cronier, P. Bizot, and P. Massin, "Treatment of complex fractures of the distal radius: A prospective randomised comparison of external fixation 'versus' locked volar plating," *Injury*, vol. 43, no. 2, pp. 174–179, 2012.

[14] H. J. Kreder, D. P. Hanel, J. Agel et al., "Indirect reduction and percutaneous fixation versus open reduction and internal fixation for displaced intra-articular fractures of the distal radius: a randomised, controlled trial," *The Journal of Bone & Joint Surgery—British Volume*, vol. 87, no. 6, pp. 829–836, 2005.

[15] D. J. Slutsky, "Nonbridging external fixation of intra-articular distal radius fractures," *Hand Clinics*, vol. 21, no. 3, pp. 381–394, 2005.

[16] C. Lin, J. S. Sun, and S. M. Hou, "External fixation with or without supplementary intramedullary Kirschner wires in the treatment of distal radial fractures," *Canadian Journal of Surgery*, vol. 47, no. 6, pp. 631–637, 2004.

[17] T. S. Axelrod and R. Y. McMurtry, "Open reduction and internal fixation of comminuted, intraarticular fractures of the distal radius," *Journal of Hand Surgery*, vol. 15, no. 1, pp. 1–11, 1990.

[18] T. F. Higgins, S. D. Dodds, and S. W. Wolfe, "A biomechanical analysis of fixation of intra-articular distal radial fractures with calcium-phosphate bone cement," *The Journal of Bone & Joint Surgery*, vol. 84, no. 9, pp. 1579–1586, 2002.

[19] J. L. Knirk and J. B. Jupiter, "Intra-articular fractures of the distal end of the radius in young adults," *The Journal of Bone & Joint Surgery*, vol. 68, no. 5, pp. 647–659, 1986.

[20] R. Arora, M. Lutz, C. Deml, D. Krappinger, L. Haug, and M. Gabl, "A Prospective Randomized Trial Comparing Nonoperative Treatment with Volar Locking Plate Fixation for Displaced and Unstable Distal Radial Fractures in Patients Sixty-five Years of Age and Older," *The Journal of Bone and Joint Surgery-American Volume*, vol. 93, no. 23, pp. 2146–2153, 2011.

[21] D. S. Lee and D. R. Weikert, "Complications of Distal Radius Fixation," *Orthopedic Clinics of North America*, vol. 47, no. 2, pp. 415–424, 2016.

15

Biomechanical Assessment of Three Osteosynthesis Constructs by Periprosthetic Humerus Fractures

Afif Harb ⓘ,[1] **Bastian Welke,**[2] **Emmanouil Liodakis,**[1] **Sam Razaeian,**[1] **Dafang Zhang,**[3] **Christian Krettek** ⓘ,[1] **Christof Hurschler,**[2] **and Nael Hawi**[1]

[1]*Trauma Department, Hannover Medical School (MHH), Carl-Neuberg-Str. 1, Hannover 30625, Germany*
[2]*Laboratory for Biomechanics and Biomaterials, Department of Orthopaedic Surgery, Hannover Medical School, Hannover, Germany*
[3]*Department of Orthopaedic Surgery, Brigham and Women's Hospital, 75 Francis St, Boston, MA 02115, USA*

Correspondence should be addressed to Afif Harb; harb.afif@mh-hannover.de

Academic Editor: Benjamin Blondel

Background. Biomechanical stability assessment of 3 different constructs for proximal fixation of a locking compression plate (LCP) in treating a Worland type C periprosthetic fracture after total shoulder arthroplasty. *Methods.* 27 Worland type C fractures after shoulder arthroplasty in synthetic humeri were treated with 14-hole LCP that is proximally fixed using the following: (1) 1×1.5 mm cerclage wires and 2x unicortical-locking screws, (2) 3×1.5 mm cerclage wires, or (3) 2x bicortical-locking attachment plates. Torsional stiffness was assessed by applying an internal rotation moment of 5 Nm and then after unloading the specimen, an external rotation moment of 5 Nm at the same rate was applied. Axial stiffness was assessed by applying a 50 N preload, and then applying a cyclic load of 250 N, then increasing the load by 50 N each time, until a maximum axial load of 2500 N was reached or specimen failure occurred. *Results.* With regard to internal as well as external rotational stiffness, group 1 showed a mean stiffness of 0.37 Nm/deg and 0.57 Nm/deg, respectively, group 2 had a mean stiffness of 0.51 Nm/deg and 0.39 Nm/deg, respectively, while group 3 had a mean stiffness of 1.34 Nm/deg and 1.31 Nm/deg, respectively. Concerning axial stiffness, group 1 showed an average stiffness of 451.0 N/mm, group 2 had a mean stiffness of 737.5 N/mm, whereas group 3 had a mean stiffness of 715.8 N/mm. *Conclusion.* Group 3 displayed a significantly higher torsional stiffness while a comparable axial stiffness to group 2.

1. Introduction

Periprosthetic fractures occur in approximately 0.6% to 3% of all total shoulder arthroplasties (TSA) [1]. Since periprosthetic fractures are heterogeneous in nature, several classification systems have been developed to guide their treatment. In our study, we used the Worland classification [2], which classifies periprosthetic humerus fractures into three types, A, B, and C, based on the fracture location and stability of the prosthetic stem. Given the wide-ranging variations in the nature of periprosthetic humerus fractures, a wide array of treatment recommendations exist, either for conservative or surgical treatment [3]. Within the realm of surgical treatment, stabilization of the proximal segment in itself presents a technical challenge due to the presence of the prosthetic stem with or without a cement mantle. This has

led to the emergence of an array of options for proximal plate fixation, including cerclage wires or cables, locking or nonlocking unicortical screws, allograft struts, and more recently, plate designs that allow bicortical fixation by directing offset locking screws tangentially around either side of the prosthesis stem [4]. The objective of our study was to perform a biomechanical assessment of torsional and axial stability of the proximal plate fixation in a Worland type C periprosthetic humerus fracture after total shoulder arthroplasty using three different fixation constructs.

2. Materials and Methods

2.1. Specimens. 27 synthetic humeri with left-sided geometry (#3404, 4th generation, Sawbones, Pacific Research Laboratories Inc., Vashon, WA, USA) were used for this biomechanical study. An anatomical total shoulder prosthesis (Univers™ II, Arthrex, Florida, USA) was implanted according to the operating instructions of the manufacturer. Each prosthesis was fixed using 40 g of Refobacin Bone Cement (Zimmer Biomet GmbH, France). After allowing for the cement to harden, a 14-hole 3.5 mm metaphyseal locking compression plate (LCP) (DePuy Synthes, Switzerland) was positioned along the lateral surface of the humeral shaft. The plate was proximally attached to the synthetic bone using three different fixation constructs. Thereafter, the specimens were divided into three different groups with nine specimens in each group:

(i) LCP attached to the proximal humerus using 1×1.5 mm cerclage wires and 2x locking unicortical screws (Figure 1(a))

(ii) LCP attached to the proximal humerus using 3×1.5 mm cerclage wires (Figure 1(b))

(iii) LCP attached to the proximal humerus using 2x locking attachment plates allowing bicortical fixation by directing offset locking screws tangentially around either side of the prosthesis stem (Figure 1(c))

Following fixation of the LCP onto the proximal segment of the humerus, we performed a 90° transverse osteotomy in the humeral mid-diaphysis 5 cm distal to the end of the prosthesis, simulating a Worland type C periprosthetic fracture and ensuring a stable prosthesis. To focus on the proximal plate fixation and to simulate an unstable fracture situation, only the proximal part of the artificial humerus was used (Figure 2).

2.2. Mechanical Testing. The biomechanical investigations were carried out on a servo-hydraulic material testing machine (MTS MiniBionix I, Model 858, Eden Prairie, Minneapolis) and a custom-made experimental setup. The synthetic humeri were mounted between two universal joints (Figure 3). The distal part of the specimen was directly attached to a mounting block with the LCP. At the proximal end, the specimen was fixed to the upper Cardan joint by means of the taper of the shoulder prosthesis. The loads were applied to the specimen from the proximal end by the actuator of the material testing machine.

2.3. Torsional Stiffness Testing. The specimens were axially loaded with a static force (compression) of 5 N with a loading rate of 0.5 N/s. Afterwards, an internal rotation moment of 5 Nm was applied at a rate of 0.5 Nm/s. After reaching the maximum moment, the specimen was unloaded and an external rotation moment of 5 Nm at the same rate was applied. Finally, the machine adjusted the axial torque back to 0 Nm. The specimens were not damaged during the test. The protocol was carried out in load and torque control. Time, cycles, angle, torque, and force were recorded with a sampling rate of 1 kHz.

2.4. Axial Stiffness Testing. The axial stiffness investigation was carried out in a cyclic test. Initially, the specimens were loaded with a preload of 50 N. In the first loading stage, a cyclic load with 1 Hz was applied in the sinusoidal form up to a load of 250 N. The lower load in all stages was 0 N, and ten cycles were carried out in each stage. In the following stages, the upper load limit was increased by 50 N each time. Thereafter, the upper load was increased until a maximum axial load of 2,500 N was reached or until the specimen sustained irreversible damage. The protocol was carried out in load and torque control. Time, cycles, angle, torque, and force were recorded with a sampling rate of 1 kHz. Load to failure was assessed by measuring the amount of axial force exerted at the time where the proximal fixation fails.

2.5. Load to Failure of the Locking Compression Plate (LCP). This test was performed to assess the maximum axial load capacity that the LCP could withstand. This test was a pure assessment of the LCP with no additional component attached to it. The plates were fixed in the assembly so that the load being applied onto the plate was identical to the load previously being applied onto both the plate with the humerus fixed to it. In total, three plates were tested with the identical load protocol as for the axial stiffness testing as well as load to failure.

2.6. Statistics. Statistical analysis was performed using SPSS software (IBM SPSS Statistics 26.0, SPSS Inc., Chicago, IL). The significance of differences between all three groups was tested using the Kruskal–Wallis test. Significant differences between the two groups were assessed using the Mann–Whitney U test. The significance level of $\alpha = 0.05$ was employed.

3. Results

3.1. Torsional Stiffness. After applying a 5 N axial load, the specimens that were treated with 1×1.5 mm cerclage wires and 2x locking unicortical screws showed a mean internal torsional stiffness of 0.37 ± 0.15 Nm/deg (mean ± standard deviation), while the specimens treated with 3×1.5 mm cerclage wires showed an average internal torsional stiffness of 0.51 ± 0.33 Nm/deg, and those treated with 2x locking attachment plates with bicortical screws showed a mean internal torsional stiffness of 1.34 ± 0.16 Nm/deg (Figure 4(a)). The differences between the groups with the specimens treated with 1×1.5 mm cerclage wires and 2x locking unicortical screws and the specimens with the 2x locking attachment plates with bicortical screws were statistically significant ($p < 0.001$). Furthermore, the difference between the specimens treated with 3×1.5 mm cerclage wires and those with the 2x locking attachment plates with bicortical screws were statistically significant ($p < 0.001$) (Table 1).

After reaching the maximum moment of each specimen in each group and adjusting the axial torque back to 0 Nm, an external torsional stress was applied allowing for the measurement of external torsional stiffness. The mean external torsional stiffness was 0.57 ± 0.20 Nm/deg for the specimens treated with 1×1.5 mm cerclage wires and 2x locking unicortical screws, 0.39 ± 0.24 Nm/deg for the group

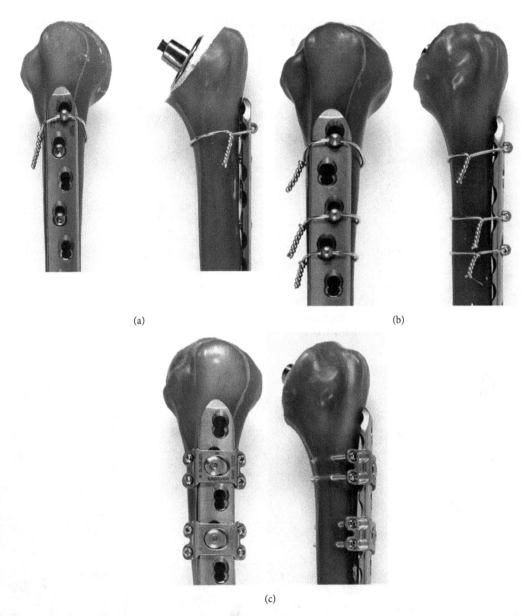

(a)   (b)

(c)

FIGURE 1: (a). LCP plate fixed on the humerus using 1×1.5 mm cerclage wires placed at the level of the 1st hole and 2x unicortical locking screws placed at the levels of the 3rd and 4th holes. (b) LCP plate fixed on the humerus using 3×1.5 mm cerclage wires placed at the levels of the 1st, 3rd, and 4th holes. (c) LCP plate fixed on the humerus using 2x locking attachment plates allowing bicortical fixation placed at the levels of the 2nd and 4th holes.

treated with 3×1.5 mm cerclage wires, and 1.31 ± 0.24 Nm/ deg for the group treated with 2x locking attachment plates with bicortical screws (Figure 4(b)). The differences between the groups with the specimens treated with 1×1.5 mm cerclage wires and 2x locking unicortical screws and the specimens with the 2x locking attachment plates with bicortical screws were statistically significant ($p < 0.001$). Furthermore, the difference between the specimens treated with 3×1.5 mm cerclage wires and the specimens with the 2x locking attachment plates with bicortical screws were statistically significant ($p < 0.001$). The difference between the groups treated with 1×1.5 mm cerclage wires and 2x locking unicortical screws and 3×1.5 mm cerclage wires were statistically significant ($p = 0.043$).

3.2. Axial Stiffness Testing. Axial stiffness was assessed by implementing a cyclical axial load to reach a maximum of 2,500 N or until the construct failed after applying an initial axial preload of 50 N. The specimens that were treated with 1×1.5 mm cerclage wires and 2x locking unicortical screws showed a mean axial stiffness of 451.0 ± 41.6 N/mm, while the specimens treated with 3×1.5 mm cerclage wires showed a mean axial stiffness of 737.5 ± 146.7 N/mm, and the specimens treated with 2x locking attachment plates with bicortical screws showed an average axial stiffness of 715.8 ± 357.7 N/ mm (Figure 4(c)). The difference between the group treated with 1×1.5 mm cerclage wires and 2x locking unicortical screws and the group treated with 3×1.5 mm cerclage wires were statistically significant ($p = 0.001$).

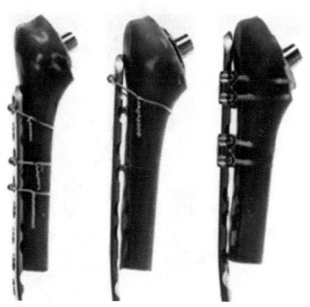

FIGURE 2: Humerus-LCP construct after performing the transverse osteotomy 5 cm distal to the end of the prosthesis, with the irreversibly bent LCP after performing the biomechanical stability testing.

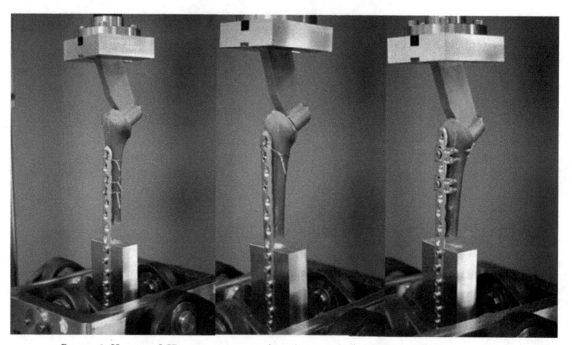

FIGURE 3: Humerus-LCP construct mounted on the servo-hydraulic material testing machine.

3.3. Patterns of Proximal Fixation or Experimental Setup Failure. When assessing the three LCPs without any humerus attached, the mechanical axial load limit of the LCPs was 1,190 N. From this axial load on, the LCPs were irreversibly deformed. When the specimens with the humeri reached this load limit, the LCPs themselves and not the proximal fixation constructs failed. However, the tests were not completed at this point. The loads were increased further until failure of the proximal shoulder implants or the proximal LCP fixation occurred. In the group where the plates were proximally fixed with 1×1.5 mm cerclage wires and 2x locking unicortical screws, the LCPs were irreversibly

bent in two specimens, the unicortical screws loosened in five specimens, and the attachment between the shoulder prostheses and the servo-hydraulic material testing machine was disrupted in two specimens. In the group with the 3×1.5 mm cerclage wires, cerclage wire loosening or rupture occurred in five specimens, the LCPs were irreversibly bent in three specimens, and the distal part of the humerus came into contact with the base of the servo-hydraulic material testing machine in one specimen. In the group with the 2x locking attachment plates with bicortical screws, the LCP was irreversibly bent in eight specimens, and the distal part of the humerus came into contact with the base of the servo-

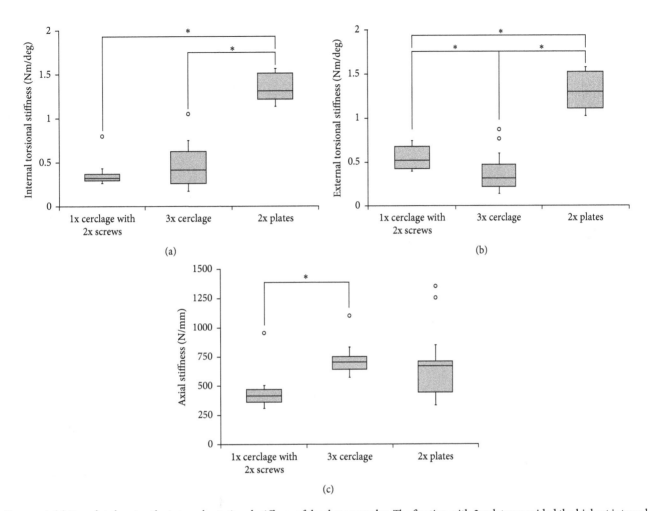

FIGURE 4: (a) Box plot showing the internal rotational stiffness of the three samples. The fixation with 2x plates provided the highest internal rotational stiffness, followed by both that with 3x cerclage wires and that with 1x cerclage and 2x screws which in turn displayed a somewhat similar stiffness, where the difference between groups 1 and 3 as well as those between 2 and 3 were statistically significant. (b) Box plot showing the external rotational stiffness of the three samples. The fixation with 2x plates provided the highest external rotational stiffness, followed by that with 3x cerclage wires and then by that with 1x cerclage and 2x screws, where the difference between groups 1 and 2, groups 2 and 3, and groups 1 and 3 were statistically significant. (c) Box plot showing the axial stiffness of the three samples. The fixation with 3x cerclage wires provided the highest axial stiffness, followed by that with 2x plates and then by that with 1x cerclage and 2x screws, where the difference between groups 1 and 2 were statistically significant.

TABLE 1: An overview table of the results in terms of mean value and standard deviation for each of the three groups.

	Cerclage + unicortical locking screws	Cerlcage	Plate + bicortical locking screws
Internal torsional stiffness (Nm/°) Mean ± SD	0.37 ± 0.15	0.51 ± 0.33	1.34 ± 0.16
External torsional stiffness (Nm/°) Mean ± SD	0.57 ± 0.20	0.39 ± 0.24	1.31 ± 0.24
Axial stiffness (N/mm) Mean ± SD	451.0 ± 41.6	737.5 ± 146.7	715.8 ± 357.7

hydraulic material testing machine in one specimen (Table 2).

4. Discussion

Given the heterogeneous nature of these fractures, various surgical techniques have been suggested and used to treat these injuries, including cerclage wiring, plating, and interfragmentary screw insertion. There seems to be a general inclination and recommendation leaning towards surgically treating periprosthetic fractures distal to the prosthetic stem when the prosthesis is stable in order to optimize rates of healing, return to function, and painless mobilization. This strategy has been supported by the works of Bonutti and Hawkins and Boyd et al. in their case series of four and seven patients, respectively, with periprosthetic

TABLE 2: An overview of the mechanisms of failure in each of the three groups.

	Cerclage + unicortical locking screws	Cerclage	Plate + bicortical locking screws
Loosening or rupture of the cerclage wire		5	
Irreversibly bent plate	2	3	8
Loosening or screw pullout	5		
Loosening or damage of the prosthesis	2		
Distal humerus end in contact with the hydraulic machine		1	1

humeral shaft fractures after TSA [5, 6]. However, despite the general agreement that surgery is the treatment of choice for these injuries, there is no consensus on the best surgical technique. To the knowledge of the authors, there has been no systematic testing of the strength of biomechanical constructs in simulated models of periprosthetic fractures distal to a stable TSA prosthesis to show that one construct is superior to another. In the present study, we have performed a biomechanical assessment of three commonly used surgical constructs for treating Worland type C periprosthetic fractures after TSA.

Multiple biomechanical studies of periprosthetic proximal femur fracture have mechanically loaded both the proximal and distal bone attachment segments together, with many failures occurring during these tests at the level of the distal fixation [7–9]. Distal failures, in turn, make it difficult to draw conclusions about construct stability at the level of the proximal fixation. To address this issue, in the present study, the attachment of the plate to the proximal fragment was tested in isolation, an approach previously described by Lenz et al. [10].

When comparing torsional stiffness, both internal and external, the group treated with the 2x locking attachment plates with bicortical screws displayed significantly higher stability and stiffness compared with the other two groups ($p < 0.05$). This supports the results of Gregory et al. where bicortical screws showed significantly higher torsional strength compared to unicortical screws or cerclage wires alone in the treatment of periprosthetic femur fractures [4]. The groups treated with cerclage wires and unicortical screws and the group treated with cerclage wires alone showed a comparable torsional stability for both internal and external torsional stresses ($p < 0.05$). This result contrasts with the findings of Dennis et al. and Fulkerson et al., which demonstrated that periprosthetic femur fractures treated with unicortical screws displayed a significantly higher torsional stability compared to fractures treated with cerclage wires alone [11, 12].

When comparing axial stiffness, the groups treated with 2x locking attachment plates and bicortical screws and the group treated with cerclage wires alone displayed comparable axial stiffness, both of which were higher than the group treated with cerclage wires and unicortical screws; however, only the difference between the group with both cerclage wires and screws and the group treated with cerclage wires alone was found to be statistically significant ($p = 0.001$). Our findings contrast with the findings of Lenz et al. showed that plates with bicortical screws displayed

higher axial stability when compared to cerclage wires in periprosthetic fractures of the femur [10]. We believe that this phenomenon could be simply explained by the fact that an initial 50 N axial load was applied on all specimens before initiating the cyclical axial load testing. After this initial load, it was visible to the experimenters that the constructs treated with the cerclage wires in isolation showed a small displacement in which the humeri were moved caudally several mm until the cerclage wires were fixed at a more cranial location on the humeri, where the circumference was in fact larger than the initial circumference at the beginning of the testing process. This may have provided the constructs treated with cerclage wires improved stability at the level of the LCP-humerus interface. Interestingly, in our study, the fractures were treated with cerclage wires alone showed a higher axial stiffness when compared to the fractures treated with both cerclage wires and unicortical screws. This finding contrasts with the findings of Lenz et al., where periprosthetic femur fractures treated with 1 cerclage cable and multiple unicortical screws displayed higher axial stability compared with fractures treated with cerclage cables alone [13].

It is worth mentioning that, in our study, the group treated with 2x locking attachment plates and bicortical screws displayed a wider SD range when assessing axial stiffness compared to that of the other two groups. This phenomenon may be due in part to differences in the distance between the humeral transverse osteotomy and the proximal edge of the servo-hydraulic press across specimens, which in turn may be resulted in variable lever arms and a wider standard deviation than expected.

The present study has several limitations in addition to the small sample size. Experiments were conducted on synthetic humeri, whose properties differ from those of *in vivo* samples. Some complexities in humeral loading were not considered. Loads not acting through the shoulder joint, from muscles and other soft tissues, were, for example, not assessed. The distal segment of the humerus was not considered in the model, precluding failures of this segment in the testing. Moreover, we did not assess the amount of displacement that each fixation method may have displayed before the failure of the setup. Nonetheless, this study provided novel information that was scarcely assessed previously; while biomechanical testing has been previously performed in models of periprosthetic fractures of the femur after total hip arthroplasty, research on periprosthetic humerus fractures after TSA is almost nonexistent. This might be due to the fact that hip arthroplasties have been present since 1925 when the American surgeon Marius Smith-Petersen created the first mold arthroplasty out of glass [14]. Even though the first-ever reported TSA took place in France in 1893 by the French surgeon Jules Emile Péan [15], it is only recently that both surgeons and patients have accepted TSA as a good therapeutic option. Accordingly, TSA usage is increasingly growing, allowing the implants and implantation techniques to evolve, and the number of TSA as well as periprosthetic fractures after TSA to increase. Accordingly, it is the opinion of the authors that more biomechanical studies are needed to guide optimal construct choice and surgical treatment for periprosthetic fractures after TSA.

5. Conclusion

Locking attachment plates with bicortical locking screws provide significantly better torsional stability compared with cerclage wires alone or cerclage wires in combination with locking unicortical screws in the treatment of Worland type C periprosthetic fractures of the humerus after TSA. However, cerclage wires alone provide an economically cheaper alternative while providing comparable axial stability to its more expensive locking plate counterpart. Nonetheless, further biomechanical studies on periprosthetic humerus fractures after TSA are needed to help guide treatment of this increasingly common and challenging injury.

Disclosure

This work was performed at the Hannover Medical School, Hannover, Germany.

Acknowledgments

Funding for this study was awarded by Alwin Jäger Stiftung (Aschaffenburg, Germany). The funds were used to purchase all the materials required for performing this experimental study (sawbones-plates-screws-implants-bone cement).

References

[1] E. R. Wagner, M. T. Houdek, B. T. Elhassan, J. Sanchez-Sotelo, R. H. Cofield, and J. W. Sperling, "What are risk factors for intraoperative humerus fractures during revision reverse shoulder arthroplasty and do they influence outcomes?" *Clinical Orthopaedics and Related Research*, vol. 473, no. 10, pp. 3228–3234, 2015.

[2] R, L. Worland, D. Y. Kim, and J. Arredondo, "Periprosthetic humeral fractures: management and classification," *Journal of Shoulder and Elbow Surgery*, vol. 8, no. 6, pp. 590–594, 1999.

[3] C. Garcia-Fernandez, Y. Lopiz-Morales, A. Rodriguez, L. Lopez-Duran, and F. M. Martinez, "Periprosthetic humeral fractures associated with reverse total shoulder arthroplasty: incidence and management," *International Orthopaedics*, vol. 39, no. 10, pp. 1965–1969, 2015.

[4] G. S. Lewis, C. T. Caroom, H Wee et al., "Tangential bicortical locked fixation improves stability in vancouver b1 peri-

[5] P. M. Bonutti and R. J. Hawkins, "Fracture of the humeral shaft associated with total replacement arthroplasty of the shoulder. a case report," *Journal of Bone and Joint Surgery American Volume*, vol. 74, no. 4, pp. 617-618, 1992.

[6] A. D. Boyd, T. S. Thornhill, and C. L. Barnes, "Fractures adjacent to humeral prostheses," *Journal of Bone and Joint Surgery American Volume*, vol. 74, no. 10, pp. 1498–1504, 1992.

[7] L. Konstantinidis, O. Hauschild, N. A. Beckmann, A. Hirschmuller, N. P. Sudkamp, and P. Helwig, "Treatment of periprosthetic femoral fractures with two different minimal invasive angle-stable plates: biomechanical comparison studies on cadaveric bones," *Injury*, vol. 41, no. 12, pp. 1256–1261, 2010.

[8] R. Zdero, R. Walker, J. P. Waddell, and E. H. Schemitsch, "Biomechanical evaluation of periprosthetic femoral fracture fixation," *Journal of Bone and Joint Surgery American Volume*, vol. 90, no. 5, pp. 1068–1077, 2008.

[9] J. D. Pletka, D. Marsland, S. M. Belkoff, S. C. Mears, and S. L. Kates, "Biomechanical comparison of 2 different locking plate fixation methods in vancouver b1 periprosthetic femur fractures," *Geriatric Orthopaedic Surgery and Rehabilitation*, vol. 2, no. 2, pp. 51-55, 2011.

[10] M. Lenz, M. Windolf, T Muckley et al., "The locking attachment plate for proximal fixation of periprosthetic femur fractures--a biomechanical comparison of two techniques," *International Orthopaedics*, vol. 36, no. 9, pp. 1915–1921, 2012.

[11] M. G. Dennis, J. A. Simon, F. J. Kummer, K. J. Koval, and P. E. DiCesare, "Fixation of periprosthetic femoral shaft fractures occurring at the tip of the stem: a biomechanical study of 5 techniques," *Journal of Arthroplasty*, vol. 15, no. 4, pp. 523–528, 2000.

[12] E. Fulkerson, K. Koval, C. F. Preston, K. Iesaka, F. J. Kummer, and K. A. Egol, "Fixation of periprosthetic femoral shaft fractures associated with cemented femoral stems: a biomechanical comparison of locked plating and conventional cable plates," *Journal of Orthopaedic Trauma*, vol. 20, no. 2, pp. 89–93, 2002.

[13] M. Lenz, S. M. Perren, B Gueorguiev et al., "A biomechanical study on proximal plate fixation techniques in periprosthetic femur fractures," *Injury*, vol. 45, no. 1, pp. S71–S75, 2014.

[14] M. N. Smith-Petersen, "The classic: evolution of mould arthroplasty of the hip joint by M. N. Smith-Petersen," *Journal of Bone and Joint Surgery: Clinical Orthopaedics and Related Research*, vol. 134, pp. 5–11, 1978.

[15] T. Lugli, "Artificial shoulder joint by Pean (1893): the facts of an exceptional intervention and the prosthetic method," *Clinical Orthopaedics and Related Research*, vol. 133, pp. 215–218, 1978.

prosthetic femur fractures: a biomechanical study," *Journal of Orthopaedic Trauma*, vol. 29, no. 10, pp. e364–e370, 2015.

16

Efficacy of the Combined Administration of Systemic and Intra-Articular Tranexamic Acid in Total Hip Arthroplasty Secondary to Femoral Neck Fracture

Joseph Maalouly ⓘ,[1] Antonios Tawk,[2] Rami Ayoubi ⓘ,[1] Georges Katoul Al Rahbani,[2] Aida Metri,[2] Elias Saidy,[1] Gerard El-Hajj ⓘ,[3] and Alexandre Nehme ⓘ[1]

[1]Department of Orthopedic Surgery and Traumatology, Saint George Hospital University Medical Center, Balamand University, P.O. Box 166378, Achrafieh, Beirut 1100 2807, Lebanon
[2]Faculty of Medicine and Medical Sciences, University of Balamand, Aschrafieh, Beirut, Lebanon
[3]Department of Medical Imaging and Radiology, Saint George Hospital University Medical Center, Balamand University, P.O. Box 166378, Achrafieh, Beirut 1100 2807, Lebanon

Correspondence should be addressed to Joseph Maalouly; josephmaalouly2@gmail.com

Academic Editor: Allen L. Carl

Background. Total hip arthroplasty (THA) is associated with substantial blood loss in the postoperative course. Tranexamic acid (TXA) is a potent antifibrinolytic agent, routinely administered by intravenous (IV) and topical (intra-articular, IA) route, which can possibly interrupt the cascade of events due to hemostatic irregularities close to the source of bleeding. However, scientific evidence of combined administration of TXA in THA secondary to a femoral neck fracture is still meagre. The present study aims to compare the patients who were administered combined IV and topical TXA with a control group in terms of blood loss, transfusion rate, and incidence of deep vein thrombosis (DVT) and thromboembolism (TE). *Patients and Methods*. 195 patients with femoral neck fracture underwent THA and were placed into two groups: (1) IV and IA TXA group which had 58 patients and (2) no TXA control group which had 137 patients. In the TXA group, 1 g IV TXA was administered 30 minutes before incision, and 1 g IA TXA was administered intraoperatively after fascia closure. No drains were placed, and soft spica was applied to the hip. *Results*. Combined usage of IV and IA TXA showed better results when compared to the control group in terms of blood transfusion rate (31%) and hemoglobin drop (28%). No cases of DVT or TE were noted among the two study groups. *Conclusion*. Combined use of IV and IA TXA provided significantly better results compared to no TXA use with respect to all variables related to postoperative blood loss in THA. Moreover, TXA use is safe in terms of incidence of symptomatic DVT and TE.

1. Introduction

Large amounts of perioperative blood loss and large transfusion rates are associated with total joint replacement surgeries. Total hip arthroplasty (THA) patients are transfused at rates of 16–37% [1]. Femoral neck fractures are pathological entities associated with high mortality and morbidity and are projected to reach more than 6 million cases in the next 30 years [2]. When compared to hemiarthroplasty, THA is associated with better functional outcome scores and decreased reported pain throughout the postoperative course. However, there is an increased risk in THA regarding blood loss, surgery time, and risk of dislocation [3]. The perioperative blood loss in THA may lead to hematomas formation and in certain cases to acute anemia, subsequently resulting in blood transfusions with their associated risks (cardiopulmonary events and transfusion reactions) and health care costs [4]. In addition, allogeneic blood transfusions can also raise the patient's risk of adverse immunological reaction, disease transmission, and postoperative infection [5]. Therefore, every operation stimulates the fibrinolytic process transiently [6]. There is no replacement, of course, for effective surgical technique and local hemostasis intraoperatively. Nevertheless, through various means such as hypotensive anesthesia [7], drain clamping [8], preoperative autologous blood donation [9], and the use of antifibrinolytic agents, a surgeon can reduce the risk of blood loss.

Tranexamic acid (TXA) is a potent antifibrinolytic agent, which may interrupt the cascade of events due to hemostatic irregularities close to the bleeding source. Tranexamic acid, a synthetic analogue of amino acid lysine, prevents fibrinolysis by competitively blocking plasminogen lysine-binding sites, resulting in reduced proteolytic activity on fibrin monomers and fibrinogen, resulting in clot stabilization. [10]. It reaches a concentration of 90%–100% in joints compared with its plasma concentration [11]. In addition, TXA concentrations of up to 10 mg/mL of blood do not influence platelet counts, coagulation times, or various coagulation factors in whole blood or citrated blood from healthy subjects [12].

However, isolated case reports of thrombus formation have been reported, leading to concerns about the risk of thromboembolic complications in a patient population that is already at high risk for deep vein thrombosis (DVT) and pulmonary embolism (PE). This prevented widespread acceptance of IV antifibrinolytics in full joint replacement operations [13, 14].

Furthermore, multiple studies [15–17] including a meta-analysis [18] showed the potential of topical (IA) TXA to be equivalent or even better than intravenous (IV) TXA. In addition, a recent study by Lin et al. [19] found that the efficacy of combined TXA administration is higher than topical use alone. Thus, it is imperative to say that a combined administration of TXA may prove to be more effective compared with topical or intravenous TXA use alone.

The present study was therefore conducted to compare the efficacy of the combined use of IV and IA TXA with that of no use of TXA in terms of total blood loss and allogeneic transfusion rate and to assess the safety profile of each regimen in terms of DVT and TE incidence. As the additional use of topical TXA increases the probability of enhanced antifibrinolytic activity, we hypothesized that there will be a significant difference between the group with the combined use of IV and IA TXA and the group without TXA use in terms of blood loss, allogeneic blood transfusion rate, and hemoglobin (Hb) drop.

2. Materials and Methods

For this study, written informed consent was obtained from all the patients recruited.

A retrospective study of a single institution was conducted. All patients aged 50 to 100 diagnosed with femoral neck fracture and scheduled for primary arthroplasty by the senior author were eligible. The study excluded patients with history of renal impairment, cardiovascular disease (previous myocardial infarction, atrial fibrillation), or cerebrovascular disease (previous stroke or peripheral vascular surgery). Patients with history of thromboembolic disease, allergy to TXA, bleeding disorder, or receiving anticoagulant

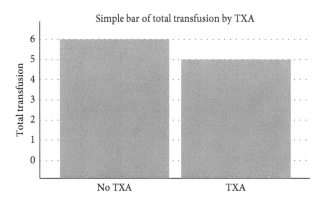

FIGURE 1: Superiority of the TXA regimen.

drug treatment were also excluded. Preoperative blood transfusions for patient preparation were not taken into account. Between January 2016 and September 2019, 195 patients (75 males and 120 females) were successfully recruited into two groups: (1) IV and IA TXA; and (2) no TXA.

30 minutes prior to incision, 1 g of IV TXA was given. All hip surgeries were operated with the standard posterolateral approach to the hip in order to decrease variability within the study, and noncemented prostheses were used. No drains were placed, and the closure of the wound was performed in a standard fashion in all cases. Soft spica was applied after dressing application. Intra-articular tranexamic acid 1 g in 20 mL NaCl was used after fascia closure in all surgeries. Postoperatively, all patients underwent a standard institution thromboembolic prophylaxis protocol. Pneumatic calf pumps were given immediately postoperatively until the patient started ambulating. As per the National Institute for Health and Care Excellence (NICE) recommendation, subcutaneous lovenox (enoxaparin sodium) 40 mg once daily (Sanofi, Paris, France) was given to all patients on the first postoperative day (POD) and continued until discharge from the hospital around 6 days postoperatively. Anticoagulation therapy was continued at home for a total of 35 days from the operation. All patients underwent inpatient postoperative physiotherapy with the aim of early mobilization. No screening for deep vein thrombosis was done in the postoperative period to detect asymptomatic occurrence. For symptomatic patients, evaluation with ultrasonography of the lower limb deep veins and CT scan of the chest (PE protocol) was done.

The primary outcomes of this study were transfusion incidences, postoperative drop in serum hemoglobin level while the secondary outcomes include duration of surgery, length of hospital stay, wound complications, and thromboembolic events within 30 days of surgery. Outcomes such as total blood loss, intraoperative blood, and hidden blood loss were not taken into account in this study.

At the institution where this study was performed, a serum hemoglobin level of less than 8.0 g/dl was considered the transfusion trigger. For patients presenting with anemic symptoms or any anemia-related organ dysfunctions, the transfusion trigger was less than 10.0 g/dl.

TABLE 1: The demographics of the studied population in the current study.

Group statistics	Group	N	Mean	Std. deviation	Std. error mean
Pre-op Hgb	No TXA	137	12.133	1.9545	0.1670
	TXA	58	12.224	1.5226	0.1999
D1 PO Hgb	No TXA	137	10.560	1.3907	0.1188
	TXA	58	11.048	1.3806	0.1813
D5 PO Hgb	No TXA	137	10.251	1.0346	0.0884
	TXA	57	10.309	1.0863	0.1439
Total transfusion	No TXA	137	1.58	1.443	0.123
	TXA	58	1.10	1.209	0.159
Age	No TXA	137	70.42	16.478	1.408
	TXA	58	73.76	13.187	1.732
Hb preop-Hb postop1	No TXA	58	1.573	0.56	0.05
Hb preop-Hb postop1	TXA	137	1.176	0.15	0.02

TABLE 2: Correlation between TXA use and hemoglobin levels and total transfusion.

Correlations		Total transfusion	TXA	D5 PO Hgb	Pre-op Hgb	D1 PO Hgb
Total transfusion	Pearson correlation	1	−0.158*	−0.200**	−0.599**	−0.450**
	Sig. (2-tailed)		0.027	0.005	0.000	0.000
	N	195	195	194	195	195
TXA	Pearson correlation	−0.158*	1	0.025	0.023	0.160*
	Sig. (2-tailed)	0.027		0.726	0.751	0.026
	N	195	195	194	195	195
D5 PO Hgb	Pearson correlation	−0.200**	0.025	1	0.277**	0.436**
	Sig. (2-tailed)	0.005	0.726		0.000	0.000
	N	194	194	194	194	194
Pre-op Hgb	Pearson correlation	−0.599**	0.023	0.277**	1	0.474**
	Sig. (2-tailed)	0.000	0.751	0.000		0.000
	N	195	195	194	195	195
D1 PO Hgb	Pearson correlation	−0.450**	0.160*	0.436**	0.474**	1
	Sig. (2-tailed)	0.000	0.026	0.000	0.000	
	N	195	195	194	195	195

*Correlation is significant at the 0.05 level (2-tailed). **Correlation is significant at the 0.01 level (2-tailed). Pre-op = preoperative, Hgb = hemoglobin, D = day, PO = postoperative.

3. Statistical Analysis

Statistical analysis was carried out in consultation with the in-house biostatistician, using SPSS® 25.0 (IBM, Armonk, New York, United States). Statistical significance was defined as a p value of ≤ 0.05. Testing for normality was done with the Shapiro-Wilk test. We used Levene's test for equality of variances and Student's t-test for equality of means.

4. Results

Our results show a decrease in the transfusion rate in the TXA group as seen in Figure 1. No statistically significant difference was found between the two studied groups in matter of age (Table 1) and BMI. Table 2 shows that there is a significant negative Pearson correlation between TXA and blood transfusions ($p < 0.05$) and a positive Pearson correlation between TXA and hemoglobin levels on the first postoperative day. This is interpreted as tranexamic acid use decreases blood transfusions and leads to higher first day hemoglobin levels. Furthermore, a negative Pearson correlation is present between hemoglobin levels preoperatively and blood transfusions ($p < 0.01$), and a positive correlation between hemoglobin

preoperatively and hemoglobin levels at day 1 and day 5 postoperatively ($p < 0.01$). This suggests that a higher preoperative hemoglobin reduces the need for transfusions and these patients have higher hemoglobin levels postoperatively. Levene's test was used for equality of variances and Student's t-test for equality of means as shown in Table 3. Our findings show no statistically significant difference in terms of preoperative hemoglobin levels and hemoglobin levels at day 5 postoperatively, while statistically significant difference between the two groups was noted in terms of day 1 postoperative hemoglobin levels and total amount of transfusions used intraoperatively and postoperatively. Since $p < 0.05$ is less than our chosen significance level $\alpha = 0.05$, we can reject the null hypothesis and conclude that statistically significant difference is present between the TXA group and the control group in terms of day 1 postoperative hemoglobin levels and total amount of transfusion.

5. Discussion

In the current study, the primary endpoint is the decrease in the hemoglobin drop and the decrease in transfusion rate seen with IV and IA administration of TXA in THA. The

TABLE 3: t-test for the TXA group and the control group.

		Independent samples test							
		Levene's test for equality of variances		t-test for equality of means						
		F	Sig.	T	Df	Sig. (2-tailed)	Mean difference	Std. error difference	95% confidence interval of the difference	
									Lower	Upper
Pre-op Hgb	Equal variances assumed	4.680	0.032	−0.317	193	0.751	−0.0913	0.2879	−0.6591	0.4765
	Equal variances not assumed			−0.350	136.438	0.727	−0.0913	0.2605	−0.6064	0.4238
D1 PO Hgb	Equal variances assumed	0.000	0.988	−2.247	193	0.026	−0.4884	0.2174	−0.9172	−0.0597
	Equal variances not assumed			−2.253	108.127	0.026	−0.4884	0.2167	−0.9180	−0.0588
D5 PO Hgb	Equal variances assumed	0.486	0.487	−0.351	192	0.726	−0.0580	0.1655	−0.3844	0.2684
	Equal variances not assumed			−0.344	100.365	0.732	−0.0580	0.1689	−0.3930	0.2770
Total transfusion	Equal variances assumed	1.450	0.230	2.225	193	0.027	0.480	0.216	0.055	0.906
	Equal variances not assumed			2.390	127.083	0.018	0.480	0.201	0.083	0.878
Age	Equal variances assumed	1.707	0.193	−1.367	193	0.173	−3.335	2.440	−8.149	1.478
	Equal variances not assumed			−1.495	132.919	0.137	−3.335	2.232	−7.749	1.079

Pre-op = preoperative, Hgb = hemoglobin, D = day, PO = postoperative.

drop in hemoglobin (Hgb) was 28% lower in THA when TXA was used. This translated into a much lower risk of requiring a blood transfusion in the THA patients in which TXA was used. The patients with TXA required 31% less transfusion on average than the control group. The protocol used in this study consisted of 1 g IV tranexamic acid 30 minutes before incision and 1 g injection after fascia closure without placing any drains and with soft spica application looks to be effective and safe. There was no reported symptomatic thromboembolic event.

Currently, TXA is FDA approved only for tooth extraction in hemophilia patients. TXA distributes widely in the extracellular and intracellular compartments when given IV [20]. It spreads rapidly into the synovial fluid until the TXA concentration in the synovial fluid reaches the serum concentration [21]. Its biological half-life in the joint fluid is three hours, and glomerular filtration eliminates 90% within 24 hours [22, 23]. Compared to IV administration, intra-articular TXA advocates believe that the benefits include easy administration, maximum concentration at the bleeding site, and minimal systemic absorption. The objective of both delivery systems is to achieve a concentration of approximately 10 mg/mL [20].

Antifibrinolytics have been in use since the 1960s as a class of drugs [22]. TXA is an amino acid lysine analogue. It competitively inhibits the activation of plasminogen and the binding of plasmin to fibrin, inhibiting the degradation of fibrin [13]. Since it works by increasing the breakdown of fibrin when created, it is not necessarily a procoagulant but promotes coagulation already in progress. This makes TXA potentially suitable for use in reducing postoperative bleeding, where surgical hemostasis has been achieved and fibrinolytic activity needs to be suppressed to help maintain hemostasis without promoting the formation of venous thrombus.

In a meta-analysis of all operations, tranexamic acid has been shown to reduce the risk of transfusion by a third [23]. It was used successfully through an intravenous route in orthopedic surgery, with several studies showing significant reductions in bleeding and transfusion risk following THA [24]. Nevertheless, the possibility of thromboembolic complications following systemic administration remains a concern [13, 14].

Kagoma et al. [25] studied the impact of antifibrinolytics on blood transfusion reduction, showing a decrease in blood transfusion rate, after total knee and hip arthroplasties.

Rajesparan et al. reported less blood loss in the TXA group in a study of 73 patients undergoing THA [26]. Gill and Rosenstein found that the use of IV TXA in different doses significantly reduced intraoperative and total blood loss during the review of 13 randomized controlled trials [27].

Zhou et al. meta-analysis of 19 randomized control experiments using different doses of IV TXA in THA found marked reductions in total, intraoperative, postoperative, and secret blood loss in the TXA group compared to the control group [28].

No significant difference in safety between the different methods was noted after a comprehensive review of the literature [29]. For THA, Amin et al. suggested administering a dose of 15 mg/kg IV given 10 minutes before incision and 3 g in 100 mL of saline soak as defined intraoperatively by Melvin [30].

Based on the evidence in the literature, Hayes et al. recommend a regimen consisting of a 1 g IV dose of TXA to be administered before incision or tourniquet inflation with an additional 1 g IV dose given at closure [31].

Based on the current evidence-based medicine, clinicians and patients need to know the possible clinical benefits and risks of TXA, when deciding on their therapy management following THA. Regarding efficacy and safety, our study suggests that TXA should be indicated in patients undergoing THA secondary to femoral neck fracture. In view of our data, our protocol of 1 g IV tranexamic acid 30 minutes before incision and 1 g injection after fascia closure seems to be effective and safe. The dosing regimen appears to be one of the lowest reported dose in the literature with a good safety profile and efficiency.

6. Conclusion

After thorough review of the literature and according to our data, it is our recommendation that 1 g of TXA in IV be given 30 minutes prior to incision and 1 g TXA intra-articular after fascia closure without drains and with the application of a soft spica, as this is seen to be beneficial in terms of blood loss, blood transfusions, and postoperative hemoglobin drop. This seems important as it decreases hospital costs and risks to the patient from the transfusion and anemia. Our protocol appears safe and effective and may be the safest effective dosing regimen.

6.1. Limitations. This study has several limitations. First, the participants included in our study excluded high risk patients. These included patients with a history of cardiovascular disease, cerebrovascular disease, thromboembolic events, renal failure, allergy to TXA, bleeding diathesis, and those on anticoagulation therapy. Second, differences in surgical techniques and blood transfusion protocol are likely to have contributed to the differences observed among studies. Third, this is a retrospective study. Few studies reported the type of surgical hemostasis utilized; these techniques are known to reduce bleeding during surgery [31].

References

[1] B. E. Bierbaum, J. J. Callaghan, J. O. Galante, H. E. Rubash, R. E. Tooms, and R. B. Welch, "An analysis of blood management in patients having a total hip or knee arthroplasty," *The Journal of Bone & Joint Surgery*, vol. 81, no. 1, pp. 2–10, 1999.

[2] P. Kannus, H. Haapasalo, M. Sankelo et al., "Possibility to increase women's bone mass by physical activity wanes rapidly after puberty," *Bone*, vol. 18, no. 1, pp. S113–S63, 1996.

[3] M. Maceroli, L. E. Nikkel, B. Mahmood et al., "Total hip arthroplasty for femoral neck fractures," *Journal of Orthopaedic Trauma*, vol. 30, no. 11, pp. 597–604, 2016.

[4] J. E. Ollivier, S. Van Driessche, F. Billuart, J. Beldame, and J. Matsoukis, "Tranexamic acid and total hip arthroplasty: optimizing the administration method," *Annals of Translational Medicine*, vol. 4, no. 24, 2016.

[5] K. Charoencholvanich and P. Siriwattanasakul, "Tranexamic acid reduces blood loss and blood transfusion after TKA: a prospective randomized controlled trial," *Clinical Orthopaedics and Related Research*, vol. 469, no. 10, pp. 2874–2880, 2011.

[6] B. Risberg, "The response of the fibrinolytic system in trauma," *Acta Chirurgica Scandinavica. Supplementum*, vol. 522, pp. 245–271, 1985.

[7] N. E. Sharrock and E. A. Salvati, "Hypotensive epidural anesthesia for total hip arthroplasty: a review," *Acta Orthopaedica Scandinavica*, vol. 67, no. 1, pp. 91–107, 1996.

[8] P. Zan, J. J. Yao, L. Fan et al., "Efficacy of a four-hour drainage clamping technique in the reduction of blood loss following total hip arthroplasty: a prospective cohort study," *Medical Science Monitor*, vol. 23, pp. 2708–2714, 2017.

[9] Z. Haien, J. Yong, M. Baoan, G. Mingjun, and F. Qingyu, "Post-operative auto-transfusion in total hip or knee arthroplasty: a meta-analysis of randomized controlled trials," *PLoS One*, vol. 8, no. 1, Article ID e55073, 2013.

[10] C. J. Dunn and K. L. Goa, "Tranexamic acid," *Drugs*, vol. 57, no. 6, pp. 1005–1032, 1999.

[11] B. Åstedt, "Clinical pharmacology of tranexamic acid," *Scandinavian Journal of Gastroenterology*, vol. 22, no. 137, pp. 22–25, 1987.

[12] Pfizer, product information, cyklokapron (tranexamic acid); 2011.

[13] P. M. Mannucci, "Hemostatic drugs," *New England Journal of Medicine*, vol. 339, no. 4, pp. 245–253, 1998.

[14] R. Raveendran and J. Wong, "Tranexamic acid reduces blood transfusion in surgical patients while its effects on thromboembolic events and mortality are uncertain," *Evidence Based Medicine*, vol. 18, no. 2, pp. 65-66, 2013.

[15] S. Alshryda, J. Mason, M. Vaghela et al., "Topical (intra-articular) tranexamic acid reduces blood loss and transfusion rates following total knee replacement," *The Journal of Bone and Joint Surgery-American Volume*, vol. 95, no. 21, pp. 1961–1968, 2013.

[16] R. N. Maniar, G. Kumar, T. Singhi, R. M. Nayak, and P. R. Maniar, "Most effective regimen of tranexamic acid in knee arthroplasty: a prospective randomized controlled study in 240 patients," *Clinical Orthopaedics and Related Research*, vol. 470, no. 9, pp. 2605–2612, 2012.

[17] J.-G. Seo, Y.-W. Moon, S.-H. Park, S.-M. Kim, and K.-R. Ko, "The comparative efficacies of intra-articular and IV tranexamic acid for reducing blood loss during total knee arthroplasty," *Knee Surgery, Sports Traumatology, Arthroscopy*, vol. 21, no. 8, pp. 1869–1874, 2013.

[18] M. Panteli, C. Papakostidis, Z. Dahabreh, and P. V. Giannoudis, "Topical tranexamic acid in total knee replacement: a systematic review and meta-analysis," *The Knee*, vol. 20, no. 5, pp. 300–309, 2013.

[19] S.-Y. Lin, C.-H. Chen, Y.-C. Fu, P.-J. Huang, J.-K. Chang, and H.-T. Huang, "The efficacy of combined use of intraarticular and intravenous tranexamic acid on reducing blood loss and transfusion rate in total knee arthroplasty," *The Journal of Arthroplasty*, vol. 30, no. 5, pp. 776–780, 2015.

[20] I. M. Nilsson, "Clinical pharmacology of aminocaproic and tranexamic acids," *Journal of Clinical Pathology*, vol. 33, no. 1, pp. 41–47, 1980.

[21] A. Ahlberg, O. Eriksson, and H. Kjellman, "Diffusion of tranexamic acid to the joint," *Acta Orthopaedica Scandinavica*, vol. 47, no. 5, pp. 486–488, 1976.

[22] J. D. Eubanks, "Antifibrinolytics in major orthopaedic surgery," *American Academy of Orthopaedic Surgeon*, vol. 18, no. 3, pp. 132–138, 2010.

[23] K. Ker, P. Edwards, P. Perel, H. Shakur, and I. Roberts, "Effect of tranexamic acid on surgical bleeding: systematic review and cumulative meta-analysis," *BMJ*, vol. 344, Article ID e3054, 2012.

[24] J. J. Callaghan, M. R. O'Rourke, and S. S. Liu, "Blood management," *The Journal of Arthroplasty*, vol. 20, no. 4, pp. 51–54, 2005.

[25] Y. K. Kagoma, M. A. Crowther, J. Douketis, M. Bhandari, J. Eikelboom, and W. Lim, "Use of antifibrinolytic therapy to reduce transfusion in patients undergoing orthopedic surgery: a systematic review of randomized trials," *Thrombosis Research*, vol. 123, no. 5, pp. 687–696, 2009.

[26] K. Rajesparan, L. C. Biant, M. Ahmad, and R. E. Field, "The effect of an intravenous bolus of tranexamic acid on blood loss in total hip replacement," *The Journal of Bone and Joint Surgery. British Volume*, vol. 91-B, no. 6, pp. 776–783, 2009.

[27] J. B. Gill and A. Rosenstein, "The use of antifibrinolytic agents in total hip arthroplasty," *The Journal of Arthroplasty*, vol. 21, no. 6, pp. 869–873, 2006.

[28] X.-D. Zhou, L.-J. Tao, J. Li, and L.-D. Wu, "Do we really need tranexamic acid in total hip arthroplasty? a meta-analysis of nineteen randomized controlled trials," *Archives of Orthopaedic and Trauma Surgery*, vol. 133, no. 7, pp. 1017–1027, 2013.

[29] N. H. Amin, T. S. Scudday, and F. D. Cushner, "Systemic versus topical tranexamic acid," *Techniques in Orthopaedics*, vol. 32, no. 1, pp. 23–27, 2017.

[30] J. S. Melvin, L. S. Stryker, and R. J. Sierra, "Tranexamic acid in hip and knee arthroplasty," *Journal of the American Academy of Orthopaedic Surgeons*, vol. 23, no. 12, pp. 732–740, 2015.

[31] A. Hayes, D. B. Murphy, and M. McCarroll, "The efficacy of single-dose aprotinin 2 million KIU in reducing blood loss and its impact on the incidence of deep venous thrombosis in patients undergoing total hip replacement surgery," *Journal of Clinical Anesthesia*, vol. 8, no. 5, pp. 357–360, 1996.

17

Influence of Timing on Surgical Outcomes for Acute Humeral Shaft Fractures

Ryogo Furuhata ⓘ, Yusaku Kamata, Aki Kono, Yasuhiro Kiyota, and Hideo Morioka

Department of Orthopedic Surgery, National Hospital Organization Tokyo Medical Center, 2-5-1, Higashigaoka, Meguro-ku, Tokyo 152-8902, Japan

Correspondence should be addressed to Ryogo Furuhata; ryogo4kenbisha@gmail.com

Academic Editor: Allen L. Carl

Surgical treatment for humeral shaft fractures has been reported to yield satisfactory results; however, there may be complications, such as delayed bone union, nonunion, iatrogenic radial nerve injury, and infection. The risk factors for postoperative complications remain largely unknown. This study aimed to investigate the influence of timing of surgery on the incidence of postoperative complications of acute humeral shaft fractures. We retrospectively reviewed 43 patients who underwent osteosynthesis for acute humeral shaft fractures between 2006 and 2020. The patients were divided into early (21 patients) and delayed (22 patients) treatment groups based on the timing of the surgical intervention (within or after four days). Outcomes were the incidences of complications (delayed union, nonunion, iatrogenic radial nerve injury, and infection) and postoperative fracture gaps. We evaluated the outcomes using plain radiographs and clinical notes. In addition, we performed subgroup analyses on outcomes in a subgroup of patients who underwent intramedullary nailing and one who underwent plate fixation. The frequency of delayed union was significantly higher in the delayed group ($P = 0.046$), and the postoperative fracture gap size was also significantly greater in the delayed group ($P = 0.007$). The subgroup analyses demonstrated a significant association between the increased incidence of delayed union and delayed surgical interventions only in the intramedullary nailing subgroup ($P = 0.017$). This study suggests that performing surgery within four days after acute humeral shaft fracture is recommended to reduce the occurrence of delayed union, particularly in cases requiring intramedullary nailing fixation.

1. Introduction

Surgical treatment of humeral shaft fractures has been reported to yield relatively satisfactory results compared to conservative treatment; however, there are complications, such as delayed bone union, nonunion, iatrogenic radial nerve injury, and infection [1–3]. To date, little has been reported on the factors affecting postoperative complications of humeral shaft fractures [3, 4]. Furthermore, the effects of the timing of surgery on the clinical outcomes for acute humeral shaft fractures remain unsolved.

This study aimed to investigate the influence of time from injury to surgery on the incidence of postoperative complications following acute humeral shaft fractures.

2. Materials and Methods

2.1. Patient Selection. This was a retrospective study in patients who underwent osteosynthesis for humeral shaft fractures between April 2006 and March 2020. All the patients were treated at a single general hospital, and surgeries were performed by eight surgeons. We included patients with acute humeral shaft fractures within three weeks of injury. Patients in whom the postoperative follow-up could not be performed adequately were excluded. Based on a previous study investigating the effects of timing of surgery for acute proximal humeral fractures [5], patients who met the above criteria were divided into patients who underwent surgery within four days after injury (early group) and those who were treated five or more days after injury (delayed group).

During the study period, 46 patients underwent osteo-synthesis for acute humeral shaft fractures. Of these patients, two in the early group and one in the delayed group were excluded due to inadequate follow-up. Finally, 27 male and 16 female patients were included, and their mean age at the time of surgery was 45.2 ± 22.4 years (range: 15–89 years). Nineteen patients had a fracture in the right humerus, while 24 patients had a fracture in the left humerus. Fourteen patients (33%) were smokers. There were six patients with preoperative radial nerve palsy and one with an open fracture. The fracture types according to the Arbeitsge-meinschaft für Osteosynthesefragen (AO) classification [6] were type A in 27 patients (63%), B in 14 patients (33%), and C in two patients (4.7%). Four patients (9.3%) had proximal third fractures, and 15 patients (35%) had distal third fractures. Fixation procedures used were intramedullary nailing in 20 patients, plate fixation in 20 patients, fixation using Kirschner wire alone in one patient, and fixation using lag screws alone in two patients.

2.2. Outcomes.

The outcomes were complications (delayed union, nonunion, iatrogenic radial nerve injury, and infection) and postoperative fracture gaps. According to a previous report [3], union was defined as "bone bridging the fracture site across both cortices on radiographs taken in two planes," and delayed union was defined as "union occurring after 26 weeks" (Figures 1(a) and 1(b)) A single examiner assessed postoperative plain radiographs. Iatrogenic radial nerve injuries were assessed based on medical records, and infections were assessed based on medical records and the use of antibiotics. Fracture gap immediately after surgery was measured on plain radiographs taken immediately after surgery as the shortest distance between the proximal and distal bone fragments, according to a previous report [7].

Subsequently, subgroup analyses were performed on outcomes in a subgroup of patients who underwent intra-medullary nailing and a subgroup of patients who under-went plate fixation.

2.3. Statistical Analysis.

All statistical analyses were con-ducted using SPSS software program (version 26.0, IBM, Armonk, NY, USA). We used the Mann–Whitney U test to compare the average of continuous values (age, time from injury to surgery, and postoperative fracture gap) and Fischer's exact test to compare the proportion of variables (sex, the side of injury, smoking, preoperative radial nerve injury, fracture type, fixation procedures, delayed union, nonunion, iatrogenic nerve injury, and infection) between the two groups. Continuous data are presented as mean-$\pm$ standard deviation (SD). The threshold for significance was $P < 0.05$.

3. Results

Twenty-one patients who underwent surgery within four days after the injury were included in the early group, and 22 patients who underwent surgery five or more days after the injury were included in the delayed group. There was a

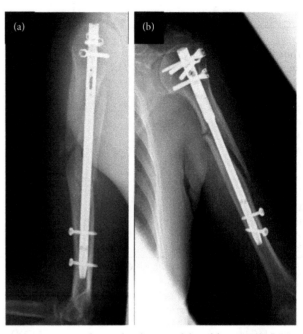

FIGURE 1: X-ray radiographs showing delayed bone union. A 70-year-old man sustained a humeral shaft fracture (AO type A1) and underwent an intramedullary nailing eight days after injury. A plain radiograph performed 26 weeks postoperation showed a visible fracture line (a). An 80-year-old woman sustained a humeral shaft fracture (AO type A2) and underwent an intramedullary nailing 11 days after injury. A plain radiograph performed 30 weeks postoperation revealed a visible fracture line and loosening distal screws (b).

significant difference in the time from injury to surgery between the early and delayed groups ($P < 0.05$); however, no significant differences were found in age, sex, injured side, percentage of smokers, the prevalence of preoperative radial nerve injury, fracture type distribution, or fixation procedures (Table 1).

In this study, eight (19%), two (4.7%), one (2.3%), and one (2.3%) patients experienced delayed union, nonunion, iatrogenic radial nerve injury, and infection, respectively. The frequency of delayed union was significantly higher in the delayed group ($P = 0.046$). No significant differences between the two groups were noted in the rates of nonunion, iatrogenic radial injury, and infection. The postoperative fracture gap was significantly greater in the delayed group: 1.2 ± 1.7 mm in the early group and 3.5 ± 3.3 mm in the delayed group ($P = 0.007$) (Table 2).

In addition, subgroup analyses were performed in a subgroup of patients who underwent plate fixation and a subgroup of patients who underwent intramedullary nailing. In the plate fixation subgroup, the incidence of delayed union was not significantly different between the early and delayed groups, whereas in the intramedullary nailing subgroup, delayed union occurred only in the delayed group at a significantly higher frequency ($P = 0.017$). Similarly, the fracture gap size immediately after surgery was also significantly greater in the delayed group only in the intramedullary nailing subgroup ($P = 0.017$) (Table 3).

TABLE 1: Patient demographics.

	Early group ($n = 21$)	Delayed group ($n = 22$)	P value
Time from injury to surgery (days)	2.5 ± 1.3	7.0 ± 1.8	<0.001*
Age (years)	43.1 ± 21.8	51.8 ± 22.2	0.21
Male/female	12/9	15/7	0.54
Side of injury, right/left	8/13	11/11	0.54
Smoker/nonsmoker	6/15	8/14	0.75
Preoperative radial nerve injury	3	3	1.0
AO type A	12	15	0.54
AO type B	8	6	0.52
AO type C	1	1	1.0
Proximal 1/3	1	3	0.61
Middle 1/3	11	12	1.0
Distal 1/3	9	6	0.35
Intramedullary nailing	7	13	0.13
Plate fixation	12	8	0.23
Kirschner wire or lag screw	2	1	0.61

*$P < 0.001$. AO: Arbeitsgemeinschaft für Osteosynthesefragen.

TABLE 2: Comparison of incidence of postoperative complications and postoperative fracture gap (early group vs. delayed group).

	Early group ($n = 21$)	Delayed group ($n = 22$)	P value
Delayed union	1 (4.8%)	7 (32%)	0.046*
Nonunion	0 (0%)	2 (9.1%)	0.49
Iatrogenic radial nerve injury	1 (4.8%)	0 (0%)	0.49
Infection	0 (0%)	1 (4.5%)	1.0
Postoperative fracture gap	1.2 ± 1.7	3.5 ± 3.3	0.007*

*$P < 0.05$.

TABLE 3: Subgroup analysis of the incidence of postoperative complications and postoperative fracture gap in intramedullary nailing group or plate fixation group.

Intramedullary nailing	Early group ($n = 7$)	Delayed group ($n = 13$)	P value
Delayed union	0 (0%)	7 (54%)	0.017*
Nonunion	0 (0%)	2 (15%)	0.51
Postoperative fracture gap (mm)	1.9 ± 1.4	4.8 ± 3.3	0.017*
Plate fixation	Early group ($n = 12$)	Delayed group ($n = 8$)	P value
Delayed union	1 (8.3%)	0 (0%)	1.0
Nonunion	0 (0%)	0 (0%)	—
Postoperative fracture gap (mm)	0.5 ± 0.7	1.9 ± 2.4	0.172

*$P < 0.05$.

4. Discussion

In this study, we investigated the influence of timing of surgery on the incidence of postoperative complications of acute humeral shaft fractures. As a result, we made two important clinical observations. First, surgical interventions for acute humeral shaft fractures five or more days after the injury were significantly associated with an increased incidence of delayed union. Second, this association between delayed surgical interventions and incidence of delayed union was observed only in a subgroup of patients who underwent intramedullary nailing.

First, the present study showed a significantly increased incidence of delayed union in the delayed group of patients with acute humeral shaft fractures compared with those in the early group. Although the difference in frequency was not significant, nonunion was observed only in the delayed group. The previously reported incidence rates of delayed union and nonunion after surgery for humeral shaft fractures are 33% [3] and 0–8.7% [1–3], respectively, and the results of this study were similar to these rates. According to a previous cohort study on humeral shaft fracture, initial surgical management without conservative treatment had a significantly higher union rate than delayed surgical management, which was initially treated using conservative management without achieving union and subsequently converted to surgical management [3]. These data suggest that delayed surgical intervention for humeral shaft fracture may be a risk factor for delayed union or nonunion; however, in acute fracture, the effects of time from injury to surgery on the union remain unclear. For acute proximal humeral fractures, surgery within five days after the injury has been recommended because postoperative complications significantly increased in patients who underwent surgery six or more days after the injury [5]; this result is similar to ours. Delayed surgical intervention is thought to complicate the anatomical fracture reduction and increase soft tissue dissection, which may result in a longer fracture union time [8, 9]. In this study, the fracture gap immediately after surgery is significantly greater in the delayed group, which supports this hypothesis that delayed surgical intervention makes the anatomical reduction difficult [8, 9]. The difficulty in an anatomical reduction in the delayed group may explain our result of a higher delayed union rate. Meanwhile, the incidence of iatrogenic radial nerve injuries did not differ significantly between the early and delayed groups in this study; this is analogous to a previously reported finding that delayed intervention for humeral shaft fractures did not increase the risk for radial nerve palsy [4]. The rate of postoperative infection in this study was 2.3%, which was similar to the rate of 3–5% reported in previous studies [10, 11]. In particular, postoperative deep wound infection is a serious complication that might be a risk factor for nonunion [12], and in this study, patients with postoperative deep wound infection had delayed bone union. However, the risk factors of postoperative infection have not been fully elucidated. The incidence of infection after plate fixation has been reported to be four times higher than after intramedullary fixation [13], which suggest that plate fixation can be a risk factor for postoperative infection; however, in this study, the only patient who developed postoperative infection underwent intramedullary nail fixation. In addition, the results of this study demonstrated that the delayed surgical intervention had no significant effect on the rate of postoperative infection.

Second, in this study, all except one patient with delayed union or nonunion were in the intramedullary nailing group, and the subgroup analyses demonstrated a significant association between the increased incidence of delayed union and delayed surgical intervention only in the intramedullary nailing subgroup, and not in the plate fixation subgroup. With respect to bone union, many reports have shown no significant differences between the patients who underwent intramedullary nailing and the patients who underwent plate fixation [3, 10, 14, 15]. However, one report showed that bone union tended to be earlier in the plate fixation group [11]; thus, the issue remains controversial. The results of the present study suggest that the incidence of delayed union may be affected by the time from injury to surgery only in patients who underwent intramedullary nailing. In addition, a significant difference in the postoperative fracture gap between the early and delayed groups was also observed only in the intramedullary nailing subgroup. The greater fracture gap size of delayed surgical intervention in the intramedullary nailing subgroup is presumably because closed reduction without opening the fracture site was performed in most patients in this subgroup; however, the fracture site was directly opened and reduced/fixed in most patients in the plate fixation subgroup. Given a previous report on conservative treatment for humeral shaft fractures identifying the magnitude of the fracture gap as a risk factor for subsequent fracture instability and nonunion [7], our findings suggest that the residual

fracture gaps immediately after surgery could have affected the incidence of delayed union in patients who underwent the delayed treatment using intramedullary nails. In this study, closed reduction in most patients who underwent intramedullary nailing may have caused the inadequate axis loading at the fracture sites in the intramedullary nailing subgroup.

This study has three major limitations. First, the sample size in this study was small; only 43 cases were included in the study. If a greater number of patients were included, significant differences between the early and delayed groups might have been observed in the incidence rates of postoperative complications. Second, because this was an observational study, biases from unobserved differences may have affected the results. For example, the surgeries in this study were performed by eight surgeons; however, the effects of competencies of the surgeons or surgical assistants were not evaluated. In contrast, female sex, smoking, and proximal third fractures have been reported to be risk factors for fracture instability in a report on conservative treatment for humeral shaft fractures [7]; the frequencies of these risk factors were not changed between the early and delayed groups in this study. Finally, questionnaire surveys on pain, range of motion, and function were not included in this study; thus, more objective functional outcome scoring was not feasible.

5. Conclusions

This study provides new information on the timing of surgery for acute humeral fractures. Delayed surgical intervention five or more days after the injury was significantly associated with postoperative delayed union of humeral shaft fractures. Moreover, the subgroup analysis in this study suggests that plate fixation is more advantageous than intramedullary nailing in patients who fail to undergo surgical treatment within four days after injury, considering bone union.

References

[1] A. Denard Jr, J. E. Richards, W. T. Obremskey, M. C. Tucker, M. Floyd, and G. A. Herzog, "Outcome of nonoperative vs operative treatment of humeral shaft fractures: a retrospective study of 213 patients," Orthopedics, vol. 33, no. 8, 2010.

[2] F. T. Matsunaga, M. J. S. Tamaoki, M. H. Matsumoto, N. A. Netto, F. Faloppa, and J. C. Belloti, "Minimally invasive osteosynthesis with a bridge plate versus a functional brace for humeral shaft fractures," Journal of Bone and Joint Surgery, vol. 99, no. 7, pp. 583–592, 2017.

[3] F. E. Harkin and R. J. Large, "Humeral shaft fractures: union outcomes in a large cohort," Journal of Shoulder and Elbow Surgery, vol. 26, no. 11, pp. 1881–1888, 2017.

[4] K. Shoji, M. Heng, M. B. Harris, P. T. Appleton, M. S. Vrahas, and M. J. Weaver, "Time from injury to surgical fixation of diaphyseal humerus fractures is not associated with an increased risk of iatrogenic radial nerve palsy," Journal of Orthopaedic Trauma, vol. 31, no. 9, pp. 491–496, 2017.

[5] G. Siebenbürger, D. Van Delden, T. Helfen et al., "Timing of surgery for open reduction and internal fixation of displaced proximal humeral fractures," *Injury*, vol. 46, no. 4, pp. S58–S62, 2015.

[6] J. L. Marsh, T. F. Slongo, J. Agel et al., "Fracture and dislocation classification compendium-2007: orthopaedic Trauma Association classification, database and outcomes committee," *Journal of Orthopaedic Trauma*, vol. 21, no. 10, pp. S1–S133, 2007.

[7] V. Neuhaus, M. Menendez, J. C. Kurylo, G. S. Dyer, A. Jawa, and D. Ring, "Risk factors for fracture mobility six weeks after initiation of brace treatment of mid-diaphyseal humeral fractures," *Journal of Bone and Joint Surgery*, vol. 96, no. 5, pp. 403–407, 2014.

[8] X. Tang, L. Liu, C.-Q. Tu, J. Li, Q. Li, and F.-X. Pei, "Comparison of early and delayed open reduction and internal fixation for treating closed tibial pilon fractures," *Foot & Ankle International*, vol. 35, no. 7, pp. 657–664, 2014.

[9] R. Furuhata, M. Takahashi, T. Hayashi et al., "Treatment of distal clavicle fractures using a Scorpion plate and influence of timing on surgical outcomes: a retrospective cohort study of 105 cases," *BMC Musculoskeletal Disorders*, vol. 21, Article ID 146, 2020.

[10] R. G. McCormack, D. Brien, R. E. Buckley, M. D. McKee, J. Powell, and E. H. Schemitsch, "Fixation of fractures of the shaft of the humerus by dynamic compression plate or intramedullary nail," *The Journal of Bone and Joint Surgery*, vol. 82-B, no. 3, pp. 336–339, 2000.

[11] K. Singisetti and M. Ambedkar, "Nailing versus plating in humerus shaft fractures: a prospective comparative study," *International Orthopaedics*, vol. 34, no. 4, pp. 571–576, 2010.

[12] J. J. Olson, V. Entezari, and H. A. Vallier, "Risk factors for nonunion after traumatic humeral shaft fractures in adults," *JSES International*, vol. 4, no. 4, pp. 734–738, 2020.

[13] M. Changulani, U. K. Jain, and T. Keswani, "Comparison of the use of the humerus intramedullary nail and dynamic compression plate for the management of diaphyseal fractures of the humerus. A randomised controlled study," *International Orthopaedics*, vol. 31, no. 3, pp. 391–395, 2007.

[14] J. R. Chapman, M. B. Henley, J. Agel, and P. J. Benca, "Randomized prospective study of humeral shaft fracture fixation: intramedullary nails versus plates," *Journal of Orthopaedic Trauma*, vol. 14, no. 3, pp. 162–166, 2000.

[15] A. B. Putti, R. B. Uppin, and B. B. Putti, "Locked intramedullary nailing versus dynamic compression plating for humeral shaft fractures," *Journal of Orthopaedic Surgery*, vol. 17, no. 2, pp. 139–141, 2009.

18

Incidence and Clinical Outcomes of Hip Fractures Involving Both the Subcapital Area and the Trochanteric or Subtrochanteric Area

Takayuki Tani ⓘ,[1] **Hiroaki Kijima** ⓘ,[1,2] **Natsuo Konishi,**[1] **Hitoshi Kubota,**[1]
Shin Yamada ⓘ,[1] **Hiroshi Tazawa,**[1] **Norio Suzuki,**[1] **Keiji Kamo,**[1] **Yoshihiko Okudera** ⓘ,[1]
Masashi Fujii,[1,2] **Ken Sasaki,**[1] **Tetsuya Kawano** ⓘ,[1] **Yosuke Iwamoto,**[1,2] **Itsuki Nagahata,**[1,2]
Naohisa Miyakoshi ⓘ,[2] **and Yoichi Shimada**[1,2]

[1]*Akita Hip Research Group, Akita 010-8543, Japan*
[2]*Department of Orthopedic Surgery, Akita University Graduate School of Medicine, Hondo, Akita 010-8543, Japan*

Correspondence should be addressed to Hiroaki Kijima; h-kijima@gd5.so-net.ne.jp

Academic Editor: Benjamin Blondel

Purpose. Proximal femoral fractures involving both the subcapital area and the trochanteric or subtrochanteric area have rarely been reported, but they are not uncommon. However, few studies have reported the incidence or clinical outcomes of such fractures. This study investigated such fractures. *Methods.* In area classification, the proximal femur is divided into 4 areas by 3 boundary planes: the first plane is the center of femoral neck; the second plane is the border between femoral neck and femoral trochanter; and the third plane links the inferior borders of greater and lesser trochanters. A fracture only in the first area is classified as a Type 1 fracture; one in the first and second areas is classified as a Type 1-2 fracture. Therefore, proximal femoral fractures involving both the subcapital area and the trochanteric area are classified as Type 1-2-3, and those involving both the subcapital area and the subtrochanteric area are classified as Type 1-2-3-4. In this study, a total of 1042 femoral proximal fractures were classified by area classification, and the treatment methods and the failure rates were investigated only for Types 1-2-3 and 1-2-3-4 cases. The failure rate was defined as the incidence of internal fixator cut-out or telescoping >10 mm. *Results.* Types 1-2-3 and 1-2-3-4 fractures accounted for 1.72%. Surgical treatment was performed for 89%. Of these, 56% underwent osteosynthesis, but the failure rate was 33%. The other patients (44%) underwent prosthetic replacement. Fracture lines of all these fractures were present along trochanteric fossa to intertrochanteric fossa in posterior aspect and just below the femoral head in anterior aspect. *Conclusion.* Fracture involving the subcapital area to the trochanteric or subtrochanteric area was found in approximately 2%. In patients for whom prosthetic replacement was selected, good results were obtained. However, 1/3 of patients who underwent osteosynthesis had poor results.

1. Introduction

Fractures of the proximal femur are classified into femoral neck fractures, femoral trochanteric fractures, or basicervical fractures. However, fractures rarely involve the subcapital area to the trochanteric or subtrochanteric area [1–3]. Although such fractures are difficult to treat, few studies have investigated the treatment methods and clinical results of these fractures, because almost all classifications of proximal femoral fractures cannot classify these fractures.

The area classification is a comprehensive classification of proximal femoral fractures that facilitates classification based on three-dimensional computed tomography (3D-CT) findings. It is also possible to detect fractures involving the subcapital area to the trochanteric or subtrochanteric region by using this classification. In addition, this classification is reliable and useful for selecting therapeutic strategies [4, 5].

In the area classification, the proximal femur is divided into 4 areas using 3 borders: the center of the femoral neck, the border between the femoral neck and the trochanteric region, and the plane linking the inferior borders of the

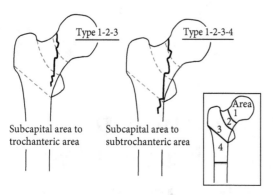

FIGURE 1: Type 1-2-3 fractures involving the area below the femoral head (area classification: Area 1) to the trochanteric area (Area 3) and Type 1-2-3-4 fractures involving Area 1 to the subtrochanteric area (Area 4).

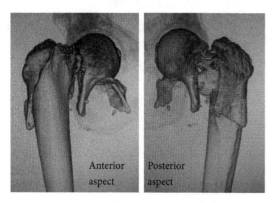

FIGURE 2: Anterior fracture line and posterior fracture line of Type 1-2-3-4 fractures. Fracture lines are present along the trochanteric fossa to the intertrochanteric fossa in the posterior region and below the femoral head in the anterior region.

greater and lesser trochanters. The subcapital area is defined as Area 1, the base of the femoral neck area is defined as Area 2, the trochanteric area is defined as Area 3, and the subtrochanteric area is defined as Area 4. Then, a fracture line that exists only in Area 1 is classified as a Type 1 fracture, and one in Area 1 and Area 2 is classified as a Type 1-2 fracture [5].

Thus, fractures involving the subcapital area to the trochanteric or subtrochanteric area are classified as Type 1-2-3 or Type 1-2-3-4 fractures, in which the fracture line involves an extensive area: Area 1 to Area 3 or Area 4 according to the area classification (Figures 1 and 2).

Therefore, in this study, the incidence, the 3-dimensional features of the fracture lines, and the clinical results of Type 1-2-3 and 1-2-3-4 fractures, which may be markedly unstable and require careful surgery for osteosynthesis, were investigated.

2. Subjects and Methods

The subjects were 1,042 patients (209 males, 833 females) with proximal femoral fractures who were treated at 8 general hospitals between January 2014 and December 2015. Their mean age was 82 years (range, 26-108 years). The

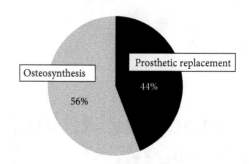

FIGURE 3: Of 1,042 patients with fracture of the proximal femur, Type 1-2-3(-4) fractures account for 1.72%, with osteosynthesis performed for 56% and prosthetic replacement performed for 44%.

type of fracture was retrospectively evaluated using the area classification [4, 5] based on X-ray films and 3D-CT images.

Subsequently, patients in whom the type of fracture were evaluated as Type 1-2-3 or 1-2-3-4, which refers to fractures involving the subcapital area to the trochanter or subtrochanteric region based on area classification, were selected, and 3D-CT images were examined from the anterior and posterior sides for all patients.

Furthermore, internal fixation materials used to treat these types of fractures and the presence of lag screw cut-out and ≥10 mm telescoping on the final assessment were investigated. Patients with cut-out or telescoping ≥10 mm of the internal fixator were assigned to the failure group (Group F). The incidence of Group F was defined as the failure rate (F rate).

In addition, when the prosthetic replacement was selected as the treatment for these cases the dislocation or the infection cases were assigned to the failure.

3. Results

Of 1,042 patients with fracture of the proximal femur, 18 (1.72%) had a Type 1-2-3 or 1-2-3-4 fracture (278 had Type 1, 235 had Type 2-3, 227 had Type 3, 100 had Type 1-2, 87 had Type 3-4, 66 had Type 2-3-4, 17 had Type 4, 10 had Type 2, and 4 cases were unclear). The average follow-up period is 5.4 months (1-18 months).

In 17 of the 18 patients, fracture lines on 3D-CT were present along the trochanteric fossa to the intertrochanteric fossa in the posterior region and the subcapital area in the anterior region (Figure 2).

Of these, conservative treatment was performed for 2 (11%), and surgical treatment was selected for the other 16 (89%). Of the 16 patients, osteosynthesis was selected for 9 (56%) (Figure 3). Of these, a short femoral nail (SFN) was used in 5 (56%), a compression hip screw (CHS) was used in 3 (33%), and a long femoral nail was used in 1 (11%). Of the 5 SFN-treated patients, the use of two lag screws was selected for 3 (60%). Of the 3 CHS-treated patients, the use of two lag screws was selected for 2 (67%), whereas an antirotation screw was added in 1 (33%) (Figure 4).

Of the 9 patients treated by osteosynthesis, ≥10 mm lag screw telescoping was observed in 3 (33%); thus, the F rate was 33%. Of the 3 patients, an SFN with a single lag screw

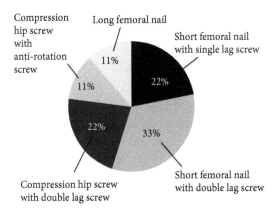

FIGURE 4: Of patients who underwent osteosynthesis for Type 1-2-3(-4) fractures, treatment consisted of a short femoral nail with single lag screw in 22%, a short femoral nail with double lag screw in 33%, a compression hip screw with double lag screw in 22%, a compression hip screw with antirotation screw in 11%, and a long femoral nail in 11%.

was used in 1, an SFN with two lag screws was used in 1, and a CHS with two lag screws was used in 1. Cut-out of the internal fixator was not observed in this study.

For the remaining 7 patients (44%), prosthetic replacement (femoral head replacement) was selected, and there was no failure in any patient with prosthetic replacement.

4. Discussion

Fractures involving the subcapital area to the trochanteric or subtrochanteric region are impossible to classify other than by Area classification of proximal femoral fractures. Therefore, it is impossible to survey the results of treatment for fractures involving the subcapital area to the trochanteric or subtrochanteric region without using the area classification. This study is the first to investigate the incidence, courses of fracture lines, and clinical results of fractures involving the subcapital area to the trochanteric or subtrochanteric region using area classification.

In the present study, such fractures were found in 1.72% of all proximal femoral fractures. Furthermore, the survey using 3D-CT images showed that the fracture lines were present along the trochanteric fossa to the intertrochanteric fossa in the posterior aspect and the subcapital area in the anterior aspect in almost all patients. Of patients who underwent osteosynthesis, more than 30% had poor results.

Most fractures of the proximal femur can be classified as cervical/trochanteric fractures. Regarding the respective types of fractures, several classifications, such as the AO/OTA classification, have been used. However, in some patients, a continuous fracture line involving the area just below the femoral head to the trochanteric or subtrochanteric region is present, extending over the border of classification. These fractures are impossible to classify other than by area classification. Such fractures have been reported as "simultaneous ipsilateral or rare fractures", but a consensus regarding imaging findings, appropriate treatment, or treatment results has not been reached [1–3, 6, 7].

In this study, proximal femoral fractures were evaluated using 3D-CT in more than 1,000 patients, and the incidence of fracture involving the subcapital area to the trochanteric or subtrochanteric region (area classification Type 1-2-3 or 1-2-3-4) was approximately 2%, indicating that this type of fracture frequently causes postosteosynthesis complications.

In almost all patients, fracture lines were present along the trochanteric fossa to the intertrochanteric fossa in the posterior aspect and below the femoral head proximal to the intertrochanteric line (area classification: Area 1) in the anterior aspect. Briefly, in the posterior aspect, the fracture line was consistent with that of a trochanteric fracture, and in the anterior aspect, it was consistent with that of a cervical fracture. According to a recent study that examined basicervical femoral fracture using 3D-CT, it is a subtype of trochanteric fracture in which the fracture line in the posterior cervix is consistent with that of a trochanteric fracture, whereas that in the anterior cervix differs [8]. This is consistent with the fracture lines observed in the present study.

Since a basicervical fracture is similar to a trochanteric fracture in blood supply for femoral head, osteosynthesis is frequently selected. However, previous studies reported a high incidence of complications related to instability [9–11]. In this study, more than 30% of patients who underwent osteosynthesis had poor results. On the other hand, the results of prosthetic replacement were good.

One limitation of this study is that the therapeutic strategies were not standardized among institutions. Therefore, details regarding cases in which osteosynthesis were possible, whether internal fixation materials appropriate for osteosynthesis were used, and procedure-related limitations were not obtained. However, in the future, an optimal strategy to treat fractures involving the subcapital area to the trochanteric or subtrochanteric region may be selected by classifying proximal femoral fractures using area classification and focusing on Type 1-2-3 or 1-2-3-4 fractures through continued surveys. This study presents important findings for this purpose.

Disclosure

The authors, their immediate families, and any research foundation with which they are affiliated did not receive any financial payments or other benefits from any commercial entity related to the subject of this article.

References

[1] H. S. An, J. M. Wojcieszek, R. F. Cooke, R. Limbird, and W. T. Jackson, "Simultaneous ipsilateral intertrochanteric and subcapital fracture of the hip. A case report," *Orthopedics*, vol. 12, no. 5, pp. 721–723, 1989.

[2] C. Isaacs and B. Lawrence, "Concomitant ipsilateral intertrochanteric and subcapital fracture of the hip," *Journal of Orthopaedic Trauma*, vol. 7, no. 2, pp. 146–148, 1993.

[3] I. Cohen and V. Rzetelny, "Simultaneous ipsilateral pertrochant-

eric and subcapital fractures," *Orthopedics*, vol. 22, no. 5, pp. 535–536, 1999.

[4] H. Kijima, S. Yamada, N. Konishi et al., "The choice of internal fixator for fractures around the femoral trochanter depends on area classification," *SpringerPlus*, vol. 5, no. 1, article no. 1512, 2016.

[5] H. Kijima, S. Yamada, N. Konishi et al., "The reliability of classifications of proximal femoral fractures with 3-dimensional computed tomography: the new concept of comprehensive classification," *Advances in Orthopedics*, vol. 2014, Article ID 359689, 5 pages, 2014.

[6] B. Blair, K. J. Koval, F. Kummer, and J. D. Zuckerman, "Basicervical fractures of the proximal femur. A biomechanical study of 3 internal fixation techniques," *Clinical Orthopaedics and Related Research*, no. 306, pp. 256–263, 1994.

[7] I. Saarenpää, J. Partanen, and P. Jalovaara, "Basicervical fracture-a rare type of hip fracture," *Archives of Orthopaedic and Trauma Surgery*, vol. 122, no. 2, pp. 69–72, 2002.

[8] T. Hisatome, T. Kanou, T. Oomoto, T. Maehara, and H. Teramoto, "Classification and diagnosis of basicervical fracture of the femur using three dimensional computed tomography," *Journal of Japanese Society for Fracture Repair*, vol. 38, no. 4, pp. 1043–1049, 2016.

[9] T. J. Bray, "Femoral neck fracture fixation: Clinical decision making," *Clinical Orthopaedics and Related Research*, vol. 339, pp. 20–31, 1997.

[10] F. K. Richard, J. E. Thomas, and C. T. David, "Surgical treatment of intertrochanteric hip fractures with associated femoral neck fractures using a sliding hip screw," *Journal of Orthopaedic Trauma*, vol. 19, no. 1, pp. 1–4, 2005.

[11] S. T. Watson, T. M. Schaller, S. L. Tanner, J. D. Adams, and K. J. Jeray, "Outcomes of low-energy basicervical proximal femoral fractures treated with cephalomedullary fixation," *Journal of Bone and Joint Surgery*, vol. 98, no. 13, pp. 1097–1102, 2016.

19

A Single Intramedullary K-Wire is Sufficient for the Management of Nonthumb Metacarpal Shaft Fractures

Mohamed I. Abulsoud ⓘ,[1] Mohammed Elmarghany ⓘ,[1] Tharwat Abdelghany ⓘ,[1] Mohamed Abdelaal ⓘ,[1] Mohamed F. Elhalawany ⓘ,[1] and Ahmed R. Zakaria ⓘ[2]

[1]Department of Orthopedic Surgery, Faculty of Medicine, Al-Azhar University, Cairo, Egypt
[2]Department of Orthopedic Surgery, Helwan University, Helwan, Egypt

Correspondence should be addressed to Mohamed I. Abulsoud; mohamedabulsoud@azhar.edu.eg

Academic Editor: Francesco Liuzza

Objective. This study aims to evaluate the outcome after the internal fixation of diaphyseal metacarpal fractures by a single intramedullary K-wire. *Methods.* In this prospective case series study, conducted from July 2017 to June 2019 in 23 adult patients with a single, unstable, diaphyseal metacarpal fracture, outcomes after internal surgical fixation using a single antegrade intramedullary K-wire were evaluated. The outcomes were evaluated by union rate, time to union, handgrip measurements at 6 and 12 months, and the modified Disabilities of the Arm, Shoulder, and Hand (DASH) score at 12 months. *Results.* The study population consisted of 17 males and 6 females, with a mean patient age of 28.4 ± 8.5 years (range, 16–45 years). The median time to final follow-up was 14 ± 1.8 months (range: 12–24 months). The mean duration of the union was 7.3 ± 1.6 weeks (range: 5–11 weeks), with a union rate of 95.7% (22 cases). The mean handgrip strength was $68\% \pm 12.8\%$ of the strength of the uninjured hand after 6 months and $92.7\% \pm 6.9\%$ after 12 months. The mean modified DASH score was 2.6 ± 0.26 after 12 months (range: 0–5.8). There were no cases of malrotation or infection. In conclusion, using a single 1.8–2.0 mm K-wire gives excellent functional outcomes and union rate without significant complications when used to treat an unstable metacarpal shaft fracture.

1. Introduction

Metacarpal fractures are the third most common upper limb injury in young adults. when combined with phalangeal fractures, they are the most common upper limb injury [1, 2]. Men and young adults are more vulnerable to these injuries, as are people of low socioeconomic status [1]. The leading mechanisms of injury are direct trauma and sports trauma [1, 2]. Diaphyseal metacarpal fractures cause marked angulation and shortening, impeding the function of extensor and flexor tendons [3–5]. Even small degrees of malrotation are poorly tolerated, leading to digital overlap and impairments of hand functions [6], as the deep transverse metacarpal ligament helps in maintaining shortening and rotation [7]. Metacarpal fractures are more easily tolerated and can be treated nonoperatively if they occur more ulnarly and distally [8]. Surgical options for treatment show wide variabilities without a preference for the fixation method [9, 10].

As early as 1953, Vom [11] described intramedullary fixation of metacarpal fracture and introduced a K-wire through the head of the metacarpal. Foucher's [12] bouquet technique is the most popular approach for antegrade K-wire fixation; it was initially restricted to the neck of fifth metacarpal fractures, but has been applied to diaphyseal fractures with different modifications [13–17]. In surgical practice, ad hoc technological instruments (e.g., plates) often are preferred as opposed to K-wires because they are supposed to fix the fracture better. However, in adult upper limb fractures, a safe and effective fixation can be obtained with smooth wires and rods with very good functional outcome [18–20].

1.1. Specific Aim and Hypothesis. This study aims to evaluate outcomes after internal fixation of diaphyseal metacarpal fractures using a single intramedullary K-wire.

We hypothesized that a single intramedullary K-wire is enough to fixate a displaced metacarpal fracture, leading to full union and a satisfactory outcome without major complications.

2. Methods

A case series study was conducted to evaluate the outcome of single antegrade intramedullary K-wire fixation on displaced metacarpal fractures within 2 weeks of the initial injury. This study included 23 consecutive patients treated from July 2017 to June 2019.

To be included, a patient had to be an adult older than 16 years with a single unstable diaphyseal fracture of the metacarpal. Unstable fractures were defined as having angulation >40°, shortening >2 mm, or malrotation.

Cases were excluded from the study if the patient had an open fracture, associated compartment syndrome of the hand, intraarticular extension, multiple metacarpal fractures, or severe comminution (AO/OTA types 77. 3.2C2 and 77. 3.2C3), or if the patient was <16 years.

All patients received a thorough clinical evaluation that included general and local examinations and X-rays from two different views to ensure there were no other fractures and to ensure patency of the medullary canal (Figure 1). All cases were treated with internal fixation by a single antegrade intramedullary K-wire.

The STROBE guidelines for cohort studies have been followed.

All patients gave consent for participation in the study. The study was approved by the institutional ethics committee.

2.1. Surgical Technique. All surgeries were performed under general anesthesia, used fluoroscopic control, did not use a tourniquet, and had an antibiotic (1 g cefotaxime) administered while inducing anesthesia.

After adequate disinfection of the skin and draping, the patient's hand was positioned on a radiolucent table. The base of the metacarpal was determined with a syringe needle to avoid an inappropriate incision (Figure 2(a)). A 2-3 cm skin incision was made on the dorsal side of the base of the involved metacarpal, allowing for good visualization of the base of the metacarpal as an entry point. The surgeon dissected the subcutaneous tissue and identified the extensor tendons, protecting them throughout the procedure by retracting them ulnarly.

With a sleeve in place in the center of the base of the dorsum to protect the extensor tendon of the involved metacarpal, a 2.5 mm drill bit was used to open the dorsal cortex at an angle of about 45° cranially while taking care not to violate the volar cortex (Figure 2(b)).

After cutting the trocar tip of a prebent 1.8–2.0 mm K-wire, a T-handle device was used to introduce the wire inside the metacarpal shaft (Figure 2(c)).

Next, the rotation was assessed clinically and radiographically, with adjustments made until any malrotation was addressed and appropriate reduction had been achieved. During this process, the K-wire was advanced into the distal segment until it reached the metacarpal head where it was adjusted to achieve the principle of three-point fixation. Violation of the articular surface of the metacarpophalangeal joint was carefully avoided. To allow skin closure, the K-wire was cut short proximally. To avoid any friction, which could lead to tendon rupture or could limit the range of motion in the finger, the bend in the K-wire was positioned away from the track of the extensor tendon (Figure 3).

The skin incision was closed with simple stitches, and a splint was applied below the elbow for 2 weeks.

2.2. Postoperative Program. Patients visited the outpatient clinic 2 weeks postoperatively to have the stitches and splint removed. X-rays were taken to ensure adequate reduction and fixation. The patient was encouraged to move all joints of the hand actively and passively. Regular follow-up visits were scheduled until full union had been achieved.

2.3. Hardware Removal. The K-wires were removed between 3 and 12 months postoperatively. Removals were performed under either general or local anesthesia after the anesthesia team discussed both options with the patient (Figures 4 and 5).

2.4. Statistical Analysis. Data were analyzed using Statistical Program for Social Science (SPSS), version 15.0 (SPSS Inc., Chicago, Illinois). Quantitative data were expressed as means ± standard deviations after confirmation of normal distribution. Data that were not distributed normally were expressed as medians and interquartile ranges. Qualitative data were expressed as frequencies and percentages. P value <0.05 was statistically significant.

3. Results

The study treated 23 metacarpal fractures in 23 patients (17 males and 6 females). All fractures were closed, unstable single fractures.

There were eight patients with a fractured second metacarpal, three with a fractured third metacarpal, four with a fractured fourth metacarpal, and eight with a fractured fifth metacarpal (Table 1).

The mean patient age was 28.4 ± 8.5 years (range: 16–45 years). The median time to final follow-up was 14 ± 1.8 months (range: 12–24 months).

The mean time to union was 7.3 ± 1.6 weeks (range: 5–11 weeks), with a union rate of 95.7% (22 cases). Only one patient failed to develop union, due to the use of a small-diameter K-wire. This patient was subsequently treated by open reduction and internal fixation using a plate and screw and an autologous bone graft.

At 6 and 12 months postoperatively, each patients' handgrip was assessed using the CAMRY Digital Hand

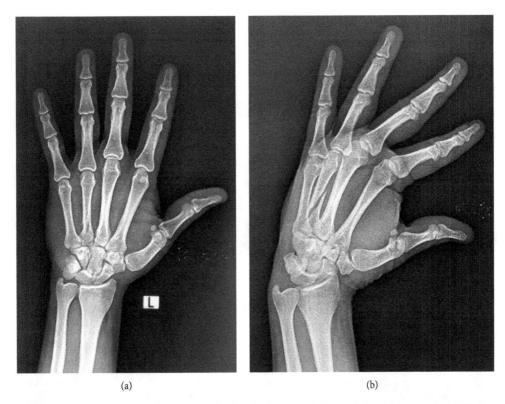

(a)   (b)

FIGURE 1: A 30-year-old male patient with spiral fracture at the fourth metacarpal: the medulla of the second and third metacarpal bones is too narrow, while the medulla of the fourth metacarpal is patent which allows intramedullary fixation.

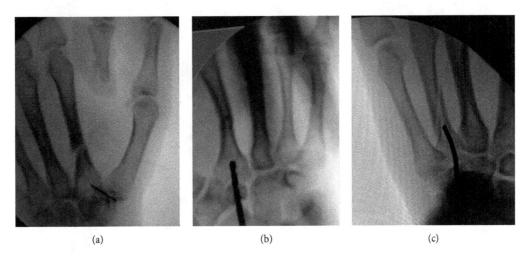

(a)   (b)   (c)

FIGURE 2: (a) Fluoroscopic photo showing the identification of the incision site by a syringe needle. (b) Fluoroscopic photo for antegrade fixation of a fracture of the second metacarpal shaft. A 2.5 drill bit is used for drilling of the dorsal cortex. (c) Fluoroscopic photo shows the advancement of the blunt-tipped prebent K-wire through the entry hole in the dorsal cortex.

Dynamometer Grip Strength Measurement, measuring capacity of 198 lbs/90 kgs by comparing the injured and uninjured hands. The mean handgrip strength of the injured hand was 68% ± 12.8% of the strength of the uninjured hand after 6 months and 92.7% ± 6.9% of the strength of the uninjured hand after 12 months.

The functional outcome was assessed according to the modified Disabilities of the Arm, Shoulder, and Hand (DASH) score, with scores ranging from 0 (best possible score) to 100 (worst possible score). The DASH score measures the severity of symptoms, including pain, stiffness, weakness, and tingling, as well as the ability to perform activities of daily living, including opening a jar, turning a key, writing, pushing a door, washing, dressing, and completing household tasks. The mean score was 2.6 ± 0.26 after 12 months (range: 0–5.8; Table 2).

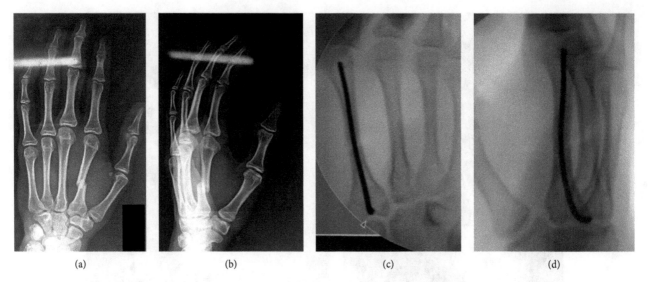

(a)   (b)   (c)   (d)

FIGURE 3: A 17-year-old male patient whose X-rays of anteroposterior and oblique views of the hand show a displaced diaphyseal fracture of the second metacarpal. Fluoroscopic photos show the final fixation of the displaced second metacarpal fracture with the three-point fixation of the intramedullary K-wire.

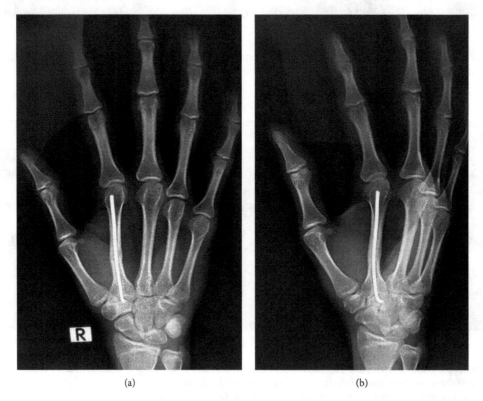

(a)   (b)

FIGURE 4: X-ray showing the 6-month follow-up of the patient, prior to K-wire removal.

Three patients (13%) developed stiffness of the interphalangeal joint due to not completing hand exercises at home. These patients received physical therapy and improved by the end of the follow-up.

None of our patients developed malrotation or wound infection. There were two patients (8.6%) who developed joint penetration of the metacarpophalangeal joint during follow-up, although this did not affect the outcome (Table 3).

4. Discussion

The study shows that a single antegrade K-wire can be used to treat an unstable metacarpal shaft fracture, with excellent functional outcomes and a low complication rate.

Although plate fixation is an attractive option in the treatment of metacarpal shaft fractures due to its stable fixation and biomechanical stability [21], it has a relatively

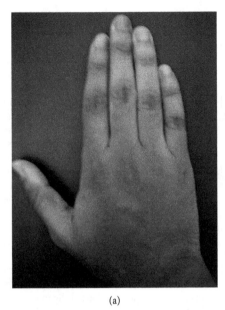

(a)

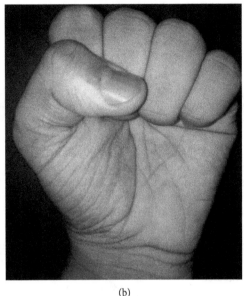

(b)

FIGURE 5: Functional outcome after K-wire removal with full range of motion and excellent functional outcome.

TABLE 1: Demographic data.

Characteristics	Value
Age (years)	
Minimum	16
Maximum	45
Mean (SD)	28.4 8.5
Gender	
Male	19
Female	6
Involved bone	
Second metacarpal	8
Third metacarpal	4
Fourth metacarpal	3
Fifth metacarpal	8

TABLE 2: Results.

Characteristics	Value
Time to union (weeks)	
Minimum	5
Maximum	11
Mean (SD)	7.3 ± 1.6
Union rate	22/23 (95.7%)
Handgrip strength (6 m)	19
Minimum	6
Maximum	
Mean (SD)	$68 \pm 12.8\%$
Handgrip strength (12 m)	
Minimum	3
Maximum	8
Mean (SD)	$92.7 \pm 6.9\%$
DASH score (12 m)	
Minimum	0
Maximum	5.8
Mean (SD)	2.6 ± 0.26

high complication rate of up to one-third of cases [22]. In a study, plate fixation resulted in functional impairments that required secondary surgery in 17% of cases [23]. Even in a study using modern, low-profile plates, various complications led to plate removal in 40% of cases within 9.6 months after surgery [24].

To the best of our knowledge, this is the first study to describe and investigate outcomes of fixation of midshaft metacarpal fractures using a single, buried K-wire. To reduce the confounders, multiple metacarpal fractures, metacarpal neck fractures, and highly comminuted fractures were excluded from the study. In 23 cases with strict inclusion criteria, the functional outcomes were excellent. The mean modified DASH score was 2.6 ± 0.26 at 12 months postoperatively, and the mean handgrip strength was $68\% \pm 12.8\%$ after 6 months and $92.7\% \pm 6.9\%$ after 12 months. These outcomes are comparable to those of most other studies treating such fractures.

The union rate was excellent (95.7%). The one case of nonunion was due to the use of a thin K-wire (1.2 mm), so we recommend using 1.8–2 mm K-wires. No cases of clinical malrotation were reported in our study. This indicates that insertion of a single intramedullary K-wire with the use of a splint for 2 weeks can maintain rotational stability in fracture types 77. 3.2A and 77. 3.2B.

In a recent study using CT to measure the diameter of the nonthumb metacarpal shaft, the narrowest point of the medullary canal was found to be between 2.6 and 3.7 mm [25], supporting the observations from our study that the use of a single intramedullary K-wire with a diameter up to 2 mm gives very good stability.

No cases of infection were detected in this study of the buried K-wire technique, although with an exposed K-wire, the infection rate is about 6% [26]. This is in line with results published by Ridley and colleagues [27] showing that the risk

Table 3: Complications.

Nonunion	Stiffness	MPJ penetration
1 (4.3%)	3 (13%)	2 (8.6%)

of infection is higher in exposed K-wires than in buried K-wires, especially in the treatment of metacarpal fractures.

The percutaneous antegrade intramedullary fixation has been described by Landi et al. [18]. The use of the blunt tip of the K-wire has been described previously by Rocchi et al. [28]. Their large sample included single and multiple K-wires and cases with both shaft and neck fractures but obtained excellent results with minimal complications. However, both techniques used unburied K-wires without focusing on the use of a single K-wire.

Although two cases of metacarpophalangeal joint penetration were observed during follow-up, the final functional outcome was not affected.

Despite the short immobilization time in our study (2 weeks), three patients reported stiffness in the corresponding interphalangeal joint during follow-up. These symptoms were improved by physiotherapy, and the patients had no limitation of motion at the final follow-up. Note that these cases of stiffness and the joint penetration cases were in different patients.

Various retrograde and antegrade techniques have been described over 70 years for intramedullary K-wire fixation of metacarpal fractures, but no technique has been proven to be definitively superior [29]. A biomechanical study concluded that using a single 1.6 mm K-wire results in significantly more stiffness than three 0.8 K-wires [30]. Smooth and unlocked fixation devices are not out of date, but they should be used in the right way. The recent literature continues to prove it. The three-point intramedullary fixation system could be superior to the rigid interfragmentary fixation and it does not hinder the movement [19, 20].

However, the study has some limitations. First, it lacks a comparison group using other techniques. Second, it required a second procedure to remove the K-wire, although most of the patients did not report major complaints during follow-up. Finally, all patients in the study were young and healthy, and the validity of this technique needs to be tested in an older age group and those with osteoporosis.

In conclusion, the use of a single 1.8–2.0 mm K-wire and immobilization for 2 weeks to treat a displaced metacarpal shaft fracture results in excellent functional outcomes and an excellent union rate without significant complications. The technique should be further validated in cases of multiple fractures or open fractures but should be used with caution in cases of osteoporotic fractures.

References

[1] J. W. Karl, P. R. Olson, and M. P. Rosenwasser, "The epidemiology of upper extremity fractures in the United States, 2009," *Journal of Orthopaedic Trauma*, vol. 29, no. 8, pp. e242–e244, 2015.

[2] M. Ameri, K. Aghakhani, E. Ameri, S. Mehrpisheh, and A. Memarian, "Epidemiology of the upper extremity trauma in a traumatic center in Iran," *Global Journal of Health Science*, vol. 9, no. 4, pp. 97–105, 2017.

[3] R. J. Strauch, M. P. Rosenwasser, and J. G. Lunt, "Metacarpal shaft fractures: the effect of shortening on the extensor tendon mechanism," *The Journal of Hand Surgery*, vol. 23, no. 3, pp. 519–523, 1998.

[4] C. K. Low, H. C. Wong, Y. P. Low, and H. P. Wong, "A cadaver study of the effects of dorsal angulation and shortening of the metacarpal shaft on the extension and flexion force ratios of the index and little fingers," *Journal of Hand Surgery*, vol. 20, no. 5, pp. 609–613, 1995.

[5] M. S. Birndorf, R. Daley, and D. P. Greenwald, "Metacarpal fracture angulation decreases flexor mechanical efficiency in human hands," *Plastic and Reconstructive Surgery*, vol. 99, no. 4, pp. 1079–1083, 1997.

[6] W. A. Eglseder, "Metacarpal fractures," in *Atlas of Upper Extremity Trauma*, W. A. Eglseder, Ed., Springer International Publishing, Berlin, Germany, 2018.

[7] A. Khan and G. Giddins, "The outcome of conservative treatment of spiral metacarpal fractures and the role of the deep transverse metacarpal ligaments in stabilizing these injuries," *Journal of Hand Surgery (European Volume)*, vol. 40, no. 1, pp. 59–62, 2015.

[8] V. W. Wong and J. P. Higgins, "Evidence-Based medicine," *Plastic and Reconstructive Surgery*, vol. 140, no. 1, pp. 140e–151e, 2017.

[9] M. H. Henry, "Fractures of the proximal phalanx and metacarpals in the hand: preferred methods of stabilization," *Journal of the American Academy of Orthopaedic Surgeons*, vol. 16, no. 10, pp. 586–595, 2008.

[10] J. B. Friedrich and N. B. Vedder, "An evidence-based approach to metacarpal fractures," *Plastic and Reconstructive Surgery*, vol. 126, no. 6, pp. 2205–2209, 2010.

[11] S. A. A. L. F. H. VOM, "Intramedullary fixation in fractures of the hand and fingers," *Journal of Bone & Joint Surgery*, vol. 35-A, no. 1, 1953.

[12] G. Foucher, ""Bouquet" osteosynthesis in metacarpal neck fractures: a series of 66 patients," *The Journal of Hand Surgery*, vol. 20, no. 3, pp. S86–S90, 1995.

[13] A. A. Faraj and T. R. C. Davis, "Percutaneous intramedullary fixation of metacarpal shaft fractures," *Journal of Hand Surgery*, vol. 24, no. 1, pp. 76–79, 1999.

[14] B. J. Mockford, N. S. Thompson, P. C. Nolan, and J. W. Calderwood, "Antegrade intramedullary fixation of displaced metacarpal fractures: a new technique," *Plastic and Reconstructive Surgery*, vol. 111, no. 1, pp. 351–354, 2003.

[15] N. D. Downing and T. R. C. Davis, "Intramedullary fixation of unstable metacarpal fractures," *Hand Clinics*, vol. 22, no. 3, pp. 269–277, 2006.

[16] B. J. Zirgibel and W. S. Macksoud, "Self-correcting intramedullary Kirschner wire fixation of metacarpal shaft fractures," *Techniques in Hand & Upper Extremity Surgery*, vol. 17, no. 2, pp. 87–90, 2013.

[17] E. M. Van Bussel, R. M. Houwert, T. J. M. Kootstra et al., "Antegrade intramedullary Kirschner-wire fixation of displaced metacarpal shaft fractures," *European Journal of Trauma and Emergency Surgery*, vol. 45, no. 1, pp. 65–71, 2019.

[18] A. Landi, R. Luchetti, F. Catalano, and M. Altissimi, *Trattato di Chirurgia della mano*, Verduci, Rome, Italy, chapter 18, 2007.

[19] R. De Vitis, M. Passiatore, V. Cilli, J. Maffeis, G. Milano, and G. Taccardo, "Intramedullary nailing for treatment of forearm non-union: is it useful?-a case series," *Journal of Orthopaedics*, vol. 20, pp. 97–104, 2020.

[20] M. Passiatore, R. De Vitis, A. Perna, M. D'Orio, V. Cilli, and G. Taccardo, "Extraphyseal distal radius fracture in children: is the cast always needed? A retrospective analysis comparing Epibloc system and K-wire pinning," *European Journal of Orthopaedic Surgery & Traumatology*, vol. 30, no. 7, pp. 1243–1250, 2020.

[21] B. D. Curtis, O. Fajolu, M. E. Ruff, and A. S. Litsky, "Fixation of metacarpal shaft fractures: biomechanical comparison of intramedullary nail crossed K-wires and plate-screw constructs," *Orthopaedic Surgery*, vol. 7, no. 3, pp. 256–260, 2015.

[22] C. Fusetti, H. Meyer, N. Borisch, R. Stern, D. D. Santa, and M. Papaloïzos, "Complications of plate fixation in metacarpal fractures," *The Journal of Trauma: Injury, Infection, and Critical Care*, vol. 52, no. 3, pp. 535–539, 2002.

[23] A. P. A. Greeven, S. Bezstarosti, P. Krijnen, and I. B. Schipper, "Open reduction and internal fixation versus percutaneous transverse Kirschner wire fixation for single, closed second to fifth metacarpal shaft fractures: a systematic review," *European Journal of Trauma and Emergency Surgery*, vol. 42, no. 2, pp. 169–175, 2016.

[24] S. M. Cha, H. D. Shin, and Y. K. Kim, "Comparison of low-profile locking plate fixation versus antegrade intramedullary nailing for unstable metacarpal shaft fractures--A prospective comparative study," *Injury*, vol. 50, no. 12, pp. 2252–2258, 2019.

[25] M. L. Dunleavy, X. Candela, and M. Darowish, "Morphological analysis of metacarpal shafts with respect to retrograde intramedullary headless screw fixation," *Hand*, Article ID 1558944720937362, 2020.

[26] L. P. Hsu, E. G. Schwartz, D. M. Kalainov, F. Chen, and R. L. Makowiec, "Complications of K-wire fixation in procedures involving the hand and wrist," *The Journal of Hand Surgery*, vol. 36, no. 4, pp. 610–616, 2011.

[27] T. J. Ridley, W. Freking, L. O. Erickson, and C. M. Ward, "Incidence of treatment for infection of buried versus exposed kirschner wires in phalangeal, metacarpal, and distal radial fractures," *The Journal of Hand Surgery*, vol. 42, no. 7, pp. 525–531, 2017.

[28] L. Rocchi, G. Merendi, L. Mingarelli, and F. Fanfani, "Antegrade percutaneous intramedullary fixation technique for metacarpal fractures: prospective study on 150 cases," *Techniques in Hand & Upper Extremity Surgery*, vol. 22, no. 3, pp. 104–109, 2018.

[29] J. P. Corkum, P. G. Davison, and D. H. Lalonde, "Systematic review of the best evidence in intramedullary fixation for metacarpal fractures," *Hand*, vol. 8, no. 3, pp. 253–260, 2013.

[30] S. V. Hiatt, M. T. Begonia, G. Thiagarajan, and R. L. Hutchison, "Biomechanical comparison of 2 methods of intramedullary K-wire fixation of transverse metacarpal shaft fractures," *The Journal of Hand Surgery*, vol. 40, no. 8, pp. 1586–1590, 2015.

20

Quality of Life and Clinical Evaluation of Calcaneoplasty with a Balloon System for Calcaneal Fracture at 5 Years of Follow-Up

Giuseppe Maccagnano ⓘ,[1] Giovanni Noia ⓘ,[1] Giuseppe Danilo Cassano,[2]
Antonio Luciano Sarni,[1] Raffaele Quitadamo,[1] Costantino Stigliani,[1] Francesco Liuzza,[3]
Raffaele Vitiello,[3] and Vito Pesce[1]

[1]Orthopaedics Unit, Department of Clinical and Experimental Medicine, Faculty of Medicine and Surgery, University of Foggia,
  Policlinico Riuniti di Foggia, Foggia, Italy
[2]Orthopaedics Unit, Department of Basic Medical Science, Neuroscience and Sensory Organs, Faculty of Medicine and Surgery,
  University of Bari, Policlinico di Bari, Bari, Italy
[3]Fondazione Policlinico Universitario A. Gemelli IRCCS, Rome, Italy

Correspondence should be addressed to Giovanni Noia; giovanni.noia@live.com

Academic Editor: Venkata Sreekanth Arikatla

Calcaneal fractures are a challenging clinical problem. Management of this type of injury remains controversial, especially in the context of intra-articular fractures. Surgical treatment with open reduction and internal synthesis (ORIF) is considered the standard treatment for CF, but it is associated with many complications. Several minimally invasive techniques such as balloon-assisted reduction, pin fixation, and tricalcium phosphate augmentation have been proposed to avoid the frequent and recurrent postoperative problems related to these fractures. We retrospectively examined 20 patients (mean age was 54.5), all undergoing minimally invasive calcaneoplasty surgery at our Department of Orthopaedics and Traumatology between 2012 and 2016. X-ray and CT scan were performed preoperatively and at 5 years of follow-up (57.9 ± 6 months). The American Orthopaedic Foot and Ankle Society (AOFAS) score was used for clinical examination, and the Short-Form (36) Health Survey (SF-36) score and Visual Analogue Scale (VAS) were used to assess the Health-Related Quality of Life (HRQoL). All 20 patients were available at the final follow-up. The mean AOFAS score was 82.25/100. The VAS results attest an overall average of 2.7/10 (0–9). The average of the parameters "Physical Health" and "Mental Health" was, respectively, 81.25 and 83.55. In terms of postoperative complications, we observed no cases of superficial or deep infections. Clinical response after balloon-assisted reduction, pin fixation, and tricalcium phosphate augmentation has shown a comparable or better outcome according to the AOFAS and VAS score. Quality-of-life scores, obtained according to the SF-36 questionnaire, are considered high. From both a clinical and quality-of-life point of view, our study highlights that there is not gender distinction. Further comparative studies with a higher number of patients are needed which assess the quality of life in the various techniques used to treat calcaneal fractures.

1. Introduction

Calcaneal fractures (CF) are common injuries of the lower extremity, accounting for 2% of all fractures and 60% of all tarsal bone fractures. [1] These types of fractures are generally caused by high-energy trauma, such as a fall from heights or a car incident, and may be extra-articular or intra-articular.

The economic impact of the injury is considerable because 80–90% of these fractures occur in men in the early years of employment. As a result, the injury negatively impacts them for several years after the injury and many are unable to return to their previous employment.

Clinically, the injuries manifest with swelling, pain (mainly located below the peroneal sheath), distal edema at the level of the calcaneus cuboid joint, and ecchymosis.

Sometimes, a deformity of the anatomical profile of the hindfoot is noticeable, and vasculonervous lesions are rare [2].

Calcaneal fractures are a challenging clinical problem because of the complex anatomy of the calcaneus, frequent involvement of the subtalar joint, and frequent joint displacement.

The management of this type of injury remains controversial, especially in the context of intra-articular fractures [3]. In the past, conservative treatment for intra-articular CF was preferred, but nowadays, it should be used only in extra-articular fractures or selected cases [4].

The main goals of the treatment are to restore the congruence of the subtalar joint and to restore the calcaneal width, height, shape, and alignment, thus avoiding medial and lateral conflict and allowing the patient to resume a normal lifestyle [5].

Surgical treatment with open reduction and internal synthesis (ORIF) [6] is considered the standard treatment for CF, but it is associated with many complications, particularly in patients with systemic diseases, such as diabetes and peripheral vascular disease.

Therefore, several minimally invasive techniques have been proposed to avoid the frequent and recurrent post-operative problems related to these fractures, to ensure good reduction with fewer complications and to reduce preoperative and hospitalization times; these techniques include arthroscopically assisted reduction and fixation, external fixation, balloon calcaneoplasty [7, 8].

Various authors have described and compared the numerous surgical techniques and outcomes [9].

Preliminary results obtained with calcaneoplasty appear to be satisfactory.

There are several studies evaluating the outcomes of calcaneoplasty at 1-year follow-up [10] or long-term follow-up [11]. Although the clinical outcome is always analyzed, the quality of life is rarely evaluated.

The aim of this study is to evaluate at a 5-year follow-up patients treated with calcaneoplasty, using clinical scales such as the AOFAS and VAS and Quality-of-Life scale (SF-36).

2. Materials and Methods

We retrospectively examined a group of twenty patients who underwent calcaneoplasty with a Balloon System (Kyphon®, Medtronic, Minneapolis, MN, USA), Tricalcium phosfate augmentation, and pin fixation for a calcaneal fracture with thalamic articular involvement, at our Department of Orthopaedics and Traumatology between 2012 and 2016. Our study sample consisted of 12 males and 8 females with a mean age of 54.5 (ranging between 43 and 72).

The mean follow-up was 57.9 ± 6 months.

Inclusion criteria were (a) age over 18 years and (b) calcaneal fracture (Sander's type II, III, and IV)

Exclusion criteria were (a) patients with a positive history of previous, concomitant, or subsequent fractures or who underwent surgery of the affected lower extremity; (b) patients with pathologies that may affect foot function, such as lumbar radiculopathy, Achilles tendinitis, and Morton's neuroma; and (c) fracture with great displacement of the sustentacular part of the calcaneus body

In the preoperative phase were performed an X-ray and CT examination.

All cases underwent surgery in the prone position, with the lateral and AP/thalamic view of a double image intensifier control. Additional techniques of reduction were often used. Using a calcaneal traction, in fact, we managed to correct varus/valgus displacement (Figure 1(a)).

Fluoroscopy was used to determine the quality of calcaneal alignment and fracture reduction. K-wires parallel to the articular surface were applied to maintain the reduction. A trocar was placed into the calcaneus (Figure 1(b)), and then, a cannula followed by the insertion of a bone tamp was attached to a digital manometer.

The balloon was inflated under fluoroscopy.

Typically, the resulting reduction force of the expanding balloon was given by the aid of K-wires, positioned distally as a palisade (see Figure 2).

Additional K-wires were used to maintain the reduction obtained. Prior to its injection into the defect, bone cement (CaPO4) was prepared and the balloon was removed.

No cast was applied. In all cases, an X-ray was performed in the immediate postoperative period, which demonstrated good reduction of postfracture calcaneal varus and restoration of calcaneal volume with satisfactory reduction of the subastragalic joint surface.

Patients were discharged on average after 2 days. Percutaneous K-wires were removed on postoperative day 7.

All patients underwent the same rehabilitation protocol, with a progressive load from the 15th day after surgery. Our study, thus, followed the impact of calcaneoplasty surgery over the years, identifying a midterm postoperative period at 5 years after surgery. At the follow up, the patient's condition in terms of foot biomechanics and quality of life was evaluated. Patients were subjected to

(i) history and objective examination according to the CRF (Case Report Form)

(ii) X-ray investigation

(iii) administration of questionnaires: (1) AOFAS (American Orthopaedic Foot and Ankle Society); (2) pain VAS (Visuo-Analogic Scale); and (3) SF-36 (Short-Form-36)

Data were recorded by two independent orthopedic surgeons (SAL and QR), and the values reported in Tables 1 and 2 are the average of the two measurements.

Student's t-test was used for statistical analysis of continuous variables, with values below 0.05 being considered significant.

3. Results

All 20 patients were available for clinical and radiographic follow-up at an average of 57.9 ± 6 months. The summary of results is shown in Tables 1 and 2.

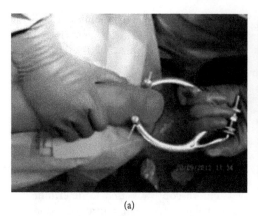
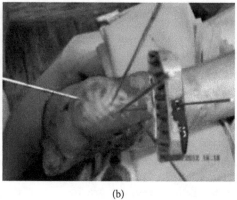

(a)   (b)

FIGURE 1: (a) Traction used to correct varus/valgus displacement. (b) Trocar insertion and K-wires positioned to maintain the reduction.

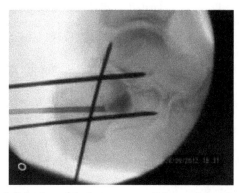

FIGURE 2: Injection of the bone cement. It is noted that the k-wires positioned distally as a palisade allow the balloon to reduce the subtalar joint.

TABLE 1: AOFAS and VAS score.

Case no.	Gender	Age	Side	AOFAS	VAS
1	M	53	Right	53	9
2	M	66	Left	100	0
3	M	37	Right	84	2
4	M	50	Right	100	0
5	M	52	Left	84	1
6	M	74	Left	80	3
7	M	59	Right	84	0
8	M	34	Left	100	0
9	M	59	Right	100	0
10	M	45	Left	100	0
11	M	64	Left	73	6
12	M	43	Right	80	3
13	F	53	Right	65	2
14	F	66	Left	73	4
15	F	64	Right	61	5
16	F	74	Right	80	5
17	F	59	Left	77	5
18	F	43	Right	77	4
19	F	45	Left	84	4
20	F	50	Right	90	1
Average		54.5		82.25	2.7

At the last follow-up, the mean AOFAS score was 82.25/100. According to AOFAS score, clinical results were excellent in 6 (30%) cases, good in 7 (35%), fair in 4 (20%), and poor in 3 patients (15%). Male patients have reached an average score of $86.5/100 \pm 14.5$ and women $75.87/100 \pm 9.51$. No gender difference emerged (p value = 0.086).

The VAS results attest an overall average of 2.7/10 (0–9), an average from the male population of 2/10 and from the female population of 3.75/10.

At the last follow-up, SF-36 was used to evaluate patients' Health-Related Quality of Life (HRQoL). The average of Physical Health (PH) and Mental Health (MH) was 81.25 ± 14.35 for PH and 83.55 ± 7.63 for MH. Our analysis revealed no significant difference in mean scores for the physical component of SF-36 between male (86.18 ± 15.57) and female (73.85 ± 8.60), p value = 0.057. However, no gender difference emerged in the comparison of the mental component of the SF-36 (male 85.07 ± 6.85, female 81.28 ± 8.61, p value = 0.288).

Regarding intraoperative complications, we had 1 (5%) case of tricalcium phosphate migration at the subtalar joint. In terms of postoperative complications, we observed no cases of superficial or deep infections. Two (10%) patients suffered from plantar fasciitis, successfully treated with physical therapy.

4. Discussion

Our study is based on the evaluation of a recently introduced treatment, calcaneoplasty, focusing on the impact it has on the patient's quality of life. The ORIF technique is still widely adopted by orthopedic surgeons [12]. It is normally performed by the conventional L-shaped lateral method, even if the soft tissues covering the lateral calcaneal wall are extremely thin and fragile, which can lead to wound problems. As a consequence, complications following calcaneal fracture are common clinical problems which cannot often be prevented, especially in patients with comorbidities such as peripheral vascular disease, a smoking habit, and diabetes mellitus [13]. Percutaneous treatment with a balloon

TABLE 2: SF-36 scale.

Case no.	Gender	Age	PF	RP	BP	GH	VT	SF	RE	MH	Average PH	Average MH
1	M	53	60	50	36.6	50	66.6	70	83.33	69.88	49.15	72.45
2	M	66	100	100	100	80	74.9	100	100	74.9	95	87.45
3	M	37	100	100	82	75	74.9	100	100	74.9	89.25	87.45
4	M	50	100	100	100	80	74.9	100	100	74.9	95	87.45
5	M	52	100	100	100	80	70.75	90	100	76.6	95	84.34
6	M	74	100	100	82	75	87.55	100	100	90.04	89.25	94.4
7	M	59	100	100	100	80	70.75	90	100	76.6	95	84.34
8	M	34	100	100	100	80	70.75	90	100	76.6	95	84.34
9	M	59	100	100	100	80	70.75	90	100	76.6	95	84.34
10	M	45	100	100	82	75	74.9	100	100	74.9	89.25	87.45
11	M	64	100	100	82	75	87.55	100	100	90.04	89.25	94.4
12	M	43	76.6	60	40.6	55	66.6	70	83.33	69.88	58.05	72.45
13	F	53	63.3	100	30	60	58.1	40	100	59.76	63.32	64.46
14	F	66	100	87.5	82	80	74.9	90	83.33	87.45	87.37	83.92
15	F	64	76.6	100	50	60	58.1	70	100	59.76	71.65	71.96
16	F	74	96.6	75	54	65	79.15	90	100	76.6	72.65	86.44
17	F	59	63.3	87.5	65	70	74.9	80	83.33	87.45	71.45	81.42
18	F	43	80	65	50	60	79.15	90	100	76.6	63.75	86.44
19	F	45	100	75	82	80	79.15	90	100	87.45	84	89.15
20	F	50	96.6	75	65	70	79.15	90	100	76.6	76.65	86.44
Average		54.5	90.65	89.47	74.16	71.5	73.67	87	96.67	76.87	81.25	83.55

reduction device can enable surgeons to treat this lesion in the first days after trauma and without wound complications associated with ORIF. The reduction is obtained using k-wires and balloon inflating. Then, the cement injection guarantees a stable construct. Various forms of bone replacements, such as PMMA by Jacquot et al. [14], tricalcium phosphate by Labbe et al. [15] and Vicenti et al. [11], and calcium phosphate by Biggi et al. [16] or calcium sulfate by Gupta et al. [8], have been used for this function. Due to its multiple characteristics and properties, tricalcium phosphate was selected in the current study.

Patients were evaluated respecting a postoperative time of at least 5 years of follow-up (57.9 months ±6). For each of them, a biphasic analysis was chosen, in which the first step imposed a clinical evaluation and in the second step, we aimed to evaluate the quality of life.

In the current study, we observed good and excellent clinical results. The mean AOFAS and VAS scores were 82.25/100- grading "good" and VAS 2.7/10- grading "low pain/mild pain," respectively. It is also important to emphasize the distinction in the AOFAS outcome between the two sexes, in favor of men with a difference of 10.62 points, but it has not statistical significance. Only 2 patients had a VAS greater than 5.

AOFAS scores presented by Chen et al. in their work are better (AOFAS 82.25 vs. 91.7) with respect to our result, and this may be due to the sample under examination since the patients analyzed by Chen et al. [17] had an average age of 31.1 years compared to that of our group in question (54.5). When we compare our results to the study of Vicenti et al. [11], they are comparable (AOFAS 82; mean age of the sample under examination 55.2).

In the study by Jacquot et al. [14], the mean AOFAS score was 84.5.

Focusing on the SF-36 evaluation, there are no studies that focus on the physical and psychological sphere of the patient treated with calcaneoplasty. Van Tetering et al. [18] show, using SF-36 scores, that patients with intra-articular calcaneus fractures had a worse quality of life than patients who had undergone surgery such as total hip or knee replacement or myocardial infarctions. Our scores of the SF-36 questionnaire are better if compared to those obtained in ORIF technique studies [19].

Our results show a good recovery both from a psychological and physical point of view, at a follow up of 5 years and do not show a gender difference in clinical results.

5. Conclusions

Although a small number of patients in our study, considering the recent introduction of balloon-assisted reduction, pin fixation and tricalcium phosphate augmentation for calcaneal fracture, have shown good clinical results, good outcomes in the PH and MH and an improvement in the clinical scores were observed. They were comparable and, in some cases, better than the most used ORIF (Open reduction and Internal Synthesis) which reported slightly lower AOFAS scores. Finally, both from a clinical and quality-of-life point of view, our study highlights that there is no gender distinction. Further comparative studies with a higher number of patients are needed which assess the quality of life in the various techniques used to treat calcaneal fractures.

Authors' Contributions

Giuseppe Maccagnano and Giovanni Noia are joint first authors.

References

[1] V. Filardi, "Stress shielding analysis on easy step staple prosthesis for calcaneus fractures," *Journal of Orthopaedics*, vol. 18, pp. 132–137, 2019.

[2] M. J. Mitchell, J. C. McKinley, and C. M. Robinson, "The epidemiology of calcaneal fractures," *The Foot*, vol. 19, no. 4, pp. 197–200, 2009.

[3] E. Guerado, M. L. Bertrand, and J. R. Cano, "Management of calcaneal fractures," *Injury*, vol. 43, no. 10, pp. 1640–1650, 2012.

[4] H. N. Mohammad and M. M. Farhad, "Operative compared to non-operative treatment of displaced intro-articular calcaneal fracture," *Journal of Research in Medical Sciences*, vol. 16, no. 8, pp. 1–3, 2011.

[5] N. Jiang, Q. R. Lin, X.-C. Lin, L. Wu, and B. Yu, "Surgical versus non surgical treatment of displaced intro-articular calcaneal fractures: a meta-analysis of current evidence base," *International Orthopaedics (SICOT)*, vol. 36, pp. 1615–1622, 2012.

[6] S. Kumar, L. G. Krishna, D. Singh, P. Kumar, S. Arora, and S. Dhaka, "Evaluation of functional outcome and complications of locking calcaneum plate for fracture calcaneum," *Journal of Clinical Orthopaedics and Trauma*, vol. 6, no. 3, pp. 147–152, 2015.

[7] A. Meraj, M. Zahid, and S. Ahmad, "Management of intra-articular calcaneal fractures by minimally invasive sinus tarsi approach-early results," *Malaysian Orthopaedic Journal*, vol. 6, no. 1, pp. 13–17, 2012.

[8] A. K. Gupta, G. S. Gluck, and S. G. Parekh, "Balloon reduction of displaced calcaneus fractures: surgical technique and case series," *Foot & Ankle International*, vol. 32, no. 2, pp. 205–210, 2011.

[9] S. Giannini, M. Cadossi, M. Mosca, G. Tedesco, A. Sambri et al., "Minimally-invasive treatment of calcaneal fractures: a review of the literature and our experience," *Injury*, vol. 47, no. Suppl 4, pp. S138–S146, 2016.

[10] D. Vittore, G. Vicenti, G. Caizzi, A. Abate, and B. Moretti, "Balloon-assisted reduction, pin fixation and tricalcium phosphate augmentation for calcanear fracture," *Injury*, vol. 45, pp. S72–S79, 2014.

[11] G. Vicenti, G. Solarino, G. Caizzi, M. Carrozzo, and G. Picca, "Balloon-assisted reduction, pin fixation and tricalcium phosphate augmentation for calcaneal fracture: a retrospective analysis of 42 patients," *Injury*, vol. 49, no. Suppl 3, pp. S94–S99, 2018 Nov.

[12] J. Bruce and A. Sutherland, "Surgical versus conservative interventions for displaced intra-articular calcaneal fractures," *Cochrane Database of Systematic Review*, no. 1, p. CD008628, 2013.

[13] X. Yu, Q.-J. Pang, L. Chen, C.-C. Yang, and X.-J. Chen, "Postoperative complications after closed calcaneus fracture treated by open reduction and internal fixation: a review," *Journal of International Medical Research*, vol. 42, pp. 17–25, 2014.

[14] F. Jacquot, T. Letellier, A. Atchabahian, L. Doursounian, and J.-M. Feron, "Balloon reduction and cement fixation in calcaneal articular fractures: a five-year experience," *International Orthopaedics*, vol. 37, pp. 905–910, 2013.

[15] J. L. Labbe, O. Peres, O. Leclair, R. Goulon, P. Scemama, and F. Jourdel, "Minimallyinvasive treatment of displaced intra-articular calcaneal fractures using the balloon kyphoplasty technique: preliminary study," *Orthopaedics & Traumatology: Surgery & Research*, vol. 99, pp. 829–836, 2013.

[16] F. Biggi, S. Di, C. Salfi, and S. Trevisani, "Percutaneous calcaneoplasty in displaced intraarticular calcaneal fractures," *Journal of Orthopaedics and Traumatology*, vol. 14, pp. 307–310, 2013.

[17] G. Vicenti, M. Carrozzo, G. Solarino et al., "Comparison of plate, calcanealplasty and external fixation in the management of calcaneal fractures," *Injury*, vol. 50, no. Suppl 4, pp. S39–S46, 2019.

[18] E. A. A. Van Tetering and R. E. Buckley, "Functional outcome (SF-36) of patients with displaced calcaneal fractures compared to SF-36 normative data," *Foot & Ankle International*, vol. 25, no. 10, pp. 733–738, 2004.

[19] M. A. Del Core, E. Mills, L. K. Cannada, and D. E. Karges, "Functional outcomes after operative treatment of calcaneal fractures: midterm review," *ournal of Surgical Orthopaedic Advances*, vol. 25, no. 3, pp. 149–156, 2016.

21

A Biomechanical Comparison of Two Techniques of Latarjet Procedure in Cadaveric Shoulders

Aditya Prinja ⓘ, Antony Raymond, and Mahesh Pimple

Whipps Cross University Hospital, London, UK

Correspondence should be addressed to Aditya Prinja; a.prinja@cantab.net

Academic Editor: Benjamin Blondel

Traumatic anterior instability of the shoulder is commonly treated with the Latarjet procedure, which involves transfer of the coracoid process with a conjoint tendon to the anterior aspect of the glenoid. The two most common techniques of the Latarjet are the classical and congruent arc techniques. The aim of this study was to evaluate the difference in force required to dislocate the shoulder after classical and congruent arc Latarjet procedures were performed. Fourteen cadaveric shoulders were dissected and osteotomised to produce a bony Bankart lesion of 25% of the articular surface leading to an "inverted pear-shaped" glenoid. An anteroinferior force was applied whilst the arm was in abduction and external rotation using a pulley system. The force needed to dislocate was noted, and then the shoulders underwent coracoid transfer with the classical and congruent arc techniques. The average force required to dislocate the shoulder after osteotomy was 123.57 N. After classical Latarjet, the average force required was 325.71 N, compared with 327.14 N after the congruent arc technique. This was not statistically significant. In this biomechanical cadaveric study, there is no difference in the force required to dislocate a shoulder after classical and congruent arc techniques of Latarjet, suggesting that both methods are equally effective at preventing anterior dislocation in the position of abduction and external rotation.

1. Introduction

Recurrent traumatic anterior instability of shoulder is best managed with operative management [1, 2]. The aim of surgery is to repair the capsule-labral soft tissue structures, and if required, the osseous defects, in order to provide anterior restraint and decrease the capsular volume [3–5]. The Bankart lesion is the most common soft tissue lesion, though variants such as anterior labrum periosteal sleeve avulsion (ALPSA) lesion have been described [6]. Recent arthroscopic techniques have results similar to open procedure with faster rehabilitation and less morbidity [7–10]. However, in the presence of a significant osseous defect, whether humeral (Hill-Sachs lesion) or glenoid (bony Bankart lesion), isolated soft tissue procedures performed either arthroscopic or open have high failure rates [11–14]. The inverse relationship between the size of glenoid defect and the stability of the shoulder has also been established by biomechanical studies [15].

In recent times, addressing the glenoid defect in an attempt to prevent recurrence has gained more attention. The defect can be addressed with a coracoid transfer (the Latarjet procedure), iliac crest bone grafting (the Eden-Hybinette procedure), or other forms of bone graft such as distal tibial allograft [16–19]. The technique of coracoid transfer, first described by Latarjet in 1954, has undergone many modifications. He described a larger (2-3 cm) piece of coracoid transferred over to the glenoid rim lengthwise and fixed with 2 screws to create a robust repair [16]. In 1958, Helfet described attaching the raw cut surface of coracoid process to the glenoid neck through the transversely sectioned subscapularis muscle [17]. He named this procedure after his mentor W. Rowley Bristow, who had taught him this surgery nearly two decades prior. Young et al. published his modifications of the procedure, which included the use of 2 screws instead of 1 to provide stable fixation of the coracoid and a subscapularis-splitting approach [20]. The technique was also modified by De Beer et al. who rotated the coracoid graft about its long axis to line up the concavity of the coracoid with the articular surface of the glenoid (the so-called "congruent arc" technique) [21].

The aim of this study was to compare the biomechanical efficacy of coracoid transfer using the two common techniques, the "classical" and "congruent arc" Laterjet. Both are well described in literature with good clinical results. We hypothesized that the force needed to dislocate the shoulder would be greater in the congruent arc technique than the classical technique because of increased contact surface area as a result of greater linear dimensions [22, 23].

2. Materials and Methods

We dissected 14 cadaveric shoulders. Deltoid and pectoralis major were detached from their clavicular attachment to improve exposure. Subscapularis and anterior capsule were also detached from their insertion on lesser tuberosity. A bony Bankart lesion was created in the anteroinferior rim of the glenoid. The bony lesions were 25% of longest diameter of the glenoid, to create an "inverted pear-shaped" glenoid (Figure 1) [15, 24]. The osteotomies were made at a 45° inclination to the long axis of glenoid, encompassing ~8 mm width defect of the inferior glenoid circle. The normal shape of glenoid is of a pear when viewed en face, with lower half significantly wider than the upper half. With a large bony Bankart lesion, the upper half become significantly wider than the lower half, resembling the shape of an inverted pear. A hook was inserted in a drill hole in the lateral humerus just inferior to surgical neck. This was passed over a pulley system incorporating a spring balance. The spring balance had a laser marker and a spirit level system attached to it to recreate the direction of force during each application (Figure 2).

The aim was to generate a force directed anteroinferiorly over the humeral head. The arm was kept in 90 degree of abduction and in maximum external rotation. The pulley system was sequentially loaded until the shoulder dislocated anteriorly. The shoulder was said to be dislocated when it would not relocate after releasing the applied force. The force needed to dislocate was noted.

The coracoid tip was then exposed. The insertion of pectoralis minor was detached. The coracoid was osteotomised at the "knee," or the junction of horizontal and vertical parts. The graft was then rigidly fixed flush to the anteroinferior glenoid using the classical technique (Figure 3(a)) with two 3.5 mm cortical screws, such that the lateral surface of coracoid became the face of the glenoid [16]. The humeral head was then loaded in a manner similar to that used for the native shoulder before coracoid transfer. The force needed to dislocate the shoulder was noted.

The graft was then removed and reoriented according to the congruent arc Latarjet technique, such that the inferior surface of the coracoid becomes the face of the glenoid [21]. Rigid fixation was confirmed with the application of two 3.5 mm cortical screws. The load was then applied in the similar manner, and the force needed to dislocate shoulder was measured again.

In alternate specimens, the congruent arc Latarjet technique was done first and tested followed by the classical

technique. This was done to minimise the effect of any cyclical loading on the biomechanical properties of the construct.

3. Results

14 cadaveric specimens were studied. The force required to dislocate uncorrected unstable shoulder was compared with the force required to dislocate the shoulder following "classical" or "congruent arc" Laterjet procedures (Table 1).

A paired t-test was used to calculate the difference in mean force needed to dislocate shoulder, before and after the coracoid transfer. The force was calculated with the formula, F (in Newton) = load × gravity.

The mean force required to dislocate the shoulder after the classical Latarjet was 325.71 N compared with 123.57 N in the uncorrected shoulder. The standard errors of mean and standard deviation were 6.51 N and 24.37 N, respectively, in uncorrected shoulders. The standard errors of mean and standard deviation were 8.30 N and 31.06 N, respectively, for the shoulders undergoing the classical technique. 95% confidence interval was from −209.00 to −195.28. The two-tailed P value was less than 0.0001, thus the difference was statistically significant.

The mean force required to dislocate the shoulder after the congruent arc Laterjet was 327.14 N compared with 123.57 N in the uncorrected shoulder. The standard errors of mean and standard deviation were 6.51 N and 24.37 N, respectively, in uncorrected shoulders, whereas, the standard errors of mean and standard deviation were 7.94 N and 29.72 N, respectively, in the shoulder treated with the congruent arc technique. 95% confidence interval was from −214.57 to −192.57. The two-tailed P value was less than 0.0001, thus the difference was statistically significant.

An unpaired t-test was performed to compare the force required to dislocate the shoulder treated with the two different techniques. Mean force required to dislocate the shoulder after the classical technique was 325.7 N compared with 327 N after the congruent arc technique. The two-tailed P value equals 0.9020 and the 95% confidence interval from −25.05 to 22.19, thus the difference was not statistically significant.

4. Discussion

The optimal strategy for surgical stabilization of the unstable glenohumeral joint remains controversial. However, there seems to be an increased awareness that an isolated soft tissue procedure alone is not always appropriate, and addressing osseous defects of a significant size is important to ensure biomechanical stability and good clinical outcomes [13, 25, 26]. The rationale for the Latarjet procedure is that firstly, it provides a "bone block" to fill the void of an anteroinferior glenoid defect and increases the contact surface area of the glenohumeral articulation. Secondly, and crucially, a sling is created by the dynamic support of the repositioned conjoint tendon which supports the humeral head and provides increased stability in abduction and external rotation (the so-called "dynamic sling effect") [27–30].

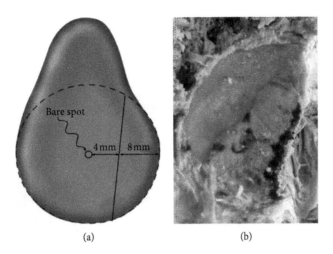

(a)   (b)

FIGURE 1: Osteotomy of cadaveric glenoid to recreate "inverted pear-shaped" anterior bony defect. (a) Posterior. (b) Anterior.

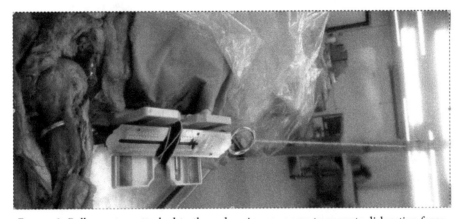

FIGURE 2: Pulley system attached to the cadaveric upper arm to recreate dislocation force.

The repair of anterior capsulolabral structures has been the standard treatment for traumatic anterior shoulder, since the essential lesion was first described by Perthes, and later by Bankart [31–33]. In Bankart's series of 27 patients, none had bony involvement, leading him to postulate that this was in fact a rare combination [32]. Later, however, Rowe showed in a series of 158 patients, almost three quarters had glenoid rim involvement [33]. The open Bankart procedure, restoring near normal anatomy with low recurrence rates, had been recognized as the gold standard treatment for many years, although the functional outcomes were sometimes reported as suboptimal [34–36]. The arthroscopic Bankart repair was subsequently introduced with the aim of decreasing the morbidity and improving functional outcomes. Despite mixed results initially, advances in arthroscopic techniques have led to widespread uptake of the procedure with good results [8,37–39]. However, several studies have shown increased rates of failures for the arthroscopic procedures, where significant osseous defects were not addressed [13, 24, 25, 40, 41]. In their study of 194 arthroscopic Bankart repairs, Burkhart et al. [13] reported a 4% recurrence rate in patients without significant bony defects compared with a 67% recurrence rate in those with a significant bony defect (7% vs.

89% in contact athletes, respectively). The study cited a failure to adequately address the glenohumeral osseous defect as the main cause of recurrence.

The glenohumeral defect can be addressed with various methods of coracoid transfer as previously mentioned. In this study, we compared the two most commonly utilised techniques, the "classical" and "congruent arc" Latarjet. In the congruent arc technique, the coracoid graft is rotated about its long axis, and the concavity is lined up with the joint surface [22]. This relatively increases the anteroposterior diameter and hence increases the surface area for anterior translation in comparison with the classic Latarjet technique, where the inferior surface of the coracoid sits on to the anterior inferior rim of glenoid. Furthermore, it has been shown that the coracoid transfer performed using the congruent arc technique restores the glenohumeral loading mechanics to intact condition, while the classical technique restores it within 5% of the intact state [23]. We hypothesized that this relative increase in surface area would make the bony block with the congruent arc technique, a more stable construct in comparison with the classical latarjet technique. This was expected to reflect as an increase in force requirement for dislocation. However, the difference in force

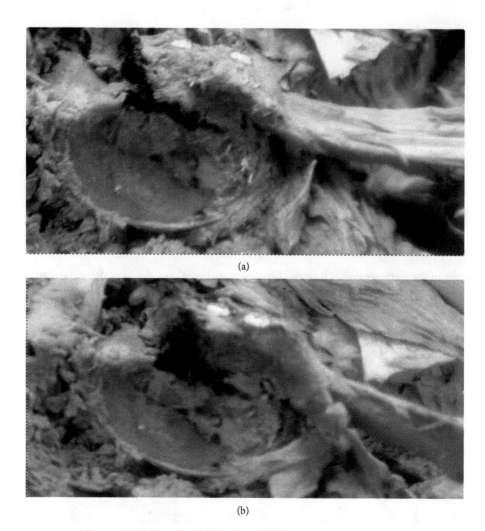

(a)

(b)

FIGURE 3: (a) The classical Latarjet. (b) The congruent arc Latarjet.

TABLE 1: Load required to dislocate the shoulder pre- and post-coracoid transfer (with the two techniques).

Cadaver	Load required to dislocate (kg)		
	After osteotomy	Classical Latarjet	Congruent arc Latarjet
1	12	32	33
2	17	39	36
3	9	29	31
4	15	36	37
5	13	32	31
6	11	28	30
7	16	37	38
8	13	33	31
9	10	30	29
10	11	32	32
11	10	30	30
12	12	33	30
13	10	31	34
14	14	34	36

needed to dislocate in these two techniques was not statistically significant to establish the superiority of one procedure over the other.

In another cadaveric study by Montgomery et al. significant different loads to failure for the two types of coracoid transfer were demonstrated [42]. They found that the congruent arc technique resulted in a lower mean failure load as compared with the classic technique; however, they were applying a tensile load to the conjoint tendon in a bid to replicate the forces experienced by the graft in the early postoperative period. They remarked that the classic technique created a larger surface area for healing to the native glenoid, whilst the congruent arc produced a greater surface area of the glenoid articular surface. They said, as a result, individual patients' anatomy should be preoperatively considered prior to selecting a technique. Giles et al. in their cadaveric comparison of the two techniques applied medially directed forces across the transferred coracoid to try and replicate the forces across the glenohumeral joint and found that the classic technique failed at a higher load than the congruent arc [43].

Mook et al. demonstrated that assessment of coracoid size preoperatively could predict outcome after Latarjet [44]. They suggested that if predicted glenoid track remained off-track with a classically performed Latarjet, a congruent arc might prove beneficial with its larger surface area. Others have said, however, that larger grafts than necessary will see higher rates of graft osteolysis, as less forces from the humeral head are applied leading to resorption in accordance with Wolff's law [45].

In this study, our results show that there is no statistically significant difference in the force required to produce an anteroinferior dislocation of the shoulder after either classical or congruent arc Latarjet. This suggests that both techniques will provide adequate bony coverage to an anterior glenoid defect and will be effective in preventing recurrent dislocation.

Limitations must be considered when interpreting our results. Firstly, this study was performed on cadavers with a mean age of 84.6 years. This is a procedure most commonly performed on patients who are much younger, and thus the effect of reduced bone mineral density of the grafted coracoid could have affected results. Furthermore, this study did not consider the effect of the conjoint tendon and the dynamic sling effect, and it may be due to the fact that tendon has differing effects according to the position, nor did it consider other soft tissue factors such as capsule-labral repair or the subscapularis split. In this study, we did not aim to address the issue of union of the coracoid, which may also be different, as the techniques differ in the area that is in contact with the glenoid. However, in this study, failure of the construct was solely due to failure of the coracoid transfer itself, and the study has clearly demonstrated that there is no difference in the performance of the transfer using the two techniques.

5. Conclusion

To conclude, both the congruent arc and classical technique of coracoid transfer are equally effective in preventing anterior shoulder dislocation in the position of abduction and external rotation in cadaveric specimens.

References

[1] T. R. Lenters, A. K. Franta, F. M. Wolf, S. S. Leopold, and F. A. Matsen III, "Arthroscopic compared with open repairs for recurrent anterior shoulder instability," *The Journal of Bone & Joint Surgery*, vol. 89, no. 2, pp. 244–254, 2007.

[2] S. Pelet, B. M. Jolles, and A. Farron, "Bankart repair for recurrent anterior glenohumeral instability: results at twenty-nine years' follow-up," *Journal of Shoulder and Elbow Surgery*, vol. 15, no. 2, pp. 203–207, 2006.

[3] D. W. Altcheck, R. F. Warren, M. J. Skyhar, and G. Ortiz, "T-plasty modification of the Bankart procedure for multidirectional instability of the anterior and inferior types," *The Journal of Bone & Joint Surgery*, vol. 73-A, pp. 105–112, 1991.

[4] C. S. Neer and C. R. Foster, "Inferior capsular shift for involuntary inferior and multidirectional instability of the shoulder. A preliminary report," *The Journal of Bone & Joint Surgery*, vol. 62, no. 6, pp. 897–908, 1980.

[5] G. Walch and P. Boileau, "Latarjet-Bristow procedure for recurrent anterior instability," *Techniques in Shoulder and Elbow Surgery*, vol. 1, no. 4, pp. 256–261, 2000.

[6] T. J. Neviaser, "The anterior labroligamentous periosteal sleeve avulsion lesion: a cause of anterior instability of the shoulder," *Arthroscopy: The Journal of Arthroscopic & Related Surgery*, vol. 9, no. 1, pp. 17–21, 1993.

[7] F. P. Tjoumakaris, J. A. Abboud, S. A. Hasan, M. L. Ramsey, G. R. Williams, and G. R. Williams, "Arthroscopic and open Bankart repairs provide similar outcomes," *Clinical Orthopaedics and Related Research*, vol. 446, pp. 227–232, 2006.

[8] C. Fabbriciani, G. Milano, A. Demontis, S. Fadda, F. Ziranu, and P. D. Mulas, "Arthroscopic versus open treatment of Bankart lesion of the shoulder: a prospective randomized study," *Arthroscopy: The Journal of Arthroscopic & Related Surgery*, vol. 20, no. 5, pp. 456–462, 2004.

[9] B. J. Cole, J. L'Insalata, J. Irrgang, and J. J. P. Warner, "Comparison of arthroscopic and open anterior shoulder stabilization," *The Journal of Bone and Joint Surgery-American Volume*, vol. 82, no. 8, pp. 1108–1114, 2000.

[10] M. R. Green and K. P. Christensen, "Arthroscopic versus open Bankart procedures: a comparison of early morbidity and complications," *Arthroscopy: The Journal of Arthroscopic & Related Surgery*, vol. 9, no. 4, pp. 371–374, 1993.

[11] P. Boileau, M. Villalba, J.-Y. Héry, F. Balg, P. Ahrens, and L. Neyton, "Risk factors for recurrence of shoulder instability after arthroscopic Bankart repair," *The Journal of Bone & Joint Surgery*, vol. 88, no. 8, pp. 1755–1763, 2006.

[12] S. S. Burkhart and S. M. Danaceau, "Articular arc length mismatch as a cause of failed bankart repair," *Arthroscopy: The Journal of Arthroscopic & Related Surgery*, vol. 16, no. 7, pp. 740–744, 2000.

[13] S. S. Burkhart and J. F. De Beer, "Traumatic glenohumeral bone defects and their relationship to failure of arthroscopic Bankart repairs," *Arthroscopy: The Journal of Arthroscopic & Related Surgery*, vol. 16, no. 7, pp. 677–694, 2000.

[14] M. Tauber, H. Resch, R. Forstner, M. Raffl, and J. Schauer, "Reasons for failure after surgical repair of anterior shoulder instability," *Journal of Shoulder and Elbow Surgery*, vol. 13, no. 3, pp. 279–285, 2004.

[15] E. Itoi, S.-B. Lee, L. J. Berglund, L. L. Berge, and K.-N. An, "The effect of a glenoid defect on anteroinferior stability of the shoulder after bankart repair: a cadaveric study," *The Journal of Bone and Joint Surgery-American Volume*, vol. 82, no. 1, pp. 35–46, 2000.

[16] M. Latarjet, "A propos du traitement des luxations récidivantes delèpaule," *Lyon Chit*, vol. 49, pp. 994–1003, 1954.

[17] A. J. Helfet, "Coracoid transplantation for recurring dislocation of the shoulder," *The Journal of Bone and Joint Surgery. British Volume*, vol. 40-B, no. 2, pp. 198–202, 1958.

[18] J. J. P. Warner, T. J. Gill, J. D. O'Hollerhan, N. Pathare, and P. J. Millett, "Anatomical glenoid reconstruction for recurrent anterior glenohumeral instability with glenoid deficiency using an autogenous tricortical iliac crest bone graft," *The American Journal of Sports Medicine*, vol. 34, no. 2, pp. 205–212, 2006.

[19] M. T. Provencher, N. Ghodadra, L. LeClere, D. J. Solomon, and A. A. Romeo, "Anatomic osteochondral glenoid reconstruction for recurrent glenohumeral instability with glenoid deficiency using a distal tibia allograft," *Arthroscopy: The Journal of Arthroscopic & Related Surgery*, vol. 25, no. 4, pp. 446–452, 2009.

[20] A. A. Young, R. Maia, J. Berhouet, and G. Walch, "Open Latarjet procedure for management of bone loss in anterior instability of the glenohumeral joint," *Journal of Shoulder and Elbow Surgery*, vol. 20, no. 2, pp. S61–S69, 2011.

[21] J. De Beer, S. S. Burkhart, C. P. Roberts, K. Van Rooyen, T. Cresswell, and D. F. Du Toit, "The congruent-arc latarjet," *Techniques in Shoulder and Elbow Surgery*, vol. 10, no. 2, pp. 62–67, 2009.

[22] C. M. Dolan, S. Hariri, N. D. Hart, and T. R. McAdams, "An anatomic study of the coracoid process as it relates to bone transfer procedures," *Journal of Shoulder and Elbow Surgery* vol. 20, no. 3, pp. 497–501, 2011.

[23] N. Ghodadra, A. Gupta, A. A. Romeo et al., "Normalization of glenohumeral articular contact pressures after Latarjet or iliac crest bone-grafting," *The Journal of Bone and Joint Surgery-American Volume*, vol. 92, no. 6, pp. 1478–1489, 2010.

[24] S. S. Burkhart, J. F. Debeer, A. M. Tehrany, and P. M. Parten, "Quantifying glenoid bone loss arthroscopically in shoulder instability," *Arthroscopy: The Journal of Arthroscopic & Related Surgery*, vol. 18, no. 5, pp. 488–491, 2002.

[25] I. K. Y. Lo, P. M. Parten, and S. S. Burkhart, "The inverted pear glenoid: an indicator of significant glenoid bone loss," *Arthroscopy: The Journal of Arthroscopic & Related Surgery* vol. 20, no. 2, pp. 169–174, 2004.

[26] W. H. Montgomery Jr., M. Wahl, C. Hettrich, E. Itoi, S. B. Lippitt, and F. A. Matsen III, "Anteroinferior bone-grafting can restore stability in osseous glenoid defects," *The Journal of Bone and Joint Surgery-American Volume*, vol. 87, no. 9, pp. 1972–1977, 2005.

[27] D. Patte, J. Bernageau, and P. Bancel, "The anteroinferior vulnerable point of the glenoid rim," in *Surgery of the Shoulder*, J. E. Bateman and R. P. Welsch, Eds., pp. 94–99, Marcel Dekker, New York, NY, USA, 1985.

[28] D. Patte and J. Debeyre, "Luxations rècidivantes de lèpaule," *Encycl Med Chir. Paris-Technique Chirurgicale. Orthop6die* vol. 44265, pp. 4–2, 1980.

[29] J. Allain, D. Goutallier, and C. Glorion, "Long-term results of the latarjet procedure for the treatment of anterior instability of the shoulder," *The Journal of Bone & Joint Surgery*, vol. 80, no. 6, pp. 841–852, 1998.

[30] T. B. Edwards, A. Boulahia, and G. Walch, "Radiographic analysis of bone defects in chronic anterior shoulder instability," *Arthroscopy: The Journal of Arthroscopic & Related Surgery*, vol. 19, no. 7, pp. 732–739, 2003.

[31] A. S. B. Bankart, "Recurrent or habitual dislocation of the shoulder," *BMJ*, vol. 2, pp. 1131–1133, 1923.

[32] A. S. B. Bankart, "The pathology and treatment of recurrent dislocation of the shoulder-joint," *British Journal of Surgery* vol. 26, no. 101, pp. 23–29, 1938.

[33] G. Perthes, "Über Operationen bei habitueller Schulterluxation," *Deutsche Zeitschrift für Chirurgie*, vol. 85, no. 1, pp. 199–227, 1906.

[34] C. R. Rowe, D. Patel, and W. W. Southmayd, "The Bankart procedure," *The Journal of Bone & Joint Surgery*, vol. 60, no. 1, pp. 1–16, 1978.

[35] T. J. Gill, L. J. Micheli, F. Gebhard, and C. Binder, "Bankart repair for anterior instability of the shoulder. Long-term outcome," *The Journal of Bone & Joint Surgery*, vol. 79, no. 6, pp. 850–857, 1997.

[36] K. B. Freedman, A. P. Smith, A. A. Romeo, B. J. Cole, and B. R. Bach, "Open Bankart repair versus arthroscopic repair with transglenoid sutures or bioabsorbable tacks for recurrent anterior instability of the shoulder," *The American Journal of Sports Medicine*, vol. 32, no. 6, pp. 1520–1527, 2004.

[37] G. M. Gartsman, T. S. Roddey, and S. M. Hammerman, "Arthroscopic treatment of bidirectional glenohumeral instability: two- to five-year follow-up," *Journal of Shoulder and Elbow Surgery*, vol. 10, no. 1, pp. 28–36, 2001.

[38] S.-H. Kim, K.-I. Ha, Y.-B. Cho, B.-D. Ryu, and I. Oh, "Arthroscopic anterior stabilization of the shoulder," *The Journal of Bone and Joint Surgery-American Volume*, vol. 85, no. 8, pp. 1511–1518, 2003.

[39] S.-H. Kim, K.-I. Ha, and S.-H. Kim, "Bankart repair in traumatic anterior shoulder instability," *Arthroscopy: The Journal of Arthroscopic & Related Surgery*, vol. 18, no. 7, pp. 755–763, 2002.

[40] L. U. Bigliani, P. M. Newton, S. P. Steinmann, P. M. Connor, and S. J. McIlveen, "Glenoid rim lesions associated with recurrent anterior dislocation of the shoulder," *The American Journal of Sports Medicine*, vol. 26, no. 1, pp. 41–45, 1998.

[41] M. D. Lazarus, J. A. Sidles, D. T. Harryman II, and F. A. Matsen III, "Effect of a chondral-labral defect on glenoid concavity and glenohumeral stability. A cadaveric model," *The Journal of Bone & Joint Surgery*, vol. 78, no. 1, pp. 94–102, 1996.

[42] S. R. Montgomery, J. C. Katthagen, J. D. Mikula et al., "Anatomic and biomechanical comparison of the classic and congruent-arc techniques of the latarjet procedure," *The American Journal of Sports Medicine*, vol. 45, no. 6, pp. 1252–1260, 2017.

[43] J. W. Giles, G. Puskas, M. Welsh, J. A. Johnson, and G. S. Athwal, "Do the traditional and modified Latarjet techniques produce equivalent reconstruction stability and strength?," *The American Journal of Sports Medicine*, vol. 40, no. 12, pp. 2801–2807, 2012.

[44] W. R. Mook, M. Petri, J. A. Greenspoon, M. P. Horan, G. J. Dornan, and P. J. Millett, "Clinical and anatomic predictors of outcomes after the Latarjet procedure for the treatment of anterior glenohumeral instability with combined glenoid and humeral bone defects," *The American Journal of Sports Medicine*, vol. 44, no. 6, pp. 1407–1416, 2016.

[45] G. Giacomo, N. de Gasperis, A. De Vita et al., "Coracoid bone graft osteolysis after Latarjet procedure: a comparison study between two screws standard technique vs mini-plate fixation," *International Journal of Shoulder Surgery*, vol. 7, no. 1, pp. 1–6, 2013.

22

Assessment of Shoulder Function after Internal Fixation of Humeral Diaphyseal Fractures in Young Adults

Hossam Fathi Mahmoud ⓘ, Ahmed Hatem Farhan ⓘ, and Fahmy Samir Fahmy ⓘ

Orthopedic Surgery Department, Faculty of Medicine, Zagazig University, Zagazig, Egypt

Correspondence should be addressed to Fahmy Samir Fahmy; fahmysamir72@yahoo.com

Academic Editor: Francesco Liuzza

Background. Humeral shaft fractures are commonly encountered in casualties. There are different methods of operative internal fixation with no consensus on the best technique. The objective of this study was to assess shoulder function and rate of complications among two different options of fixation, intramedullary nailing, and minimal invasive plate osteosynthesis (MIPO) in young adults. *Methods.* Forty-two patients with humeral shaft fractures were included in the study and divided into two equal groups: group A treated with antegrade intramedullary locked nails (IMN) and group B with MIPO. Fracture union was evaluated with serial X-rays, and shoulder function was assessed in both groups using the scale of the American Shoulder and Elbow Surgeons (ASES), University of California at Los Angeles Shoulder Scale (UCLA), and visual analog score (VAS). The mean differences between groups were recorded and considered significant if the P value was ˂0.05. *Results.* The results were reported prospectively with no significant differences in mean age, sex, side of injury, type of fracture, mechanism of injury, and the follow-up period between the groups studied. Group A had shorter operative time and minimal blood loss than group B. Regarding shoulder function scores (ASES, UCLA, and VAS), the results in the MIPO group were better than the IMN group with shorter time of union and fewer complications. *Conclusion.* Despite a shorter operative time and lower blood loss during locked intramedullary nail fixation in the management of humeral shaft fractures, MIPO enables more superior shoulder function with better fracture healing and lower morbidities.

1. Introduction

Humeral shaft fractures represent 3% of all adult fractures. Conservative management remains the main stay for treatment of stable and nondisplaced fractures, but in certain conditions, surgical intervention is needed [1–4].

Poor compliance with conservative treatment and failure to maintain reduction, as well as open fractures, segmental fractures, neurovascular insults, floating elbows, and poly-trauma patients with multiple fractures are the main indications for surgical intervention [5].

Advances in the last few decades in the design and manufacture of modern surgical implants used for fixations have helped expand the indications for operative intervention with the achievement of early fracture union and lower complications [6].

The choice of the ideal method of fixation for humeral shaft fractures remains controversial, and there is no consensus in literature about the best method. However, both locked intramedullary nail (IMN) and minimal invasive plate osteosynthesis (MIPO) are accepted surgical options that enable minimal invasive biological fracture fixation [5].

Although open dynamic compression plating (ORIF) provides more accurate anatomical reduction and rigid fixation and reduces the risks of malunions, it requires wide intraoperative exposure with more soft tissue injury. This may contribute to high infection rates and increased rates of nonunion due to violation of soft tissue at the fracture site and severance of periosteal blood supply [7].

The use of intramedullary locked nails is considered more superior to (ORIF) for fixation of humeral diaphyseal fractures because it is minimally invasive with less soft tissue stripping and results in less infection rates and rapid return to activities. The shoulder problems at the insertion site of the nail are the main concern of this fixation method, which can potentially be avoided with modern straight nail designs. Accidental injury to the rotator cuff, shoulder impingement, and accumulation of debris from reaming are the main causes of shoulder dysfunction [8, 9].

Minimal invasive plating osteosynthesis has gained popularity for the treatment of diaphyseal humeral fractures since it provides stable fixation with micromotion at the fracture site and stimulation of callus formation. It has a diminished risk of nonunion, infection, and shoulder disabilities [10].

The purpose of the current study was to assess and compare the outcomes of shoulder functions in two groups of young adult patients with humeral diaphyseal fractures treated by locked IMN and MIPO. Also, the benefits and shortcomings of each treatment method were evaluated.

2. Patients and Methods

Forty-two skeletally mature patients with closed humeral diaphyseal fractures were enrolled in this prospective cohort study. It was conducted at Zagazig University Hospitals between March 2017 and January 2021. 21 patients were managed with antegrade interlocking nail (group A) and 21 patients with MIPO (group B).

This work was conducted in accordance with the World Medical Association (Declaration of Helsinki) guidelines for studies involving humans. Informed consent from the patients and IRB approval from our ethical committee (ZU-IRB #65760/8-1-2017) were obtained prior to prospective collection of patient data.

Patients included in this comparative study were older than eighteen years of age and had closed humeral shaft fractures. Patients older than 50 and those who had fractures with articular extension, associated vascular injuries, floating elbows, delayed cases of more than three weeks, pathological fractures, open fractures, presence of radial nerve palsy, and distal level were all excluded from this study. The demographic criteria of the patients who participated in this study are listed in Table 1.

The patients were clinically assessed for soft tissue injury, integrity of radial nerves, vascular integrity, and presence of other fractures. Anteroposterior and lateral view X-ray films including shoulder and the elbow joints were requested for the injured limb to assess the fracture. Also, radiological evaluation of any other suspected injuries including the skull, neck, chest, pelvis, spine, and other limb injuries were done in polytrauma cases.

After primary management in the emergency room and splinting of the affected limb, the patients were admitted and prepared for surgery.

All patients were operated under general anesthesia by the same surgeon. A prophylactic antibiotic of 1 gm intravenous ceftriaxone was administered 30 minutes before surgery. Draping of the affected limb was done, and the arm was left free to help manipulation and reduction. All surgeries were done under the control of a C-arm image intensifier.

2.1. *Antegrade Nailing Group.* Patients were placed in a beach chair position. The site of entry was made through a small stab incision approximately 1 cm in length in front of the anterior rim of the acromion between the anterior and middle deltoid fibers with careful dissection down to the entry point, which was lateral to the articular margin and just medial to the greater tuberosity. The awl was placed over this point and verified with the C-arm to confirm its alignment with the medullary canal in the anteroposterior and lateral views. The medullary canal was opened with subsequent passage of the guide rod in the canal. The fracture was manipulated with gentle traction for reduction and passage of the guide through the distal part of the bone.

Prior to insertion, the guide wire whole length was determined, and the outer part of the wire was measured and subtracted from the whole length of the guide to assess the anticipated nail length.

Using a protective sleeve, reaming was started with sharp end-cutting reamer over the guide rod with 0.5 mm increments until the best fit diameter was reached. The ball tip wire was exchanged, and the nail was advanced through the medulla. The guide rod was removed after the nail had reached the distal end of the canal; 1 cm proximal to the olecranon fossa. The nail tip needs to be sunken 2 mm below the articular cartilage to avoid impingement.

After closing the fracture gap, proximal and distal locking screws were inserted under C-arm guidance, and subsequently the wound was closed in layers.

2.2. *Plate Group (MIPO).* Patients were placed in a supine position with their arms abducted to 90° and their forearms supinated. The C-arm was placed on the same side as the limb to be operated.

A three-centimeter-long proximal incision was made between the medial border of the deltoid and biceps muscle six centimeters distal to the acromion and dissected to the humerus. The distal incision was made along the lateral border of biceps three centimeters long just proximal to the flexion crease by five centimeters. The distal incision should be far distal to the fracture site. The biceps muscle was retracted medially to identify and protect the musculocutaneous nerve, which lies above the brachialis muscle. Then, dissection was done through brachialis retracting the musculocutaneous nerve medially, while the radial nerve was protected by the lateral half of the brachialis muscle.

An extraperiosteal tunnel was made under the brachialis muscle using a periosteal elevator from distal to proximal under brachialis muscle. A plate of suitable length was passed through the tunnel and anchored to the bone with a 'proximal and distal screw after reducing the fracture by gentle manual traction. After proper alignment and reduction were confirmed by image intensifier, the rest of the locked screws were inserted sequentially, and the wound was closed.

TABLE 1: The demographic and intraoperative data of the groups studied.

		IMN (group A) (N = 21)	MIPO (group B) (N = 21)	P value
Mean age (years)		34.8 ± 8.4	38.5 ± 8.4	0.167
Sex	Male	16 (76.2%)	15 (71.5%)	0.725
	Female	5 (28.8%)	6 (28.5%)	
Side	Right	7 (33.3%)	9 (42.9%)	0.525
	Left	14 (66.7%)	12 (57.1%)	
Mechanism of trauma	RTA	11 (52.4%)	13 (61.9%)	0.532884
	Falling	10 (47.6%)	8 (38.1%)	
AO/OTA classification	Type A	9 (42.9%)	12 (57.1%)	0.644497
	Type B	9 (42.9%)	7 (33.3%)	
	Type C	3 (14.3%)	2 (9.5%)	
Time before surgery (days)		1.9 ± 1.04	2.29 ± 1.34	0.311851
Operative time (minutes)		88.1 ± 16.9	124.05 ± 19.5	P < 0.001
Blood loss (cc)		84.29 ± 16.8	134.05 ± 31.2	P < 0.001
Follow-up period (months)		28.76 ± 6.04	31.1 ± 7.6	0.280379
Time of union (weeks)		15.48 ± 4.3	12.76 ± 3.7	0.035994

IMN: intramedullary nail; MIPO: minimal invasive plate osteosynthesis; N: number of patients in each group; RTA: road traffic accident. Sex, mechanism of injury, the affected side, and AO/OTA classification were compared by chi-square test, and the other variables were compared by independent T-test. P value less than 0.05 is considered significant.

The arm was immobilized in a sling, and antibiotic was continued for 48 hours only after surgery. Passive mobilization of the wrist, elbow, and shoulder was allowed immediately as much as could be tolerated. The stitches were removed after 14 days. Active resistance exercises were not possible until the fracture healed. Serial radiological follow-up was conducted with a monthly X-ray film until evidence of union (Figures 1 and 2). Shoulder functions were evaluated using the American Shoulder and Elbow Surgeons (ASES) score [11], University of California at Los Angeles shoulder scale (UCLA) [12], and visual analog score (VAS) [13].

2.3. Statistical Analysis. The data were analyzed using Statistical Package for Social Sciences software program version 16. The numerical values were recorded as means and standard deviation. Before comparing the means, the Kolmogorov–Smirnov test was used to check the normality of the groups analyzed. The means of quantitative variables were compared using independent t-tests, while the nominal and categorical data were compared by Chi-square and Fisher's exact tests. In all tests, P values below 0.05 were considered statistically significant. The sample size that gives 80% statistical power, α error of 0.05, and large effect size more than 0.5 was calculated using G-power software calculator version 3.1.

3. Results

No significant differences were identified among the two groups with respect to mean age, sex, mechanism of fracture, the affected side, type of fracture according to AO classification, time before operative intervention, and the follow-up time (Table 1).

The mean operative time showed significant differences between the two groups (P value <0.001), and it was shorter in the IMN group than the MIPO group by 36 minutes. Also, blood loss was less in the nail group compared with MIPO,

the difference between the two groups being significant ($P = 0.035$). The IMN group exhibited better results with respect to blood loss and operative time. According to the Radiological Union Scale, radiographic union occurs when a bridging callus with invisible fracture line (score 3) is seen in at least three of four cortices. The mean time of fracture healing was shorter in the MIPO group than the IMN group (12.76 ± 3.7 and 15.48 ± 4.3 weeks, respectively). The difference between the groups was significant. Regarding the results of shoulder functions, the last follow-up records of ASES, UCLA, and VAS were better in the MIPO than the IMN group with statistically significant differences (Table 2).

The overall complication rate was higher in the IMN group (23.8%) than the MIPO group (9.5%). There were five complications in group A (IMN); two cases of fracture nonunion were treated using augmentation plates and bone grafting, and three cases with shoulder pain (two patients with subacromial bursitis and one patient with partial cuff tear) were treated by shoulder arthroscopy (Figure 1(d)). There were no reported cases of nonunion and shoulder problems in the MIPO group. However, in the MIPO group, there were two cases of malunions (5°) without functional deficit. There were no recorded cases of infections and iatrogenic radial nerve palsy in both groups.

4. Discussion

Open reduction and internal fixation (ORIF) technique is the gold standard and most widely used operative method for treating humeral diaphyseal fractures. The major drawbacks of this technique are the need for a big skin incision, soft tissue disruption, and periosteal stripping that may predispose to higher rates of infection, radial nerve palsy, and nonunion [14].

With advances in surgical techniques, implants, and the emerging concept of biological minimal invasive fixation, both intramedullary locked nail and MIPO fixation, are commonly used nowadays for treating shaft fractures. Until

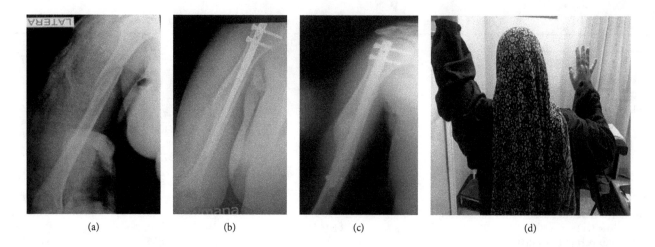

(a)   (b)   (c)   (d)

FIGURE 1: A 48-year-old female had right humeral shaft fracture AO/OTA type 12-A$_2$ as shown in the preoperative X-ray (a). She was treated by interlocking nail (b). 8 months after surgery, there was complete bone union (c), but there was limited range of shoulder motion due to impingement and secondary frozen shoulder (d).

now, there are controversies in literature regarding functional outcomes following both techniques and which of them is more superior [15].

This study was conducted keeping in mind the limited comparative studies between IMN and MIPO and focused on comparing the results of shoulder functions and the complication rate of both techniques among active young patients.

MIPO technique was developed to avoid soft tissue and periosteal violations associated with ORIF, so it has lower rate of postoperative infections and fracture nonunion and better cosmesis. However, most published studies have reported more operative time and blood loss for MIPO compared with IMN [16].

This is consistent with the results of our study. We found that the nail group had lower duration of surgery (88.1 vs. 124.05 minutes, respectively) and less blood loss (84.29 vs. 134.05 cc) than the MIPO group, which were statistically significant. This can be attributed to the time taken for fracture manipulation to achieve good reduction and proper alignment. Also, in a retrospective study, Wang et al. [16] showed that the nail group had shorter duration of operation with less exposure to radiation.

In a meta-analysis by Wen et al. [17], it was reported that the IMN had superior results in terms of postoperative infections than when plates were used. Contrary to that in our study, we had no cases of infection for both treatment groups. Also, they stated that the MIPO had better union than IMN and no significant difference in occurrence of iatrogenic radial nerve lesion, which is similar to what we found. These conclusions are different from the study of Wang et al. [16] who reported more nonunion and radial nerve lesions in the MIPO group.

The complication of malunion with the MIPO technique was more in the reviews published due to the indirect reduction methods used. We found two cases of malunion (varus deformity of five degrees) in the MIPO group, but this deformity did not affect the function of limb, and the patients were able to return to their normal activities. No

malunion was found in the nail group. Also, Wang et al. [16] reported 2 cases of malunion in 30 patients treated by MIPO.

In the current published literature, we found contrasting results regarding nonunion for both IMN and MIPO. Wang et al. [16] had shorter time of union in the nail group, while Ma et al. [18] reported no significant difference in the nonunion rate between the nail and plate. In a cross-sectional descriptive study, Kivi et al. [19] noticed that the intramedullary nail of humeral shaft fracture fixation had a high nonunion rate. Wen et al. [17] stated that the MIPO technique had better results of union than the nail group, and this was consistent to our findings.

We report lower complication rates in the MIPO group than in the IMN, and the difference between both was statistically significant. Similar to our records, Wen et al. [17] stated that MIPO is superior to the locked nail in terms of overall complication rate.

At the end of the follow-up period, the mean VAS for the MIPO group was lower than that for IMN. This may be explained by the presence of shoulder problems and nonunion in the IMN group. Other studies have reported no significant differences for both groups [16].

We assessed the shoulder function between the nail and MIPO groups using ASES and UCLA scores and found superior functional outcomes in the MIPO than the nail group, and the difference was significant. Many published studies have not shown significant differences between both methods; however, most of them compare the IMN and ORIF techniques [16, 20–22].

The main causes of shoulder pain after antegrade IMN fixation are impingement, rotator cuff injuries, and adhesive capsulitis. We encountered three (14.2%) shoulder problems in the IMN group: two cases of subacromial bursitis were treated by arthroscopic bursectomy and debridement of the accumulated debris with rotator interval release, and the other case was a partial rotator cuff tear treated by arthroscopic repair. There were no shoulder functional deficits in the MIPO group.

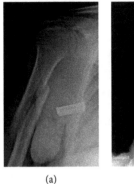 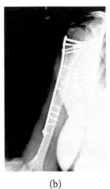 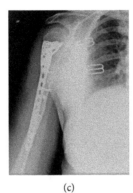 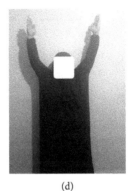 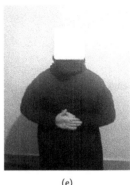

(a)   (b)   (c)   (d)   (e)

FIGURE 2: A 41-year-old female patient had humeral diaphyseal fracture due to a car accident. Preoperative X-ray shows AO/OTA type 12-B_1 (a). She was treated by MIPO technique with complete fracture union as shown in 5 months postoperative X-ray (b, c). The patient had full shoulder function and complete range of motion (d, e).

TABLE 2: The final results of shoulder scores and complications for both groups.

	Group A	Group B	P value
ASES score	87.4 ± 14.5	95.01 ± 6.9	0.03
UCLA score	31.04 ± 4.4	33.3 ± 2.2	0.04
VAS	1.1 ± 1.08	0.54 ± 0.63	0.03
Complications number	5	2	0.214193
Nonunion	2	0	0.4878
Varus deformity	0	2	0.4878
Radial nerve injury	0	0	—
Infection	0	0	—
Shoulder complications	2 cases of subacromial bursitis; 1 case of partial rotator cuff tear	0	$P < 0.001$

ASES: American Shoulder and Elbow Surgeons; UCLA: University of California at Los Angeles Shoulder, and VAS; visual analog score. They were compared by independent T-test, while the complications by chi-square test and Fisher's exact test.

In a study by Kassem et al. [23], they had two cases of shoulder impingement and limited range of motion in the nail group, which were treated by removal of the nail with no residual dysfunction. Also, Bisaccia et al. [24] described similar findings. Ouyang et al. [5] and Wang et al. [16] noticed that shoulder complications were fewer in plating, but Wen et al. [17] declared no significant difference between IMN and MIPO.

Mocini et al. [9] used an antegrade straight interlocking nail with medial entry point for fixation in their series and did not find major complications related to the nail insertion site.

All the patients in our MIPO group regained full shoulder function with satisfactory outcomes and no deficits. The rate of complications was lower than the IMN group. Davies et al. [25] compared the results of MIPO and nail groups in 30 patients, and they recommended the MIPO technique as it had less complications and better functional results.

Our study has some limitations. The sample size in our study was small, and in future studies, a larger number of patients will be needed in order to increase the confidence in the final conclusions. Also, a longer follow-up will help identify remote complications that may not appear earlier. Finally, the lack of randomization is also another weak point of this clinical study.

5. Conclusion

In conclusion, both MIPO and locked intramedullary nail are biological and effective techniques for the management of diaphyseal fractures of the humerus. However, locked IMN has shorter operative time, less bleeding, and less exposure to radiation, and MIPO on the other hand results in better shoulder function and union rate with lower complications. There are no differences between both techniques with respect to infection rates and radial nerve injury. Further long-term studies are recommended to confirm superiority of either technique.

References

[1] C.-H. Tsai, Y.-C. Fong, Y.-H. Chen, C.-J. Hsu, C.-H. Chang, and H.-C. Hsu, "The epidemiology of traumatic humeral shaft fractures in Taiwan," International Orthopaedics, vol. 33, no. 2, pp. 463–467, 2009.

[2] P. A. Cole and C. A. Wijdicks, "The operative treatment of diaphyseal humeral shaft fractures," Hand Clinics, vol. 23, no. 4, pp. 437–448, 2007.

[3] R. Ekholm, J. Adami, J. Tidermark, K. Hansson, H. Törnkvist, and S. Ponzer, "Fractures of the shaft of the humerus," Journal of Bone and Joint Surgery British Volume, vol. 88-B, no. 11, pp. 1469–1473, 2006.

[4] K. Singisetti and M. Ambedkar, "Nailing versus plating in humerus shaft fractures: a prospective comparative study," International Orthopaedics, vol. 34, no. 4, pp. 571–576, 2010.

[5] H. Ouyang, J. Xiong, P. Xiang, Z. Cui, L. Chen, and B. Yu, "Plate versus intramedullary nail fixation in the treatment of humeral shaft fractures: an updated meta-analysis," Journal of Shoulder and Elbow Surgery, vol. 22, no. 3, pp. 387–395, 2013.

[6] J.-G. Zhao, J. Wang, C. Wang, and S.-L. Kan, "Intramedullary nail versus plate fixation for humeral shaft fractures," *Medicine*, vol. 94, no. 11, p. e599, 2015.

[7] S.-H. Ko, J.-R. Cha, C. C. Lee, Y. T. Joo, and K. S. Eom, "Minimally invasive plate osteosynthesis using a screw compression method for treatment of humeral shaft fractures," *Clinical Orthopaedic Surgery*, vol. 9, no. 4, pp. 506–513, 2017.

[8] M. Changulani, U. K. Jain, and T. Keswani, "Comparison of the use of the humerus intramedullary nail and dynamic compression plate for the management of diaphyseal fractures of the humerus. A randomised controlled study," *International Orthopaedics*, vol. 31, no. 3, pp. 391–395, 2007.

[9] F. Mocini, G. Cazzato, G. Masci, G. Malerba, F. Liuzza, and G. Maccauro, "Clinical and radiographic outcomes after antegrade intramedullary nail fixation of humeral fractures," *Injury*, vol. 51, no. 3, pp. S34–S38, 2020.

[10] T. Apivatthakakul, O. Arpornchayanon, and S. Bavornratanavech, "Minimally invasive plate osteosynthesis (MIPO) of the humeral shaft fracture," *Injury*, vol. 36, no. 4, pp. 530–538, 2005.

[11] L. A. Michener, P. W. McClure, and B. J. Sennett, "American shoulder and elbow surgeons standardized shoulder assessment form, patient self-report section: reliability, validity, and responsiveness," *Journal of Shoulder and Elbow Surgery*, vol. 11, no. 6, pp. 587–594, 2002.

[12] H. C. Amstutz, A. L. Sew Hoy, and I. C. Clarke, "UCLA anatomic total shoulder arthroplasty," *Clinical Orthopaedics and Related Research*, vol. 155, pp. 7–20, 1981.

[13] D. A. Delgado, B. S. Lambert, and N. Boutris, "Validation of digital visual analog scale pain scoring with a traditional paper-based visual analog scale in adults," *The Journal of the American Academy of Orthopaedic Surgeons*, vol. 2, no. 3, pp. 1–6, 2018.

[14] M. W. Gosler, M. Testroote, J. W. Morrenhof, and H. M. Janzing, "Surgical versus non-surgical interventions for treating humeral shaft fractures in adults," *Cochrane Database of Systematic Reviews*, vol. 1, Article ID CD008832, 2012.

[15] M. S. Shetty, M. A. Kumar, K. Sujay, A. R. Kini, and K. G. Kanthi, "Minimally invasive plate osteosynthesis for humerus diaphyseal fractures," *Indian Journal of Orthopaedics*, vol. 45, no. 6, pp. 520–526, 2011.

[16] Y. Wang, H. Chen, L. Wang et al., "Comparison between osteosynthesis with interlocking nail and minimally invasive plating for proximal- and middle-thirds of humeral shaft fractures," *International Orthopaedics Published on line*, vol. 45, no. 8, pp. 2093–2102, 2020.

[17] H. Wen, S. Zhu, C. Li, Z. Chen, H. Yang, and Y. Xu, "Antegrade intramedullary nail versus plate fixation in the treatment of humeral shaft fractures: an update meta-analysis," *Medicine (Baltimore)*, vol. 98, no. 46, Article ID e17952, 2019.

[18] J. X. Ma, D. Xing, X. L. Ma et al., "Intramedullary nail versus dynamic compression plate fixation in treating humeral shaft fractures: grading the evidence through a meta-analysis," *PLoS One*, vol. 8, no. 12, Article ID e82075, 2013.

[19] M. M. Kivi, M. Soleymanha, and Z. Haghparast-Ghadim-Limudahi, "Treatment outcome of intramedullary fixation with a locked rigid nail in humeral shaft fractures," *The archives of bone and joint surgery*, vol. 4, no. 1, pp. 47–51, 2016.

[20] E. Benegas, D. T. Amódio, L. F. M. Correia et al., "Estudo comparativo prospectivo e randomizado entre o tratamento cir_urgico das fraturas diafisárias do _umero com placa em ponte e haste intramedular bloqueada (análise preliminar)," *Acta Ortopédica Brasileira*, vol. 15, pp. 87–92, 2007.

[21] A. B. Putti, R. B. Uppin, and B. B. Putti, "Locked intramedullary nailing versus dynamic compression plating for humeral shaft fractures," *Journal of Orthopaedic Surgery*, vol. 17, pp. 139–141, 2009.

[22] Y. Fan, Y. W. Li, H. B. Zhang et al., "Management of humeral shaft fractures with intramedullary interlocking nail versus locking compression plate," *Orthopedics*, vol. 38, pp. e825–9, 2015.

[23] M. S. Kassem, E. Morsi, K. L. El-Adwar, and B. A. Motawea, "Minimally invasive plate osteosynthesis versus intramedullary nailing for fixation of humeral shaft fractures in adults," *Journal of Orthopaedics and Sports Medicine*, vol. 3, pp. 019–027, 2021.

[24] M. Bisaccia, L. Meccariello, G. Rinonapoli et al., "Comparison of plate, nail and external fixation in the management of diaphyseal fractures of the humerus," *Medical Archives*, vol. 71, pp. 97–102, 2017.

[25] G. Davies, G. Yeo, M. Meta, D. Miller, E. Hohmann, and K. Tetsworth, "Case-match controlled comparison of minimally invasive plate osteosynthesis and intramedullary nailing for the stabilization of humeral shaft fractures," *Journal of Orthopaedic Trauma*, vol. 30, pp. 612–617, 2016.

23

Operative Fixation of Pediatric Forearm Fractures: Does the Fracture Location Matter?

Ahmed Elabd [ID],[1] Ramy Khalifa,[2] Zainab Alam,[2] Ehab S. Saleh,[3] Ahmed M Thabet,[2] and Amr Abdelgawad [ID][4]

[1]Department of Orthopaedic Surgery, Medstar Washington Hospital Center, Washington, DC, USA
[2]Department of Orthopaedic Surgery and Rehabilitation, TTUHSC-El Paso, Paul L. Foster SOM, Elpaso, TX, USA
[3]Department of Orthopaedic Surgery, Oakland University William Beaumont School of Medicine, Rochester, MI, USA
[4]Department of Orthopaedic Surgery, Maimonides Medical Center, Brooklyn, NY11204, USA

Correspondence should be addressed to Amr Abdelgawad; amratef@doctor.com

Academic Editor: Francesco Liuzza

Background. Flexible intramedullary nails (FNs) are successfully used to treat pediatric forearm fractures, especially midshaft fractures. Distal forearm fractures have been described as "difficult to manage" with FN insertion. The purpose of this study was to report the clinical and radiographic outcomes of using flexible nails in pediatric forearm fractures and the impact of fracture location on the outcome of the procedure. *Methods.* This is a retrospective review of pediatric patients who presented with forearm fractures that were surgically treated with flexible nails between 2009 and 2018. Patient demographics, fracture location, and classification were reported. Intraoperative and postoperative complications were reported. The primary outcomes were fracture radiographic union, intraop and postop complications, and the need for additional surgical procedures. *Results.* Fifty-nine patients were included, with a mean age of 11 years. All fractures healed with patients regaining full range of motion. The authors were able to use flexible nails successfully in 48/59 (81%) patients. In eleven cases (19%), FN fixation was not able to provide adequate fixation to maintain reduction. The method of fixation was changed from FN insertion to another method in nine cases. In two cases, FN fixation was augmented with another fixation method. Fractures within 3 inches of the distal articular surface were at a higher risk of intraoperative change/augmentation of the fixation method (29%) compared with fractures that occurred more than 3 inches from the distal articular surface (11%). *Conclusion.* The majority of pediatric forearm fractures can be treated successfully with flexible nails. Surgeons involved in treating these fractures should pay attention to distal third fractures. Stabilizing the distally located fractures using FN fixation can be challenging. Surgeons should be prepared to use an alternative fixation method when needed.

1. Introduction

Forearm fractures are common fractures among the pediatric population. They account for approximately 18% of all pediatric fractures [1]. Traditionally, these fractures have been treated with closed reduction and casting. Recently, there is an increasing trend toward operative treatment to avoid the complications associated with nonoperative treatment including malunion, loss of reduction, and limited forearm rotation [2]. The operative indications include open fractures, failure to obtain or maintain adequate closed reduction, compartment syndrome, floating elbow, and displaced fractures in older children near skeletal maturity [3].

Flexible nail (FN) has been successfully used as a fixation method for pediatric forearm fractures [4]. Schmittenbecher reported the effect on fracture location on the outcome of using FN in pediatric forearm fractures. The authors reported that the distally located pediatric forearm fractures were more prone to loss of reduction compared with the diaphyseal and proximal pediatric forearm fractures. This may be attributed to the distal radial fragment usually being too short to be sufficiently held by the nail. The larger medullary canal will not be adequately filled with the FN to maintain the reduction [5]. Other authors have proposed that FN fixation is not a good option for distal forearm fractures [6, 7]. Other alternative fixation methods include plating, percutaneous Kirschner wire (K-wire) osteosynthesis, and external fixation.

The purpose of this study was to report the clinical and radiographic outcomes of using flexible nails in pediatric forearm fractures and the effect of fracture location on the use of flexible nails in distal third fractures.

2. Materials and Methods

The study was an institutional review board (IRB) approved, retrospective chart, and radiograph review of all pediatric forearm fractures. The study included all operatively treated at forearm fractures at level I pediatric trauma center between 2009 and 2018. The study group included all patients aged between 7 and 18 years treated with surgical fixation of forearm fractures. Exclusion criteria were patients older than 18 years or those who were primarily treated with other fixation methods. The study variables included patient demographics, time to surgery, operating surgeon, and operative reports. Radiographs were reviewed for fracture characteristics: fractured bone (radius, ulna, or both); fracture location; and fracture type (open or closed). Distal third fractures were defined as fractures that occur within 3 inches from the distal articular surface. Intraoperative variables included method of fixation and type of reduction (open or closed). The majority of forearm fractures at our institution were treated nonoperatively by closed reduction and castings. Nearly all fractures in children under the age of eight years are treated by closed reduction and casting. Operative fixation was only indicated for fractures that we were unable to obtain and/or maintain acceptable reduction by closed means, most displaced fractures in patients older than 11 years in female or 13 years in male (much less remodeling potential), open fractures, and floating elbow [3].

The primary outcomes were fracture radiographic union, intraop and postop complications, and the need for additional surgical procedures. Acceptable reduction was dependent on the patient age. For patients older than 8 years, our limit for accepted reduction was 15° angulation for distal shaft fractures, 10° for more proximal fractures, and 50% apposition [8]. The need for open reduction to restore fracture alignment was reported. All operations were performed by two surgeons who were fellowship-trained in both orthopedic trauma and pediatric orthopedics.

2.1. Surgical Technique. All surgical interventions were done under general anesthesia. The entry point for the distal radius was the dorso lateral aspect of the radius just proximal to the distal radius physis (which was identified by fluoroscopy. Deep dissection was in-between the first and second dorsal compartment. A drill hole was performed proximal to the distal radius, and the hole was enlarged using an awl. A flexible nail (2 or 2.5 mm depending on the patient age/size) was introduced in a retrograde fashion. A trial of closed reduction was done by gentle traction and gentle

manipulation. If the reduction and nail passage were not achieved using few trials, open reduction of the fracture was done using a small incision centered over the fracture. Two bone clamps were used to reduce the fracture, and then the nail was passed from one side to the other. If reduction could not be maintained using FN fixation (more than 50% overlap), the surgeon either decided to add another FN to maintain better reduction, add crossing K-wire fixation, or abandon the FN and use plate fixation. This decision to augment or change the fixation method was considered "additional surgical procedure." After radius fixation, the ulnar fracture was assessed. If it was reduced and stable, it was not surgically fixed. If, on the contrary, the ulnar fracture was still displaced and/or unstable, ulnar fixation using antegrade nailing was done. Small incision was done distal to the ulnar physis (physeal sparing), and then FN was passed from the proximal to distal end of the fracture.

2.2. Statistical Analysis. Quantitative variables were described using means and standard deviations. Categorical variables were described using frequencies and proportions. Student's t-test and the chi-squared test were used to assess differences in changes of fixation methods. Linear regression models with the Poisson family and link log were used to assess the unadjusted association between change in fixation and selected cofactors. These were reported as prevalence ratios (PRs) and 95% confidence intervals (CIs). A P value < 0.05 was considered statistically significant. All analyses were conducted using Stata 15 (StataCorp LLC, College Station, Texas, USA). The statistical work was reviewed by the Statistical Department of the School of Medicine to ensure correct methodology.

3. Results

This study included 59 patients (42 male and 17 female patients) with 59 fractures. The mean patient age at the time of surgery was 11 years (range: 7–16 years). The fracture location was the distal third in 24 fractures (41%), and 35 fractures were in the middle and proximal (59%). According to the Gustilo–Anderson classification, six (10%) of the fractures were open fractures: type I (5/59) and type II (1/59). The time from injury to surgical intervention was an average of 3 days (range: 0–18 days).

Forty-eight (81%) of the 59 procedures were successfully completed using FN insertion (requiring either closed or open reduction). The surgeons' satisfaction with the reduction quality and stability was recorded in the operative reports. Among the 48 cases, 22 (46%) entailed closed reduction, and 26 (54%) required open reduction of at least one bone.

Eleven (19%) of the 59 cases who required either a change of the method of fixation or augmentation of the FN fixation of the radius were identified. Among nine of the 11 cases, the method of fixation was changed intraoperatively to plate fixation in eight cases (Figure 1) and K-wire fixation in one. In the remaining two cases, the surgeon augmented the FN fixation because the reduction continued to be displaced

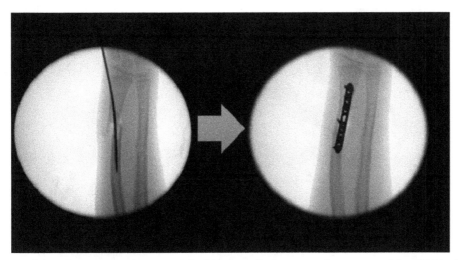

Figure 1: Intraoperative fluoroscopic images showing residual fracture displacement after passage of the FN. The fixation method was changed to plate fixation, and anatomical reduction was obtained.

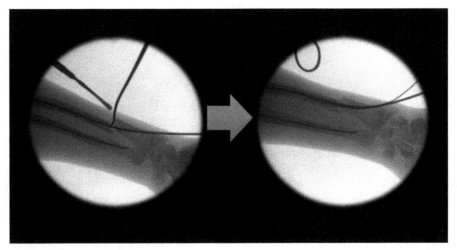

Figure 2: Intraoperative fluoroscopic images showing residual fracture displacement after passage of the FN. Augmentation of fixation was pursued with another FN.

with single FN. The augmentation was accomplished with another small nail in one case (2 nails across the fracture) (Figure 2) and with crossing K-wires in the other (Figure 3).

Seven out of these 11 cases (64%) were located at the distal third of the shaft. This represented 29% of distal forearm fractures (7 out of 24). Four of the 11 cases (34%) that required further intervention were located more than 3 inches from the distal articular surface (mid/proximal shaft fractures). These 4 cases represented only 11% of the mid/proximal shaft fractures (4 out of 35). All cases which required change/augmentation were related to the radius bone. A summary of the results is presented in Table 1.

The findings of statistical analysis of variables in relation to changing the method of fixation from FN insertion to other methods were reported as PR, 95% CI, and P values. Age and fracture classification had no statistically significant relation to intraoperative failure. Fractures within 3 inches of the distal articular surface were at a higher risk of intraoperative change/augmentation of the fixation method

(29%) compared with fractures that occurred more than 3 inches from the distal articular surface (11%) (PR = 1.28; CI: 1.06–1.56; $P = 0.012$).

4. Discussion

Forearm fractures in children are a common reason for emergency department visits [1]. Most pediatric forearm fractures are treated nonoperatively with closed reduction and immobilization with a cast or splint [9, 10]. Operative fixation is indicated for certain fractures [3, 8]. Fixation options include FN fixation, small-fragment plate fixation, and K-wire fixation [11]. FN insertion is becoming more popular because of the less invasive nature of the procedure, shorter operative time, and excellent functional outcomes [1, 4].

The current study has an important finding that the distally located fracture is more prone to reduction difficulty or even failure when fixation with FN was elected as the

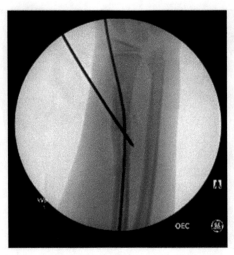

FIGURE 3: Intraoperative fluoroscopic image showing fixation augmentation with a K-wire.

TABLE 1: Summary of the results.

N	Successful	Further intervention	Total	Success (%)	Failure (%)
Distal 1/3	17	7	24	71	29
Proximal 2/3	31	4	35	89	11
Total	48	11	59	81	19

fixation method compared to other radius fractures in the pediatric population. In the current study, all fractures healed with few complications. All patients returned back to preoperative activity levels. No additional surgical procedures were needed. The majority of fractures (81%) were successfully stabilized intraoperatively with FN insertion as preoperatively planned. However, the surgeons needed to change or augment the method of fixation in approximately one-fifth of the patients, 19%. The change to different fixation methods or augmentation represents the inability of the single FN to maintain the reduction. The change of the fixation method occurred more in distal third fractures (29%). This important finding was echoed by other authors [5, 7, 12, 13]. Cai et al. [12] described the distal radial metaphyseal fractures as "difficult to manage" because of the geometry of that area. In the classic intramedullary nailing practice, the entry point is close to the fracture plane, and the elasticity of the nail usually pushes the proximal fragment toward the contralateral side, thereby potentially leading to angulation and malalignment. Additionally, Kim et al. [13] studied FN insertion as a method of fixation of distal metadiaphyseal junction forearm fractures in adolescents. They determined that the minimal distance between the fracture line and the distal articular surface should be > 3.5 cm for FN fixation to be considered. If a fracture site was located ≤3.5 cm from the physis, it was considered unsuitable for FN insertion.

The current study showed that the use of FN insertion to treat pediatric forearm fractures is not a panacea, especially for fractures of the distal part of the shaft. Inability to use the flexible nails to maintain reduction in nearly one-third of the distally located fractures (29%) was observed. By reviewing the operative reports and intraoperative fluoroscopic images, we tried to identify the possible causes of failure. In some cases, after insertion of the FN, the fracture was still notably displaced (Figures 1 and 2) with minimal apposition. The remaining displacement was because of the distal location of the fracture with a wide medulla, the progression of the fracture line from the insertion point to the original fracture, or the marked fracture comminution—either traumatic or iatrogenic—from the repeated trial of reduction and nail insertion.

Moreover, some authors have described distal forearm fractures as not optimum for FN [5, 7]. In 2005, Schmittenbecher [5] evaluated the treatment procedures, problems, complications, and final results of pediatric forearm fractures going back to 1976. Successful treatment of these fractures depends on the selection of the correct treatment modality. It is not only the decision between nonoperative and operative treatment but also the choice of the implant. Schmittenbecher indicated that the FN is the first choice for midshaft and proximal fractures; however, K-wires are often preferred in distal diaphyseal or diaphyseal-metaphyseal fractures. It is acceptable if the surgeon considers plate fixation as the primary treatment in females who have started menstrual periods and in males older than 13 years. Slongo [7] discussed the complications and failures associated with the FN technique, addressing system-related and fracture-related problems separately. The main causes of FN failure when used to treat forearm fractures were small nail diameter and lack of correct tensioning of the two nails against each other. However, the greatest problems occurred when the FN was inappropriately used for radial fractures in the distal third and metaphyseal regions. Slongo considered those fractures not ideal indications for FN insertion. Recently, Du and Han [14] introduced a new operative approach to treat irreducible distal radius fracture in

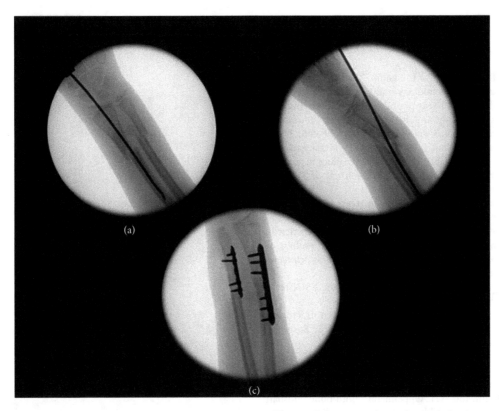

FIGURE 4: (a, b) Intraoperative fluoroscopic images showing two views of flexion deformity and translation at the fracture site induced by ulnar entry of the FN. (c) Intraoperative fluoroscopic image showing the change of the fixation method to plate osteosynthesis.

the diaphyseal-metaphyseal junction with satisfactory outcomes. They used antegrade FN technique from the proximal radius with an entry point located 2.4 cm distal to the proximal articular surface of the radius at the dorsolateral aspect (Thompson approach). The authors noted that the classic retrograde insertion of FN is not possible for distal fractures [15].

It is worth noting that the failure of FN fixation to maintain reduction of the distal forearm fracture was described in the *Nancy University Manual*, in which this form of treatment was first introduced to orthopedic surgeons [15]. The authors of the manual noted that when the FN is introduced from its usual dorsoradial entry point in a distal fracture, it displaces the fracture, very similar to our findings. For this reason, they advised against using this entry point and recommended an ulnar entry point for these distal fractures. Using the modified entry point, in our experience, did not completely solve the problem of fracture displacement in all cases because doing so can cause flexion of the distal fragment in exchange for correcting the coronal alignment problems associated with using the radial entry point (Figure 4).

All operations were performed by two surgeons who were fellowship-trained in both orthopedic trauma and pediatric orthopedics. Failure to maintain satisfactory reduction is therefore not likely to be attributable to the lack of surgical training or knowledge. Our current approach to the distal third of the radius and ulnar fractures is a single trial of fixation using an FN. If, after the passage of the nail, the fracture is still significantly displaced, plate fixation should be considered.

The main limitation of our study is the retrospective nature of the study and small number in each group. However, even with the relatively small number of each group, the authors were able to find a statistically and clinically significant impact of fractures' location on using FN in pediatric forearm fractures.

5. Conclusions

The majority of pediatric forearm fractures can be treated successfully with flexible nails. Surgeons involved in treating these fractures should pay attention to distal third fractures. Stabilizing the distally located fractures using FN fixation can be challenging. The study results show that FN fixation of distally located forearm fractures (compared with proximal and midshaft fractures) has a higher chance of inability to maintain fracture reduction requiring utilization of another fixation method. Surgeons planning to use FN in distal forearm fractures should be prepared to use an alternative fixation method.

Acknowledgments

The authors thank Dori Kelly, MA, for professional manuscript editing.

References

[1] S. M. Naranje, R. A. Erali, W. C. Warner, J. R. Sawyer, and D. M. Kelly, "Epidemiology of pediatric fractures presenting to emergency departments in the United States," *Journal of Pediatric Orthopaedics*, vol. 36, no. 4, pp. e45–e48, 2016.

[2] J. M. Flynn, K. J. Jones, M. R. Garner, and J. Goebel, "Eleven years experience in the operative management of pediatric forearm fractures," *Journal of Pediatric Orthopaedics*, vol. 30, no. 4, pp. 313–319, 2010.

[3] A. Lyman, D. Wenger, and L. Landin, "Pediatric diaphyseal forearm fractures: epidemiology and treatment in an urban population during a 10-year period, with special attention to titanium elastic nailing and its complications," *Journal of Pediatric Orthopaedics B*, vol. 25, no. 5, pp. 439–446, 2016.

[4] P. Lascombes, J. Prevot, J. N. Ligier, J. P. Metaizeau, and T. Poncelet, "Elastic stable intramedullary nailing in forearm shaft fractures in children: 85 cases," *Journal of Pediatric Orthopaedics*, vol. 10, no. 2, pp. 167–171, 1990.

[5] P. P. Schmittenbecher, "State-of-the-art treatment of forearm shaft fractures," *Injury*, vol. 36, pp. A25–A34, 2005.

[6] F. F. Fernandez, M. Langendörfer, T. Wirth, and O. Eberhardt, "Failures and complications in intramedullary nailing of children's forearm fractures," *Journal of children's orthopaedics*, vol. 4, no. 2, pp. 159–167, 2010.

[7] T. F. Slongo, "Complications and failures of the ESIN technique," *Injury*, vol. 36, pp. A78–A85, 2005.

[8] J. L. Pace, "Pediatric and adolescent forearm fractures," *Journal of the American Academy of Orthopaedic Surgeons*, vol. 24, no. 11, pp. 780–788, 2016.

[9] C. T. Price, D. S. Scott, M. E. Kurzner, and J. C. Flynn, "Malunited forearm fractures in children," *Journal of Pediatric Orthopaedics*, vol. 10, no. 6, pp. 705–712, 1990.

[10] S. Kay, C. Smith, and W. L. Oppenheim, "Both-bone midshaft forearm fractures in children," *Journal of Pediatric Orthopaedics*, vol. 6, no. 3, pp. 306–310, 1986.

[11] C. C. Franklin, J. Robinson, K. Noonan, and J. M. Flynn, "Evidence-based medicine," *Journal of Pediatric Orthopaedics*, vol. 32, pp. S131–S134, 2012.

[12] H. Cai, Z. Wang, and H. Cai, "Fixation of distal radial epiphyseal fracture: comparison of K-wire and prebent intramedullary nail," *Journal of International Medical Research*, vol. 44, no. 1, pp. 122–130, 2016.

[13] B. S. Kim, Y. S. Lee, S. Y. Park, J. H. Nho, S. G. Lee, and Y. H. Kim, "Flexible intramedullary nailing of forearm fractures at the distal metadiaphyseal junction in adolescents," *Clinics in orthopedic surgery*, vol. 9, no. 1, p. 101, 2017.

[14] M. Du and J. Han, "Antegrade elastic stable intramedullary nail fixation for paediatric distal radius diaphyseal metaphyseal junction fractures: a new operative approach," *Injury*, vol. 50, no. 2, pp. 598–601, 2019.

[15] P. Lascombes and T. Haumont, "Both-bone forearm fracture," in *Flexible Intramedullary Nailing in Children: The Nancy University Manual*, P. Lascombes, Ed., Springer, Berlin, Germany, 2010.

24

New System for the Classification of Epiphyseal Separation of the Coracoid Process: Evaluation of Nine Cases and Review of the Literature

Takamitsu Mondori ⓘ,[1] Yoshiyuki Nakagawa,[1] Shimpei Kurata,[2] Shuhei Fujii,[3] Takuya Egawa,[4] Kazuya Inoue,[2] and Yasuhito Tanaka[2]

[1]*Department of Orthopaedics, Uda City Hospital, Nara Shoulder & Elbow Center, 815 Hagiwara, Haibara, Uda, Nara 633-0298, Japan*
[2]*Department of Orthopaedics, Nara Medical University, 840 Shijyo, Kashihara, Nara 634-8521, Japan*
[3]*Department of Orthopaedics, Nara Prefecture Seiwa Medical Center, 1-14-16 Mimuro, Sangou-cho, Ikoma-gun, Nara 636-0802, Japan*
[4]*Department of Orthopaedics, Okanami General Hospital, 1734 Ueno Kuwamachi, Iga, Mie 518-0842, Japan*

Correspondence should be addressed to Takamitsu Mondori; mondori3@hotmail.com

Academic Editor: Benjamin Blondel

Objectives and Design. Epiphyseal separation of the coracoid process (CP) rarely occurs in adolescents. In this retrospective case series, we reviewed the data of nine patients treated at our center and those of 28 patients reported in the literature. This injury can be classified into three types according to the injured area: Type I, base including the area above the glenoid; Type II, center including the coracoclavicular ligament (CCL); and Type III, tip with the short head of the biceps and coracobrachialis, as well as the pectoralis minor. *Patients/Participants.* A total of 37 patients were included in the analysis. Data on sex, age, cause and mechanism of injury, separation type, concomitant injury around the shoulder girdle, treatment, and functional outcomes were obtained. *Main Outcome Measurements and Results.* Type I is the most common type. The cause of injury and associated injury around the shoulder girdle were significantly different between Type I, II, and III fractures. The associated acromioclavicular (AC) dislocation and treatment were significantly different between Type I and III fractures. Our new classification system reflects the clinical features, imaging findings, and surgical management of epiphyseal separation of the CP. Type I and II fractures are mostly associated with AC dislocation and have an associated injury around the shoulder girdle. Type III fractures are typically caused by forceful resisted flexion of the arm and elbow. Although the latter are best managed surgically, whether conservative or surgical management is optimal for Type I and II fractures remains controversial. *Conclusions.* We noted some differences in the clinical characteristics depending on the location of injury; therefore, we aimed to examine these differences to develop a new system for classifying epiphyseal separation of the CP. This would increase the clinicians' awareness regarding this injury and lead to the development of an appropriate treatment.

1. Introduction

Fractures of the coracoid process (CP) do not commonly occur, accounting for only 2%–13% of all scapular fractures and approximately 1% of all fractures [1–4]. The epiphyseal separation of the CP in the adolescent is even more uncommon [5, 6], with few cases reported in the literature [1, 4, 7–26]. This injury can complicate acromioclavicular (AC) dislocations and fractures of the coracoid in adults. Although a diagnosis of AC dislocation is easily made, the epiphyseal separation of the CP may be overlooked due to the complexity of the anatomical structures and superimposition on standard shoulder radiographs. Misdiagnosis of isolated AC dislocation, which is mainly due to damage of the coracoclavicular ligament (CCL), has a profound influence on the choice of treatment and prognosis. In order to establish an accurate diagnosis of epiphyseal separation of the CP, clinicians must have a good understanding of the pathophysiology of this injury and the location of the epiphyseal line of the CP. Therefore, the appropriate classification of this injury is necessary. Although several classification systems for coracoid fractures in adults have been proposed from previous studies, there is no available system for classifying epiphyseal separation of the CP in adolescents.

2. Objectives

The aim of this study was to examine the clinical characteristics associated with epiphyseal separation of the CP and propose a new classification system for this condition.

3. Materials and Methods

3.1. Participant Recruitment. The epiphyses of the coracoid close as the child reaches the age of 17–25 [11, 27]. Therefore, we recruited all published cases of patients aged below 17 years or over whose computed tomography (CT) images clearly revealed epiphyseal lesions as cases of adolescent epiphyseal separation of the CP. We retrospectively reviewed nine patients who were treated at our center and the data of 28 published cases, and we found that epiphyseal separation of the CP differs depending on the location of the injury. We hypothesized that each site may have its own characteristics. Nine patients with epiphyseal separation of the CP were treated immediately after obtaining an injury at our center between 1989 and 2019 (Table 1). All patients underwent follow-up examinations for >1 year and were directly examined at our center at the final observation. All patients were included in this retrospective study, regardless of treatment type or concomitant injuries. Additionally, we identified another 28 cases by review of the literature that provided sufficient case details (Table 2). All procedures performed in studies involving human participants were in accordance with the ethical standards of the 1964 Helsinki Declaration and its later amendments or comparable ethical standards. Informed consent was obtained from all study participants. This study was approved by the Ethics Committee of Uda City Hospital (approval number: R2-002).

3.2. Data Extraction and Analysis. The medical records from our center and previously published studies were retrospectively reviewed to extract the data regarding sex, age, cause and mechanism of injury, separation type, concomitant injury around the shoulder girdle, treatment, and functional outcomes.

In these 37 patients, separation occurred at the base of the CP. The separation occurred above the glenoid in 28 (76%) patients, at the center with CCL in 6 (16%), and at the tip of the short head of the biceps and coracobrachialis or the pectoralis minor in 3 (8%). The differences identified in the epiphyseal separation of the CP lesions were classified depending on the location of the injury (Figure 1): Type I,

the base including the area above the glenoid (Figure 2); Type II, the center with CCL (Figure 3); and Type III, the tip including the short head of the biceps and coracobrachialis in addition to the pectoralis minor (Figure 4).

The three types of fractures were compared statistically in terms of sex, age, cause and mechanism of injury, concomitant injury around the shoulder girdle, concomitant AC dislocation, and treatment (surgery or conservative therapy) and functional outcome (excellent, good/fair, or poor).

In this study, the method used for evaluating functional outcome was not standardized. Therefore, with regard to the clinical results at the time of final observation described in the article, the absence of (1) pain, (2) limited range of motion, and (3) inability to return to sports were considered as excellent. If one of the abovementioned items were reported by the patient, the results were considered to be good/fair. If two or more of the abovementioned items were reported by the patient, the results were considered to be poor.

3.3. Statistical Analysis. Statistical analysis was performed using the StatMate IV software for Windows (version IV; ATMS ISBN:978-4-90-430722-9, 2009, Japan). The Kruskal–Wallis test with Bonferroni/Dunn correction was used to compare sex, age, cause and mechanism of injury, concomitant injury around the shoulder girdle, concomitant AC dislocation, treatment, and functional outcomes; the chi-square test or Fisher's exact test was used to compare sex, cause and mechanism of injury, concomitant injury around the shoulder girdle, concomitant AC dislocation, treatment, and functional outcomes.

4. Results

The average age at the time of injury was 14.4 years (Type I, 14.0 years; Type II, 15.7 years; Type III, 16.7 years). Among the total population, except for one example that was not described, 33 (91.7%) were men and three (8.3%) were women. In cases of Type I injury, 21 (75%) patients had associated injuries around the shoulder girdle with the following breakdown: 19 (90.4%), AC dislocation; 1 (4.8%), clavicle distal end fracture; and 1 (4.8%), a combination of lateral clavicular epiphyseal separation and rupture of the CCL. In Type II, five patients had associated injuries around the shoulder girdle, of whom four (80%) had AC dislocation and one (20%) had double fracture of the clavicle. All Type III cases were isolated injuries.

In the Type I group, the mechanism of injury in three patients was unknown. Among the patients whose mechanism of injury was identified, 14 (56%) experienced falling on the shoulder, 8 (32%) had a direct trauma to the shoulder, and 3 (12%) had forceful resisted flexion of the arm and elbow. In Type II, the mechanism of injury was unknown in one patient; among the patients with known mechanism of injury, falling on the shoulder was reported in four (80%) and direct trauma to the shoulder in one (20%). All cases of Type III injury were caused by forceful resisted flexion of the arm and elbow. Conservative treatment was carried out in 21

TABLE 1: Characteristics of patients with epiphyseal separation of the coracoid process treated in our center.

	Location of separation	Age	Sex	Cause of injury	Mechanism of injury	Associated injury*	Treatment	Functional outcome
1	Base (I)	15	M	Fall	Fall on the shoulder	AC dislocation (II)	ACJ: K-wiring coracoid: screw fixation	Excellent
2	Base (I)	15	M	Fall from bicycle	Fall on the shoulder	AC dislocation (II)	Conservative (sling 4 weeks)	Excellent
3	Base (I)	14	M	Rugby	Direct trauma by tackle	AC dislocation (III)	Conservative (sling 4 weeks)	Excellent
4	Base (I)	11	M	Fall	Fall on the shoulder	Clavicle distal end fixation	Coracoid: screw fixation	Excellent
5	Base (I)	14	M	Soccer	Fall on the shoulder	AC dislocation (III)	ACJ: K-wiring coracoid: screw fixation	Excellent
6	Base (I)	11	F	Judo	Fall on the shoulder	AC dislocation (III)	ACJ: K-wiring coracoid: screw fixation	Excellent
7	Base (I)	16	M	Fall	Fall on the shoulder	AC dislocation (III)	Conservative (sling 4 weeks)	Excellent
8	Center (II)	16	M	Motorcycle	Fall on the shoulder	Clavicle double fixation	Clavicle: K-wire and soft wire fixation	Good after infection
9	Center (II)	17	M	Motorcycle	Fall on the shoulder	AC dislocation (II)	Conservative (sling 4 weeks)	Excellent

AC, acromioclavicular; ACJ, acromioclavicular joint; F, female; M, male. *The numbers in parentheses indicate the grade of AC dislocation (II: subluxation of AC joint; III: complete dislocation of AC joint).

TABLE 2: Characteristics of patients with epiphyseal separation of the coracoid process identified from the literature review.

	Location of separation	Publish year	Author	Age	Sex	Cause of injury	Mechanism of injury	Associated injury*	Treatment	Functional outcome
1	Tip (III)	1971	Benton J	19	M	Tennis	Overuse or forceful resisted flexion of the arm	—	Conjoined tendon reattach	Excellent
2	Base (I)	1975	Protass JJ	17	M	Football	Unknown	AC dislocation (III)	Conservative	Unknown
3	Base (I)	1975	Protass JJ	14	M	Fall off the bicycle	Unknown	AC dislocation (II)	Conservative	Unknown
4	Center (II)	1977	Montgomery SP	15	M	Football	Fall on the shoulder	AC dislocation (III)	Epiphysis reattached by a nonabsorbable suture	Excellent
5	Center (II)	1977	Montgomery SP	15	M	Bike accident	Unknown	AC dislocation (III)	Conservative (sling 4 weeks)	Poor
6	Base (I)	1982	Bernard TN	13	M	Football	Direct trauma	AC dislocation (III)	Conservative (AC immobilizer 4 weeks)	Excellent
7	Base (I)	1982	Bernard TN	15	M	Football	Fall on the shoulder	AC dislocation (III)	Conservative (AC immobilizer 6 weeks)	Excellent
8	Base (I)	1982	Bernard TN	17	M	Motorcycle	Direct trauma	AC dislocation (III)	ACJ: K-wiring, coracoid: screw fixation	Good
9	Base (I)	1986	Taga I	9	F	Unknown	Unknown	—	Conservative (Velpeau bandage 4 weeks)	Excellent
10	Base (I)	1990	Martin-Herrero T	16	M	Free skating	Forceful resisted flexion of the arm	AC dislocation (III)	Conservative (Desault bandage 4 weeks)	Excellent

Table 2: Continued.

	Location of separation	Publish year	Author	Age	Sex	Cause of injury	Mechanism of injury	Associated injury*	Treatment	Functional outcome
11	Base (I)	1990	Martin-Herrero T	17	M	Judo	Fall on the shoulder	AC dislocation (?)	Conservative (Watson–Jones bandage 3 weeks)	Excellent
12	Base (I)	1995	Combalia A	12	M	Soccer	Fall on the shoulder	AC dislocation (III)	Conservative (Robert–Jones bandage 4 weeks)	Excellent
13	Base (I)	1995	Eyres KS	17	M	Folk-lift overturn	Trapping the arm	AC dislocation (III)	Conservative (broad arm sling)	Unknown
14	Base (I)	1996	Cottalorda J	15	M	Judo	Fall on the shoulder	—	Conservative	Excellent
15	Base (I)	1998	Holst AK	13	M	Fall	Fall on the shoulder	—	Conservative (broad arm sling 2 weeks)	Excellent
16	Base (I)	1999	Naraen A	11	M	Archery	Overuse or forceful resisted flexion of the arm	—	Conservative (sling 2 weeks)	Excellent
17	Base (I)	2009	Dipaora M	15	M	American football	Direct trauma by tackle	AC dislocation (II)	Conservative (sling)	Excellent
18	Center (II)	2009	Leijnen M	16	M	Fall off motorcycle	Fall on the shoulder	—	Conservative	Excellent
19	Base (I)	2010	Jettoo P	12	M	Fall from high place	Fall on the shoulder	AC dislocation (III)	ACJ: K-wiring coracoid: screw fixation	Excellent
20	Tip (III)	2011	Nakama K	16	M	Gymnastic (frying ring)	Overuse or forceful resisted flexion of the arm	—	Coracoid: screw fixation	Excellent
21	Base (I)	2012	Alsey KJ	14	?	Rugby	Direct trauma by tackle	—	Conservative (sling 4 weeks)	Excellent
22	Base (I)	2012	Chitre AR	13	M	Ski	Fall on the shoulder	—	Conservative	Excellent
23	Base (I)	2012	Chitre AR	15	M	Wheelbarrow race	Fall on the shoulder	—	Conservative	Excellent
24	Base (I)	2014	Pedersen V	14	M	Ice-hockey	Direct trauma by tackle	AC dislocation (II)	Conservative (sling)	Excellent
25	Center (II)	2016	Ito T	15	F	Judo	Direct trauma	AC dislocation (III)	ACJ: K-wiring coracoid: soft anchor fixation	Excellent
26	Tip (III)	2016	Archik S	15	M	Cricket	Overuse or forceful resisted flexion of the arm	—	Coracoid: screw fixation	Excellent
27	Base (I)	2018	Cross GWV	15	M	Rugby tackled violently	Direct trauma by tackle	AC dislocation (III)	Conservative (sling)	Excellent
28	Base (I)	2019	Duerr RA	12	M	Scooter accident	Direct trauma to the superolateral shoulder	Epiphyseal separation of the distal clavicle, CCL tear (triple injury)	Coracoid: screw fixation CCL and ACL repair	Excellent

AC, acromioclavicular; ACJ, acromioclavicular joint; CCL, coracoclavicular ligament; F, female; M, male. *The numbers in parentheses indicate the grade of AC dislocation (II: subluxation of AC joint; III: complete dislocation of AC joint; ?: unidentified).

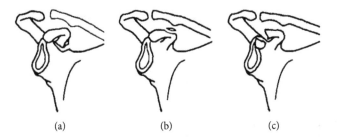

(a)   (b)   (c)

FIGURE 1: The proposed classification of epiphyseal separation of the coracoid process along with the anteroposterior radiograph and/or three-dimensional computed tomography reconstruction. Type I: the base including the area above the glenoid; Type II: the center with the coracoclavicular ligament; and Type III: the tip including the short head of the biceps and coracobrachialis, in addition to the pectoralis minor.

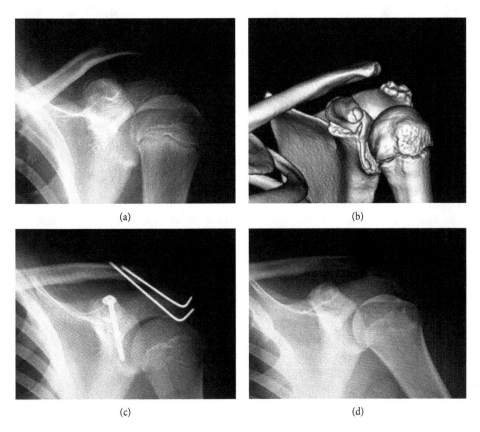

(a)   (b)

(c)   (d)

FIGURE 2: Case 6: representative anteroposterior radiograph: (a) three-dimensional computed tomography reconstruction and (b) Type I injury with an associated acromioclavicular dislocation. Anteroposterior radiograph immediately after the surgery (c) and anteroposterior radiograph three years after the surgery (d).

(75%) patients with Type I injury, and surgical therapy was administered in 7 (25%) patients. All surgical cases of Type I injury associated with AC dislocation were repaired by screw fixation of the coracoid and AC joint using a Kirschner wire (K-wire). The functional outcomes were good or excellent for both methods. For Type II injuries, conservative treatment was used in four (66.7%) patients, and surgery was performed in two (33.3%). In the Type II group, one of the four (25%) patients treated conservatively had a poor functional outcome and two (100%) patients who underwent surgery showed an excellent functional outcome. Surgical therapy was used in all patients with Type III injury, with excellent clinical results. The cause of injury and associated

injury around the shoulder girdler were significantly different between Type I, II, and III cases. The associated AC injury and treatment were significantly different between Type I and Type III cases (Table 3).

5. Discussion

Due to the rarity of epiphyseal separation of the CP, clinicians' understanding and knowledge regarding clinical management of this condition is limited [5, 6]. Although epiphyseal separations of the CP are similar to CP fractures in terms of the clinical presentation and mechanism of injury, the imaging features that lead to the diagnosis, the

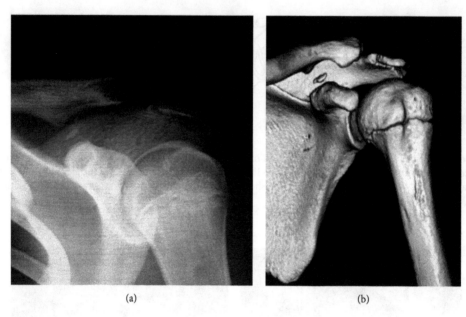

(a)   (b)

FIGURE 3: Representative anteroposterior radiograph of case 9: three-dimensional computed tomography reconstruction (a) and type II injury with an associated acromioclavicular dislocation (b).

healing form, and the prognosis differ depending on the age and the presence or absence of the epiphysis. The coracoid has four (or three) main centers where ossification can occur: the base and body of the process, the center of the process at the point of attachment of the CCL, and the tip [11, 20, 21, 23, 28]. The epiphyseal nucleus of the body of the coracoid appears 1 year after birth, and that of the base of the coracoid appears at the age of 7–10 years; soon it is in unison with the emerged scapula body; therefore, there are three epiphyseal plates between each epiphyseal nucleus [28] (Figure 5). The center of the process is the site of insertion of the CCL [29], while the tip is the site of insertion of the conjoint tendon (the short head of the biceps and coraco-brachialis, as well as the pectoralis minor). During development, the coracoid and epiphyseal plate at the base and tip fuse by the age of 17 years, while the epiphyseal plate at the center fuses by the age of 25 years [11, 27]. Prior to epiphyseal closure, the ligament and muscle attachments are often stronger than the epiphyseal plate. This means that injury to the epiphyseal plate is more common in younger individuals [4, 11, 23, 30]. In this study, three sites were damaged during the epiphyseal separations of the CP, and their positions also corresponded to the three epiphyseal plates.

A number of several classification systems for coracoid fractures in adults have been reported. In 1995, Eyres et al. classified these fractures into five types based on the location of fracture (Type I, tip or epiphyseal fracture; Type II, mid-process; Type III, basal fracture; Type IV, superior body of scapula involved; and Type V, extension into glenoid fossa) [1]. Later, Ogawa et al. proposed a new classification system dividing the CP into two distinct locations based on the CCL attachment: Type I fractures are located behind the liga-ments, while Type II fractures are located in front of the

ligaments [2]. To date, there has been no classification system proposed for epiphyseal separation of the CP in adolescents. Fractures classified as Type I according to our system are equivalent to Type I fractures of Ogawa et al. and Type III, IV, and V fractures of the classification of Eyres et al. Fractures classified as Type II by our system are equivalent to Type II fractures of the system of Ogawa et al. and Type I and II fractures of Eyres et al. However, our Type II classification is not equivalent to any type of previous systems. Although the mechanism of injury for Type II fractures combined with AC dislocation is the same as that of isolated AC dislocation, epiphyseal separation can occur rather than disruption of the CCL in adolescents because the epiphyseal plate is weaker than the CCL.

Epiphyseal separation of the CP is usually diagnosed by obtaining plain shoulder radiographs consisting of three views. Special radiograms are required in order to make a definitive diagnosis: 30° cephalad roentgenogram [7], 45° to 60° cephalad tilt [31], or abduction view that clearly scans the CP without overlapping other bone structures [9, 16]. However, CT, especially three-dimensional CT, and mag-netic resonance imaging are usually necessary because of the limitations of plain radiography [1, 14, 18]. Comparison of CT data from the healthy side may help in the accurate diagnosis of this condition. Duerr et al. [19] reported an exceedingly rare case of combined lateral clavicular epiph-yseal separation (or AC joint dislocation), the base of cor-acoid separation, and rupture of the coracoclavicular ligaments, a so-called "triple injury." In cases of injury I that involves double disruption of the superior shoulder sus-pensory complex in the case of >100% displaced distal clavicle separation, careful scrutiny of radiographs is im-portant to ensure correct identification of the CCL, AC ligament, and other sites. Thus, given the challenges in the

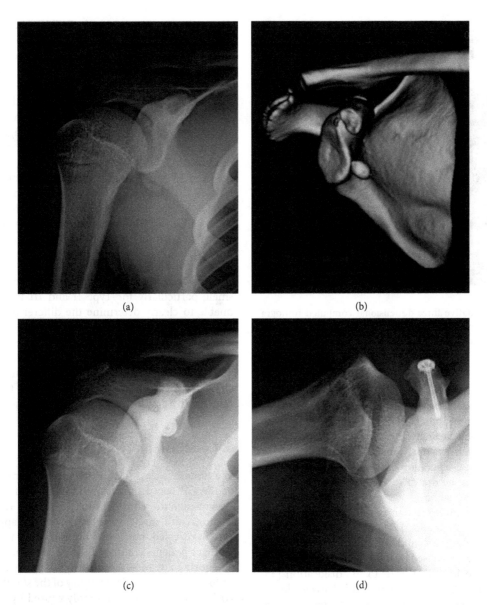

(a)

(b)

(c)

(d)

FIGURE 4: Representative anteroposterior radiograph: three-dimensional computed tomography reconstruction (a), Type III injury (b), anteroposterior radiograph two years postoperatively (c), and axillary radiograph two years postoperatively (d). This image was used with permission from Kurume University Medical Center and Dr. K. Nakama [21].

TABLE 3: Results of statistical analysis.

	Kruskal–Wallis test, Bonferroni/ Dunn correction			Chi-square test/Fisher's exact test		
	I-II	I–III	II-III	I-II	I–III	II-III
Age	NS	NS	NS	—	—	—
Sex (male/female)	NS	NS	NS	NS	NS	NS
Cause of injury	NS	$p < 0.05$	$p < 0.05$	—	—	—
Associated injury around the shoulder girdle (yes/no)	NS	$p < 0.05$	$p < 0.05$	NS	$p < 0.05$	$p < 0.05$
Associated injury AC dislocation (yes/no)	NS	NS	NS	NS	$p < 0.05$	NS
Treatment (surgery/conservative)	NS	$p < 0.05$	NS	NS	$p < 0.05$	NS
Functional outcome (excellent, good/fair, or poor)	NS	NS	NS	NS	0	NS

AC, acromioclavicular; NS, not significant.

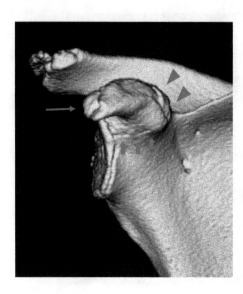

FIGURE 5: Representative three-dimensional computed tomography image of a normal epiphyseal line around the coracoid of an 11-year-old girl. A normal coronoid process has three epiphyseal lines: the base (broad arrows), center (triangular arrows), and tip (narrow arrow).

diagnosis of epiphyseal separation of the CP from imaging investigations, our proposal of classifying these fractures into three types will facilitate the correct diagnosis of this condition from such examinations. By recognizing in advance that epiphyseal separation of the CP can occur in three places, attention can be drawn to the epiphyseal line of the CP when making a diagnosis.

There have been three mechanisms of injury reported for coracoid fractures in adults [14]: direct trauma to the anterolateral aspect of the shoulder [32], direct trauma to the shoulder girdle usually caused by a fall or blow with the arm in the adducted position that leads to AC dislocation [33], and forceful resisted flexion of the arm and elbow leading to a strong pull of the muscles inserting into the coracoid, pectoralis minor, and coracobrachialis [10, 14, 26, 34]. In the present study, most Type I and II injury cases were caused by direct trauma to the anterolateral aspect of the shoulder with involvement of the shoulder girdle; AC dislocation without associated CCL tear accounted for two-thirds of the cases. Interestingly, a clear difference in the mechanism of injury of Types I and II was observed from that of Type III injury. Because Type III injuries occur from overuse or forceful resisted flexion of the arm and elbow [20–22], the factor of fatigue fracture is considered to be involved.

In our center, only Type I and Type II cases were reported. In cases with AC joint dislocation, surgical treatment is recommended because the presence of AC joint dislocation will cause a dysfunction in the future, and conservative treatment is recommended for patients who refused to undergo surgery. Hence, surgery was performed in 3 of 7 patients with AC joint dislocation. The type of surgical procedure performed was the same as that conducted in previous studies, with screw fixation of the coracoid process and percutaneous fixation of the AC joint using a Kirschner

wire. All operative cases had excellent outcomes. All Type I and II patients who have undergone surgery underwent surgical treatment to cure AC joint dislocation in previous studies. However, the review of the literature revealed no clear advantage of surgery over conservative treatment because most patients with Type I and II were treated conservatively with good/excellent outcomes [11, 26]. More studies are required to clarify the advantages or differences in outcomes between surgical treatment and conservative treatment. By contrast, all patients with Type III injuries reported in the literature were treated surgically by reattaching the fragment or conjoined tendon and had good/excellent outcomes. Surgical therapy involving rigid fixation can result in early improvements in the range of motion and return to training and normal physical or sports activities [20–22].

This study has some limitations. The sample size was small, particularly for Type II and III fractures. We were unable to clearly determine the difference between Type I and Type II cases for each item. If the number of Type II cases increases, a difference may be found. The study is retrospective in nature; hence, it was difficult to confirm all images of cases in the literature. In the future, data on the characteristics of this injury according to type must be obtained by conducting a prospective study.

6. Conclusions

We propose a classification system for epiphyseal separation of the CP based on the location of ossification. Our new system includes consideration of clinical features, imaging findings, and surgical management. The application of the system revealed that Type I injuries occur predominantly in younger patients compared with Type II and III. Type I and II injuries are most commonly associated with AC joint dislocation and associated injury of the shoulder girdle. Type III injuries are most commonly caused by forceful resisted flexion of the arm and elbow, and surgical therapy offers the best outcomes. However, the management for Type I and II injuries remains controversial because both approaches appear to be effective. Further investigations are required to ascertain the optimal method.

Acknowledgments

The authors would like to express their deep gratitude to Dr. Kenji Nakama and Dr. Masafumi Goto from the Kurume Medical Center for providing the image presented in Figure 4 and for giving permission to include it.

References

[1] K. S. Eyres, A. Brooks, and D. Stanley, "Fractures of the coracoid process," *Journal of Bone & Joint Surgery*, vol. 77, no. 3, pp. 425–428, 1995.

[2] K. Ogawa, A. Yoshida, M. Takahashi et al., "Fractures of the coracoid process," *Journal of Bone & Joint Surgery*, vol. 79,

no. 1, pp. 17–19, 1997.

[3] J. R. Ada and M. E. Miller, "Scapula fractures: analysis of 113 cases," *Clinical Orthopaedics & Related Research*, vol. 269, pp. 174–180, 1991.

[4] P. Jettoo, G. de Kiewiet, and S. England, "Base of coracoid process fracture with acromioclavicular dislocation in a child," *Journal of Orthopaedic Surgery & Research*, vol. 5, p. 77, 2010.

[5] G. B. Black, J. A. McPherson, and M. H. Reed, "Traumatic pseudodislocation of the acromioclavicular joint in children: a fifteen year review," *American Journal of Sports Medicine*, vol. 19, no. 6, pp. 644–646, 1991.

[6] A. K. Holst and J. V. Christiansen, "Epiphyseal separation of the coracoid process without acromioclavicular dislocation," *Skeletal Radiology*, vol. 27, no. 8, pp. 461-462, 1998.

[7] J. J. Protass, F. V. Stampfli, and J. C. Osmer, "Coracoid process fracture diagnosis in acromioclavicular separation," *Radiology*, vol. 116, no. 1, pp. 61–64, 1975.

[8] T. N. Bernard, M. E. Brunet, and R. J. Haddad, "Fractured coracoid process in acromioclavicular dislocations: report of four cases and review of the literature," *Clinical Orthopaedics & Related Research*, vol. 175, pp. 227–232, 1983.

[9] I. Taga, M. Yoneda, and K. Ono, "Epiphyseal separation of the coracoid process associated with acromioclavicular sprain: a case report and review of the literature," *Clinical Orthopaedics & Related Research*, vol. 207, pp. 138–141, 1986.

[10] T. Martín-Herrero, C. Rodríguez-Merchán, and L. Munuera-Martínez, "Fractures of the coracoid process: presentation of seven cases and review of the literature," *Journal of Trauma*, vol. 30, no. 12, pp. 1597–1599, 1990.

[11] A. Combalía, J. M. Arandes, X. Alemany et al., "Acromioclavicular dislocation with epiphyseal separation of the coracoid process: report of a case and review of the literature," *Journal of Trauma*, vol. 38, no. 5, pp. 812–815, 1995.

[12] J. Cottalorda, D. Allard, N. Dutour et al., "Fracture of the coracoid process in an adolescent," *Injury*, vol. 27, no. 6, pp. 436-437, 1996.

[13] A. Naraen, K. A. Giannikas, and P. J. Livesley, "Overuse epiphyseal injury of the coracoid process as a results of archery," *International Journal of Sports Medicine*, vol. 20, no. 1, pp. 53–55, 1999.

[14] M. DiPaola and P. Marchetto, "Coracoid process fracture with acromioclavicular joint separation in an american football player: a case report and literature review," *American Journal of Orthopedics*, vol. 38, no. 1, pp. 37–39, 2009.

[15] K. J. Alsey, A. N. Mahapatra, and J. H. Jessop, "Coracoid fracture in an adolescent rugby player: a case report and review of the literature," *Radiography*, vol. 18, no. 4, pp. 301-302, 2012.

[16] A. R. Chitre, H. M. Divecha, M. Hakimi et al., "Traumatic isolated coracoid fractures in the adolescent," *Case Reports in Orthopedics*, vol. 2012, Article ID 371627, 4 pages, 2012.

[17] V. Pedersen, W. C. Prall, B. Ockert et al., "Non-operative treatment of a fracture to the coracoid process with acromioclavicular dislocation in an adolescent," *Orthopedic Reviews*, vol. 6, no. 3, p. 5499, 2014.

[18] G. W. V. Cross, P. Reilly, and M. Khanna, "Salter-Harris type 1 coracoid process fracture in a rugby playing adolescent," *BJR Case Reports*, vol. 4, no. 3, p. 20180011, 2018.

[19] R. A. Duerr, P. R. Melvin, and D. J. Phillips, "Acromioclavicular "pseudo-dislocation" with concomitant coracoid process fracture and coracoclavicular ligament rupture in a 12-year-old male," *The Orthopaedic Journal at Harvard Medical School*, vol. 19, pp. 52–57, 2018.

[20] J. Benton and C. Nelson, "Avulsion of the coracoid process in athlete," *Journal of Bone & Joint Surgery*, vol. 53, no. 2, pp. 356–358, 1971.

[21] K. Nakama, M. Gotoh, Y. Mitsui et al., "Epiphyseal fracture of the coracoid process occurring at the conjoined tendon origin," *Case Reports in Orthopedics*, vol. 2011, Article ID 329745, 4 pages, 2011.

[22] S. Archik, S. N. Nanda, S. Tripathi et al., "An isolated displaced fracture of the coracoid process treated with open reduction and internal fixation-a case report and review of literature," *Journal of Orthopaedic Case Reports*, vol. 6, no. 1, pp. 37–39, 2016.

[23] S. P. Montgomery and R. D. Loyd, "Avulsion fracture of the coracoid epiphysis with acromioclavicular separation: report of two cases in adolescents and review of the literature," *Journal of Bone & Joint Surgery*, vol. 59, no. 7, pp. 963–965, 1977.

[24] M. Leijnen, P. Steenvoorde, A. D. Da Costa et al., "Isolated apophyseal avulsion of the coracoid process: case report and review of literature," *Acta Orthopaedica Belgica*, vol. 75, no. 2, pp. 262–264, 2009.

[25] T. Ito, T. Morihara, R. Furukawa et al., "A case of acromioclavicular joint dislocation with coracoid process epiphysiolysis in young judo player," *Central Japan Association Orthopaedic Surgery & Traumatology*, vol. 59, pp. 1161-1162, 2016, in Japan.

[26] O. Kose, K. Canbora, F. Guler et al., "Acromioclavicular dislocation associated with coracoid process fracture: report of two cases and review of the literature," *Case Reports in Orthopedics*, vol. 2015, Article ID 858969, 8 pages, 2015.

[27] H. Flecker, "Roentgenographic observations of the times of appearance of epiphyses and their fusion with the diaphysis," *Journal of Anatomy*, vol. 67, no. 1, pp. 118–164, 1932.

[28] Y. Nakagawa, J. Ozaki, K. Masuhara et al., "Fractures of the coracoid process of the scapula," *Orthopaedic Surgery Traumatology*, vol. 1088, no. 31, pp. 581–588, 1988, in Japan.

[29] T. Morioka, K. Ogawa, and M. Takahashi, "Avulsion fracture of the coracoid process at the coracoclavicular ligament insertion: a report of three cases," *Case Reports in Orthopedics*, vol. 2016, Article ID 1836070, 5 pages, 2016.

[30] R. B. Salter and W. R. Harris, "Injuries involving the epiphyseal plate," *Journal of Bone & Joint Surgery*, vol. 45, no. 3, pp. 587–622, 1963.

[31] A. I. Froimson, "Fracture of the coracoid process of the scapula," *Journal of Bone & Joint Surgery*, vol. 60, no. 5, pp. 710-711, 1978.

[32] D. W. Boyer Jr., "Trapshooter's shoulder: stress fracture of the coracoid process. case report, case report," *Journal of Bone & Joint Surgery*, vol. 57, no. 6, p. 862, 1975.

[33] K. M. Wilson and J. C. Colwill, "Combined acromioclavicular dislocation with coracoclavicular ligament disruption and coracoid process fracture," *American Journal of Sports Medicine*, vol. 17, no. 5, pp. 697-698, 1989.

[34] D. J. Hak and E. E. Johnson, "Avulsion fracture of the coracoid associated with acromioclavicular dislocation," *Journal of Orthopaedic Trauma*, vol. 7, no. 4, pp. 381–383, 1993.

25

Functional and Radiological Outcome Analysis of Osteoperiosteal Decortication Flap in Nonunion of Tibia

Vineet Kumar,[1] **Shah Waliullah** [ID],[2] **Sachin Avasthi** [ID],[1] **Swagat Mahapatra** [ID],[1] **Ajai Singh** [ID],[3] **and Sabir Ali** [ID][3]

[1]*Department of Orthopaedics, Dr RMLIMS, Lucknow, India*
[2]*Department of Orthopaedics, KGMU, Lucknow, India*
[3]*Department of Paediatric Orthopaedics, KGMU, Lucknow, India*

Correspondence should be addressed to Swagat Mahapatra; drswagat@gmail.com

Academic Editor: Francesco Liuzza

Introduction. The treatment of long bone shaft nonunions is challenging. The technique of osteoperiosteal decortications flap for approaching the nonunion site coupled with fixation modalities was first described by Judet in 1963. Despite promising clinical and radiological union, this technique is not popular among orthopaedic surgeons. Our study aimed to evaluate the radiological union and functional results of shaft tibia nonunions treated by the osteoperiosteal decortication approach. *Methods.* This retrospective study included all the cases with established tibial shaft nonunion following stringent inclusion and exclusion criteria and operated upon by following the principle of osteoperiosteal flap technique from April 2015 to July 2019. Further subgroups were made based on nonunions complexity based on nonunion scoring system (NUSS) score. The outcome measures included radiological union scale in tibial fractures (RUST) and lower extremity functional scale (LEFS). The preoperative scores for union and function were recorded, and the subsequent scores were obtained at three, six, and nine months and one year. Appropriate statistical analysis of the data was done. *Results.* Thirty-four cases were shortlisted for analysis, fulfilling our inclusion and exclusion criteria. There were 22 males (64.7%) and 12 females (35.3%) with a mean age of 34.17 ± 10.3 years. Subgroup analysis based on the complexity of nonunion (NUSS score) revealed 14 cases in group A, 10 cases in group B, 10 cases in group C, and 0 cases in group D. The average time from fracture to surgery in these cases was 14.6 months. The average time to achieve union was 9.6 months, with patients in groups A, B, and C, having a mean duration of 9, 10.5, and 12 months, respectively. Statistically, significant improvement was seen in both RUST scores and LEFS score. Complications included infection in seven cases, wound dehiscence in two cases, and four cases of persistent nonunion. *Conclusion.* Osteoperiosteal decortication remains a highly effective surgical technique in the management of nonunion of long bones. NUSS scoring is an essential tool for prognosticating nonunion cases. This score is inversely related to the radiological union (RUST score) of the bone and functional recovery (LEFS score) of the patient.

1. Background of the Work

The basic fracture healing process is natural, though this is a complex biological process involving bone tissue regeneration. The process of fracture union can well be considered as a variant of tissue regeneration. Under normal circumstances, this bone tissue regenerates, but sometimes it goes into nonunion [1]. The process of fracture union is hampered if there is an insult to the biology of the bone and surrounding tissue. Surgery is a planned iatrogenic insult to the soft tissues. Therefore, it becomes imperative to maintain an adequate balance between soft tissue biology and surgical technique. This balance forms the foundation for the bone regeneration process after the surgery.

Tibia fractures are one of the most typical long bone fractures to go into nonunion. The reasons for the nonunion of tibia have been extensively documented in the literature [2]. The soft tissues surrounding the bones are one of the crucial factors responsible for the fracture healing process. This factor holds even more importance in tibia fractures, as the bone is subcutaneous throughout its anterior and anteromedial aspect. A fresh fracture [3] of the tibial shaft can be managed both surgically and conservatively, but surgical intervention becomes mandatory in cases with established nonunion [4]. The anterolateral approach is the standard surgical approach for addressing the nonunion of the tibia. Several surgical techniques have been described in the literature to address this challenging situation. These techniques are often combined with one or the other bone induction methods to achieve fracture union [5, 6]. When the cause of nonunion is biological, the problem becomes even more challenging to address. The diamond concept introduced by Calori et al. says that there are three biological (growth factors, osteoconductive scaffolds, and osteogenic cells) and a mechanical factor that forms the four pillars required for adequate bone healing during the fracture union process [7, 8]. Therefore, any alteration in any of the factors directly threatens the fracture healing process.

Open surgical procedures disturb the soft tissue envelop surrounding the fracture, more so in the tibial diaphysis, which has already a precarious extraosseous blood supply [9]. The osteoperiosteal decortication flap technique effectively addresses this issue in the nonunion tibia and ensures an adequate biological environment at the nonunion site. Judet first described this technique to manage nonunions of the tibia in 1962, and the results of this technique were first published in 1972 with 92% union results [10]. The bone chips (osteoperiosteal) were denuded from the tibia shaft on either side of the fracture using the standard incision. These bone chips with their blood supply (through the muscles attached) constitute the osteoperiosteal flap. Subsequently, in 2012 Guyver et al., in their publication, demonstrated similar results with 92.3% union rates [11]. Despite promising results, this technique has not gained much popularity. Most of the data available in the literature using this technique have been on the nonunion of long bone fractures. The nonunion of the tibia was exclusively included in this study to have a comparable group on which the outcome analysis would be more justifiable. There are few articles available in the literature, which assess the union rate after Judet's technique. Therefore, we planned this study in cases of the nonunion tibia to validate this technique and assess the functional outcome in cases managed by this technique.

2. Materials and Methods

This retrospective cohort study (Figure 1) was conducted in the Departments of Orthopaedic Surgery at two tertiary care multispecialty teaching hospitals in North India. After approval of the Institutional Ethical Committee (IEC 73/20), a comprehensive data collection was done from the record section of both the institutes from April 2015 to July 2019.

The inclusion criteria comprised all cases aged 12–65 years of either gender with established tibial shaft nonunion [2, 4] operated on using the principle of osteoperiosteal flap technique with fracture stabilization using either an internal or external fixation device.

Cases with neurovascular involvement, musculoskeletal ailment, and any previous surgery in the ipsilateral limb,

pregnant females, patients with significant life-threatening comorbidities, patients on immunosuppressive therapies, and nonunion cases requiring a simultaneous plastic procedure were excluded from our study.

We included only the cases with nonunion of the tibia shaft in our series, as the tibia is more prone to go into nonunion amongst all the long bones. This is attributed to its subcutaneous location. The tibia is also more prone to injury in high-velocity injuries [12–15]. The incidence of nonunion in the tibia further increases in cases of open fracture.

The study sample was further categorized into four groups based on the complexity of nonunion, as per the Calori nonunion scoring system (NUSS) criteria devised by Calori et al. [16, 17]. NUSS is a complex scoring system with eighteen variables summing up to a maximum total score of 50. This score is then doubled to 100 and divided equally in four groups, which signify the severity of nonunion. The primary outcome measures were to analyze the radiological union and the functional status of the limb. The radiological union scale in tibial fractures (RUST) score was used for the estimation of radiological union, and the lower extremity functional scale (LEFS) was used for the assessment of functional status [18–23]. The RUST scoring system (range = 4–12) utilises X-rays in both anteroposterior and lateral views to assess union by documenting the bridging callus and visible fracture line in all four cortices. The LEFS scoring system (range = 0–80) is a questionnaire (20 questions) for assessing the functional state of the lower extremity, with each question carrying a score from 0–4.

The radiological union and function scores were recorded preoperatively and, after that, subsequently at three months, six months, nine months, and one year. The data were recorded on the excel sheet and analyzed. The results obtained were compared with the data available in the literature. The outcome analysis was also done between the groups categorized as per the Calori system to assess this procedure's efficacy. Statistical analysis of the data was done using GraphPad Prism version 7 (GraphPad Software, San Diego, CA, USA).

3. Results

We could retrieve 34 cases for analysis from the database, fulfilling our inclusion and exclusion criteria. Of these, there were 22 males (64.7%) and 12 females (35.3%), with a mean age of 34.17 ± 10.3 years, and road traffic accident (RTA) was the most common cause of primary injury (Table 1). The patients were further analyzed by categorizing them into four groups to have similarity in the fracture's complexity pattern as per the Calori scoring system. The categorization was done to minimize the bias during the analysis stage. We had 14 cases in group A, 10 cases in group B, and 10 cases in group C, while no patients were available in group D. The average time from fracture to surgery in these cases was 14.6 months ($R = 9$–24 months). The follow-up records of all the cases were obtained for one year. The average time to achieve union was 9.6 months, with patients in groups A, B, and C, having a mean duration of 9, 10.5, and 12 months, respectively ($A = 7.92 \pm 1.49$, $B = 10.5 \pm 1.58$, $C = 11.1 \pm 1.44$).

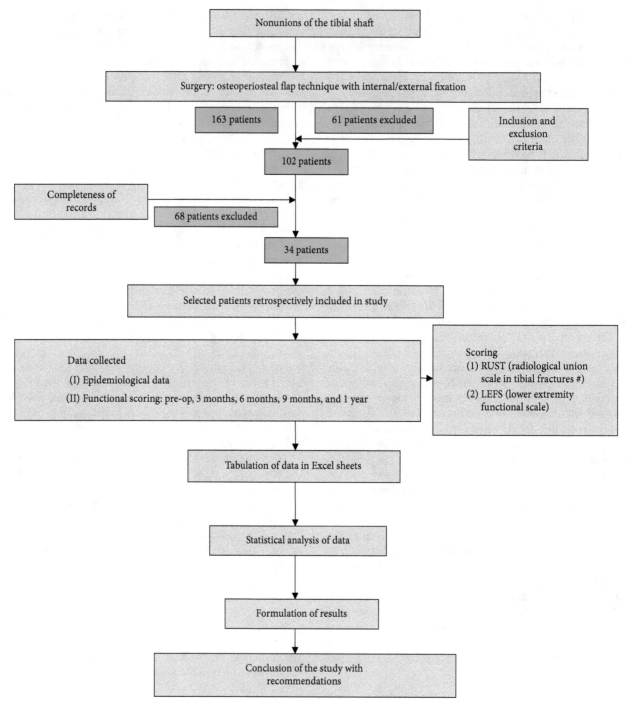

FIGURE 1: Methodology flowchart.

Data were analyzed within the respective groups using a "paired *T*-test" with 95% CI of difference of means and were recorded for their RUST score (Table 2) and LEFS score (Table 3) at the predetermined intervals.

As evaluated by the RUST score, the radiological union in groups B and C demonstrated a statistically significant improvement from six months postoperatively. In contrast, group A showed a statistically significant improvement from three months postoperatively (Table 2). The functional status in groups A and B, as evaluated by the LEFS score, demonstrated a statistically significant improvement from three

months postoperatively. In contrast, group C showed a statistically significant improvement from six months postoperatively (Table 3). Intergroup analysis of the mean RUST scores and LEFS scores using ANOVA revealed a significant improvement at each visit from three months onwards (Table 4).

The complications encountered in our study included infection, persistent nonunion, and wound dehiscence. Postoperative infection was seen in seven cases. One of them required debridement of the wound and a plastic procedure, whereas the remaining cases were successfully managed with

TABLE 1: Demographic details of the study population.

Parameters		Group A NUSS (1–25) [n = 14]	Group B NUSS (26–50) [n = 10]	Group C NUSS (51–75) [n = 10]	Total [n = 34]
Age (in years)		35 ± 10.82 35	31.6 ± 9.14 31.5	35 ± 10.94 36	34.17 ± 10.3
Sex	Male	8	6	8	22 (64.7%)
	Female	6	4	2	12 (35.3%)
Mode of injury	RTA	10	9	8	27 (79.4%)
	Assault	3	0	2	5 (14.7%)
	Fall from height	1	1	0	2 (5.9%)

TABLE 2: Comparison of RUST score at serial follow-up.

RUST score	Group A NUSS (1–25) [n = 14]		Group B NUSS (25–50) [n = 10]		Group C NUSS (51–75) [n = 10]	
	95.00% CI of diff.	P value	95.00% CI of diff.	P value	95.00% CI of diff.	P value
Pre-op vs. 3 months	−1.833 to 0.1132	0.1080	−2.129 to 0.9295	0.7980	−1.48 to 1.68	0.9998
3 months vs. 6 months	−3.473 to −1.527	<0.0001*	−2.929 to 0.1295	0.0872	−2.08 to 1.08	0.8958
6 months vs. 9 months	−3.473 to −1.527	<0.0001*	−4.029 to −0.9705	0.0003*	−3.58 to −0.4196	0.0068*
9 months vs. 12 months	−2.693 to −0.7468	<0.0001*	−3.379 to −0.3205	0.0107	−6.08 to −2.92	<0.0001*

*Significant; Student's t-test.

TABLE 3: Comparison of LEFS at serial follow-up.

LEFS score	Group A NUSS (1–25) [n = 14]		Group B NUSS (25–50) [n = 10]		Group C NUSS (51–75) [n = 10]	
	95.00% CI of diff.	P value	95.00% CI of diff.	P value	95.00% CI of diff.	P value
Pre-op vs. 3 months	−26.4 to −9.741	<0.0001*	−18.74 to 7.139	0.7083	−15.36 to 5.565	0.6740
3 months vs. 6 months	−31.12 to −14.46	<0.0001*	−30.94 to −5.061	0.0024*	−20.66 to 0.265	0.0593
6 months vs. 9 months	−30.18 to −13.52	<0.0001*	−35.84 to −9.961	<0.0001*	−23.66 to −2.735	0.0070*
9 months vs. 12 months	−25.98 to −9.321	<0.0001*	−31.64 to −5.761	0.0015*	−51.96 to −31.04	<0.0001*

*Significant; Student's t-test.

TABLE 4: Intergroup analysis of mean RUST and LEFS score.

		Group A NUSS (1–25) [n = 14]	Group B NUSS (25–50) [n = 10]	Group C NUSS (51–75) [n = 10]	P value
RUST score	Pre-op	4.42 ± 0.64 4	4.4 ± 0.96 4	4.1 ± 0.31 4	F = 0.736 P = 0.487
	3 months	5.28 ± 1.06 5	5 ± 0.81 5	4 ± 0 4	F = 7.56 P = 0.0021*
	6 months	7.78 ± 1.36 8	6.4 ± 1.57 6	4.5 ± 0.97 4	F = 17.78 P < 0.0001*
	9 months	10.28 ± 0.91 10	8.9 ± 1.28 8.5	6.5 ± 2.17 6.5	F = 19.9 P < 0.0001*
	12 months	12 ± 0 12	10.75 ± 1.25 11	11 ± 1.41 11.5	F = 5.207 P = 0.0112*
LEFS score	Pre-op	5.14 ± 6.61 2	13.1 ± 9.84 13.115.5	9.2 ± 7.22 9	F = 3.033 P = 0.0626
	3 months	23.21 ± 6.61 20	18.9 ± 8.25 20.5	14.1 ± 5.30 15	F = 5.255 P = 0.0108*
	6 months	46 ± 11.50 43.5	36.9 ± 12.35 37.5	24.3 ± 9.67	F = 28.08 P < 0.0001*
	9 months	67.85 ± 7.11 69.5	59.8 ± 13.88 62.5	37.5 ± 10.27 35.5	F = 25.63 P < 0.0001*
	12 months	85.5 ± 6.18 87.5	78.5 ± 2.88 78.5	79 ± 7.74 81	F = 5.256 P = 0.0108*

*Significant; ANOVA test.

an extended regime of antibiotics. Out of the seven infected cases, five cases were from group C. The statistical analysis of the data (chi-square test) revealed a significantly increased postoperative infection rate in group C ($P = 0.0232$). In addition, we had four cases with persistent nonunion (cases where we could not achieve union at 12 months), of which one case was from group B and three cases from group C. However, on intergroup analysis, the difference was not found to be statistically significant ($P = 0.0781$). Finally, we had two cases of wound dehiscence, one each from groups B and C (Table 5). Both of them required debridement of the wound followed by a plastic surgery procedure.

Resurgery was required in 29% (10/34) of the cases, of which eight cases were from group C and one each from groups A and B. Resurgery included plastic procedure or bone grafting. 80% (8/10) of the cases in group C required resurgery. Intergroup chi-square analysis revealed a statistically significant increase in the requirement for resurgery in group C ($P = 0.0125$) (Table 6).

Correlation analysis between NUSS versus RUST score and NUSS versus LEFS score at subsequent follow-up using Spearman r correlation showed statistically significant negative correlation, except the preoperative RUST ($P = 0.1286$) and LEFS ($P = 0.1540$) score (Table 7).

4. Discussion

Nonunions, though common, are tricky to address. Comprehensive data are available in the literature for the management of the same. The use of adjuvants and the type of implant used, rather than soft tissue biology, are usually prioritized in the management of these nonunions. The focus of the current study is the soft tissue dissection element. For orthopaedic surgeons, fresh diaphyseal tibia fractures are simple to treat, but nonunions of these fractures pose a significant challenge. Fresh diaphyseal tibial fractures have shown a good outcome in conservatively managed cases with a nonunion rate close to 1.1%. In contrast, the literature reports a nearly 5% nonunion rate in operatively managed cases [8, 24]. This calls for some insight into the blood supply of diaphysis of the tibia. The major vascularity in the tibial diaphysis is by the tibial nutrient artery (TNA), which is responsible for supplying the inner two-third of the diaphyseal cortex [9]. The extraosseous blood supply of the tibial diaphysis is poor compared with the proximal and distal metaphysic [25]. This is probably the reason for increased nonunion rates in metaphyseal areas if managed by open reduction and plating. Therefore, results are better in these cases when managed by minimally invasive percutaneous plate osteosynthesis (MIPPO), as this technique utilises the submuscular plane instead of subperiosteal dissection. In cases of established nonunion, open reduction is the only alternative. Judet's osteoperiosteal flap technique provides a possible solution for these fractures. The osteoperiosteal flap technique, described initially by Judet and Patel, has been used as a soft tissue handling technique to manage aseptic nonunions. This technique avoids the subperiosteal plane and elevates the soft tissue with the cortical bone underlying the periosteum. These flaps are with the

muscle attachments, which have a blood supply that aids in new bone production and, eventually, union at the fracture site. Judet and Patel reported a 92% success rate in their series of 1068 cases [10]. In his series, there were 290 cases of aseptic nonunion with 94.8% union rates, 126 cases of septic nonunion with 85% union rates and 108 malunion cases with 98% union rates. In his latest series of 297 cases, he reported a union rate of 99% in eight months [26].

Our surgical management protocol involved the denudation of the superficial cortical bone with a sharp osteotome along with the soft tissue flap for exposure of the nonunion site. This technique helps in retaining the vascularity of the flap and thus prevents skin necrosis. The cortical bone chips also provide a local graft at the nonunion site for enhancing union, although this bone is not considered adequate in cases of nonunion with bone defects [27]. This dissection technique also ensures that the surgical wound heals adequately and quickly. The sutures also have a firm hold due to the cortical bone chips adhered to the soft tissue envelope, thus preventing wound dehiscence despite friable and inadequate tissue at the local site. This is of importance in cases of resurgery or in cases having a previous open wound scar or a plastic procedure. However, this procedure may not be suitable to address periarticular and intra-articular fracture nonunions due to the absence of periosteal cover.

A few studies have used Judet's technique for addressing the nonunion. Ramoutar et al. [27] showed a 95% union rate in his case series using the Judet technique to treat nonunion of both upper and lower limb bones. They also advocated that proper execution of the Judet technique was associated with a decrease in the requirement of autologous bone graft for treatment of the nonunion. We considered osteoperiosteal flap as an adjunctive procedure for an extra bone graft at the nonunion site. In this series, we used autologous bone graft in almost all of our cases. We had four cases of persistent nonunion, that is, 88.2% (30/34) union rate in our series. The union rate was 100% in group A, 90% in group B, and 70% in group C. Thus, the union rates in our cases vary from 70%–100%, depending on the initial NUSS score with which the patient has presented. Thus, NUSS scoring system appears to have prognostic importance in cases of fracture nonunions. The disparity in results among the three groups underlines the need of categorizing nonunions based on their severity or complexity before prognosticating the case and estimating the likelihood of union. Guyver et al. [11] observed a 92% union rate in their study, while Raju et al. [28] showed a 100% union rate in their case series of 20 patients with tibial fracture nonunion. In both these studies, the classification of nonunion according to their severity or complexity has not been taken into consideration. Guyver observed three patients with superficial infections and two patients with deep infections [11]. In our study, we had an infection rate of 20.5% (7/34), out of which the infection rate in group A was 7% (1/14), 10% (1/10) in group B, and 50% (5/10) in group C. The infection rate was significantly higher in group C compared with groups A and B. This increased infection rate could be attributed to the factors we considered in NUSS scoring. We were able to manage infection in all the cases with an extended antibiotic regime, except in

TABLE 5: Complications.

Complications		Group A NUSS (1–25) [n = 14]	Group B NUSS (25–50) [n = 10]	Group C NUSS (51–75) [n = 10]	P value
Infection	Yes	1	1	5	χ = 7.525
	No	13	9	5	P = 0.0232*
Wound dehiscence	Yes	0	1	1	χ = 1.488
	No	14	9	9	P = 0.4753
Nonunion	Yes	0	1	3	χ = 5.1
	No	14	9	7	P = 0.0781

TABLE 6: Patients requiring resurgery.

Resurgery required	Group A NUSS (1–25) [n = 14]	Group B NUSS (25–50) [n = 10]	Group C NUSS (51–75) [n = 10]	P value
Yes	1	1	8	χ = 8.762
No	13	9	2	P = 0.0125*

*Significant. χ, chi-square test.

TABLE 7: Correlation analysis of NUSS versus RUST and LEFS at various follow-ups.

NUSS vs.	RUST score	RUST (1st FU)	RUST (2nd FU)	RUST (3rd FU)	RUST (4th FU)
Spearman r	−0.2659	−0.5558	−0.7583	−0.7951	−0.5513
95% confidence interval	−0.561 to 0.0897	−0.757 to −0.2584	−0.8751 to −0.5579	−0.8952 to −0.6186	−0.8422 to −0.01182
P (two-tailed)	0.1286	0.0006*	<0.0001*	<0.0001*	0.0444*
NUSS vs.	LEFS	LEFS (1st FU)	LEFS (2nd FU)	LEFS (3rd FU)	LEFS (4th FU)
Spearman r	0.2862	−0.5574	−0.7145	−0.7699	−0.4016
95% confidence interval	−0.067 to 0.576	−0.758 to −0.2605	−0.8507 to −0.4884	−0.8815 to −0.5767	−0.7755 to 0.1809
P (two-tailed)	0.1008	0.0006*	<0.0001*	<0.0001*	0.1540

*Significant; Spearman r correlation.

one case in group C, which required wound debridement and subsequent plastic procedure.

In the current study, the radiological union was evaluated by RUST score. The RUST scoring system, with its advent way back in 2010, has shown a formidable performance with excellent intra- and interrater reliability for grading union and predicting union in tibial shaft fractures [18–21]. For clinical evaluation, we chose the LEFS score. LEFS has been shown to have good reliability and predictive correlation in assessing lower limb. Moreover, it is a reliable and valid tool for monitoring recovery in cases with tibia shaft fractures [22, 23].

We observed that the average time taken for the radiological union was similar to the graph pattern of clinical improvement as evaluated by LEFS (Figures 2 and 3). Thus, we performed a correlation analysis. This analysis revealed a strong correlation between NUSS and RUST/LEFS score from the third month postoperatively. The lesser the NUSS score, the better the union rate and the functional outcome as interpreted by the RUST score and LEFS score. This association is best observed between three and nine postoperative months. Prognostication in terms of the time to union in relation to the NUSS score is thus well explained by the correlation analysis.

Limitations of our study included the small sample size and absence of a control group. We have used autologous bone graft in almost all cases. We, therefore, could not comment on the usefulness of local graft alone, which is created by decortication for promoting union at the nonunion site. The types of nonunion (atrophic, oligotrophic, and

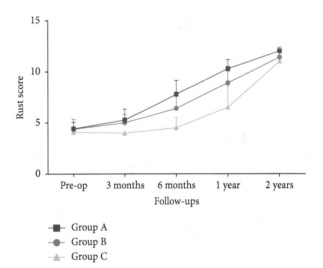

FIGURE 2: Graphical representation showing RUST score at subsequent follow-up of patients of different groups.

hypertrophic) have not been categorized and analyzed separately. They have been taken as a part of the scoring system (NUSS). Similarly, aseptic and septic cases have also not been analyzed separately. However, in our series, 71.5% (5/7) cases with clinical signs of infection landed up in group C after the NUSS score. One more important limitation of this study is that we have not considered and have not standardized the nonunion fixation or stabilization method. Standardization of the fracture fixation method could have further added new information in managing nonunion cases by this technique.

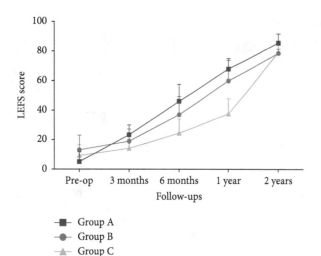

FIGURE 3: Graphical representation showing LEFS score at subsequent follow-up of patients of different groups.

5. Conclusion

Judet's technique of osteoperiosteal decortication combined with autologous corticocancellous bone grafting and internal or external fracture stabilization device is a highly effective and reproducible surgical technique in the management of diaphyseal fracture nonunion. NUSS scoring is an essential tool for prognosticating nonunion cases. This score is inversely related to the radiological union (RUST score) of the bone and functional recovery (LEFS score) of the patient.

References

[1] R. Marsell and T. A. Einhorn, "The biology of fracture healing," *Injury*, vol. 42, no. 6, pp. 551–555, 2011.

[2] A. F. Rodriguez-Buitrago and A. Jahangir, Tibia Nonunion. [Updated 2020 Jan 31]. In: StatPearls [Internet]. Treasure Island (F.L.): StatPearls Publishing; 2020 Jan. Available from: https://www.ncbi.nlm.nih.gov/books/NBK526050/, 2020.

[3] R. Zura, Z. Xu, G. J. Della Rocca, S. Mehta, R. G. Steen, and R. G. Steen, "When is a fracture not "fresh"? aligning reimbursement with patient outcome after treatment with low-intensity pulsed ultrasound," *Journal of Orthopaedic Trauma*, vol. 31, no. 5, pp. 248–251, May.

[4] K. Fong, V. Truong, C. J. Foote et al., "Predictors of nonunion and reoperation in patients with fractures of the tibia: an observational study," *BMC Musculoskeletal Disorders*, vol. 14, no. 1, p. 103, 2013.

[5] G. E. Friedlaender, C. R. Perry, J. D. Cole et al., "Osteogenic protein-1 (bone morphogenetic protein-7) in the treatment of tibialnonunions," *Journal of Bone and Joint Surgery*, vol. 83, no. A Suppl 1(Pt 2), S151-8. PMID: 11314793; PMCID: PMC1425155, 2001.

[6] P. V. Giannoudis and H. T. Dinopoulos, "Autologous bone graft: when shall we add growth factors?" *Orthopedic Clinics of North America*, vol. 41, no. 1, pp. 85–94, 2010.

[7] G. M. Calori and P. V. Giannoudis, "Enhancement of fracture healing with the diamond concept: the role of the biological chamber," *Injury*, vol. 42, no. 11, pp. 1191–1193, 2011, PubMed: 21596376.

[8] G. M. Calori, W. Albisetti, A. Agus, S. Iori, and L. Tagliabue, "Risk factors contributing to fracture non-unions," *Injury*, vol. 38, no. Suppl 2, pp. S11–S18, 2007, PubMed: 17920412.

[9] H. Almansour, J. Jacoby, H. Baumgartner, M. K. Reumann, K. Nikolaou, and F. Springer, "Injury of the tibial nutrient Artery canal during external fixation for lower extremity fractures: a computed tomography study," *Journal of Clinical Medicine*, vol. 9, no. 7, p. 2235, 2020.

[10] P. R. Judet and A. Patel, "Muscle pedicle bone grafting of long bones by osteoperiosteal decortication," *Clinical Orthopaedics and Related Research*, vol. 87, no. 9, pp. 74–80, 1972.

[11] P. Guyver, C. Wakeling, K. Naik, and M. Norton, "Judet osteoperiosteal decortication for treatment of non-union: the Cornwall experience," *Injury*, vol. 43, no. 7, pp. 1187–1192, 2012.

[12] E. Antonova, T. K. Le, R. Burge, and J. Mershon, "Tibia shaft fractures: costly burden of nonunions," *BMC Musculoskeletal Disorders*, vol. 14, no. 1, p. 42, 2013.

[13] M. Bhandari and E. H. Schemitsch, "Clinical advances in the treatment of fracture nonunion: the response to mechanical stimulation," *Current Opinion in Orthopedics*, vol. 11, no. 5, pp. 372–377, 2000.

[14] J. C. J. Webb and J. Tricker, "A review of fracture healing," *Current Orthopaedics*, vol. 14, no. 6, pp. 457–463, 2000.

[15] A. Akhtar, A. Shami, and M. Sarfraz, "Functional outcome of tibial nonunion treatment by Ilizarov fixator," *Annals of Pakistan Institute of Medical Sciences*, vol. 8, no. 3, pp. 188–191, 2012.

[16] M. van Basten Batenburg, I. B. Houben, and T. J. Blokhuis, "The Non-Union Scoring System: an interobserver reliability study," *European Journal of Trauma and Emergency Surgery*, vol. 45, no. 1, pp. 13–19, 2019.

[17] G. M. Calori, M. Colombo, E. L. Mazza et al., "Validation of the non-union scoring system in 300 long bone non-unions," *Injury*, vol. 45, no. Suppl 6, pp. S93–S97, 2014, Epub 2014 Oct 29. PMID: 25457326.

[18] M. Bhandari, B. W. Kooistra, J. Busse, S. D. Walter, P. Tornetta, and E. H. Schemitsch, "108-Radiographic Union Scale for Tibial (R.U.S.T.) fracture healing assessment: preliminary validation," *Orthopaedic Proceedings*, vol. 93-B, no. SUPP IV, Epub, 2011.

[19] E. Cekic, E. Alici, and M. Yesil, "Reliability of the radiographic union score for tibial fractures," *Acta Orthopaedica et Traumatologica Turcica*, vol. 48, no. 5, pp. 533–540, 2014.

[20] K. A. Ross, K. O'Halloran, R. C. Castillo et al., "Prediction of tibial nonunion at the 6-week time point," *Injury*, vol. 49, no. 11, pp. 2075–2082, 2018.

[21] A. V. Christiano, A. M. Goch, P. Leucht, S. R. Konda, and K. A. Egol, "Radiographic union score for tibia fractures predicts success with operative treatment of tibial nonunion," *Journal of Clinical Orthopaedics and Trauma*, vol. 10, no. 4, pp. 650–654, 2019.

[22] J. M. Binkley, P. W. Stratford, S. A. Lott, and D. L. Riddle, "The Lower Extremity Functional Scale (LEFS): scale development, measurement properties, and clinical application," *Physical Therapy*, vol. 79, no. 4, pp. 371–383, 1999.

[23] S.-L. Pan, H.-W. Liang, W.-H. Hou, and T.-S. Yeh, "Responsiveness of SF-36 and lower extremity functional scale for assessing outcomes in traumatic injuries of lower extremities," *Injury*, vol. 45, no. 11, pp. 1759–1763, 2014.

[24] J. Litrenta, P. Tornetta, H. Vallier et al., "Dynamizations and exchanges: success rates and indications," *Journal of Ortho-*

paedic Trauma, vol. 29, no. 12, pp. 569–573, 2015, PubMed.

[25] J. Borrelli, W. Prickett, E. Song, D. Becker, and W. Ricci, "Extraosseous blood supply of the Tibia and the effects of different plating techniques: a human cadaveric study," *Journal of Orthopaedic Trauma,* vol. 16, no. 10, pp. 691–695, 2002.

[26] C. Jayadev, M. Mullins, P. Piriou, and T. Judet, "The role of JudetDecirtication in the 21st century," in *Proceedings of the Presentation in 10th Effort Congress,* Vienna, Austria, June 2009.

[27] D. N. Ramoutar, J. Rodrigues, C. Quah, C. Boulton, and C. G. Moran, "Judet decortication and compression plate fixation of long bone non-union: is bone graft necessary?" *Injury,* vol. 42, no. 12, pp. 1430–1434, 2011.

[28] D. P. Raju, D. M. I. N. Ahmed, D. L. B. Hosamani, D. S. Ramachandra, and D. N. Sherikar, "Efficacy of modified Judet's technique in non union tibia, with inter locking nail as fixation device," *International Journal of Orthopaedics Sciences,* vol. 6, no. 3, pp. 78–80, 2020.

26

Anterolateral Bone Window for Revision Broken Cemented Stem of Unipolar Hemiarthroplasty

Mohamed Mosa Mohamed Mahmoud ⓘ**, Bahaaeldin Ibrahim** ⓘ**, Amr Abdelhalem Amr, and Maysara Abdelhalem Bayoumy** ⓘ

Orthopaedic and Traumatology Department, Faculty of Medicine in Assiut, Al-Azhar University, Assiut 71524, Egypt

Correspondence should be addressed to Mohamed Mosa Mohamed Mahmoud; drmohamedmosa@yahoo.com

Academic Editor: Benjamin Blondel

Background. Fractured stem of the hip prosthesis is well documented in the literature. Although it is rare, it is considered as a challenging problem. Many techniques have been described to solve this problem. *Purpose of the Study.* Evaluation of the effect of anterolateral bone window for extraction of the cemented femoral stem of hemiarthroplasty in revision total hip replacement. *Methods.* The study included eight revision hip arthroplasties in eight patients, with a broken stem of cemented (Thompson) hemiarthroplasty, which has been revised by the anterolateral proximal femoral window. All cases received cemented cups and cement-in-cement stems, except one case who received cementless long stem. Clinical follow-up of cases by Harries hip score (HHS) and X-ray. *Results.* Functional improvement of HHS of all cases, with no signs of loosening, after a mean follow-up period of 1.5 years. *Conclusion.* Extraction of broken stem is a challenging procedure. Many techniques have been described for revision of cases with a fractured stem of hip prosthesis, but we think that the anterolateral femoral bone window is a reproducible technique due to the characteristics of simplicity, short-time procedure, less invasive, not requiring extra instruments, and can be successful for most patients.

1. Introduction

Fractured stem of the hip prosthesis is well documented in the literature with an incidence rate between 0.23 and 11% [1, 2]. Three-dimensional analysis of stresses around the stem showed the highest concentration of stresses on the lateral aspect of the middle third, so fracture usually starts at the anterolateral aspect of the stem [3].

The causes of stem fracture can be categorized into patient factors: young and or overweight patients; technical factors: varus positioning of the stem or deficient cement; and implant factors: metallurgic deficiency [4, 5]. After the introduction of modern cementing techniques and the more resistant metal alloys, the incidence of stem fracture after hip replacement has been markedly reduced [1, 2]. However, there are some very few cases that may occasionally present with a broken stem especially with older designs that are used in the past such as cemented Thompson hemiarthroplasty, which is still used in some countries for fractured neck of

femur in the older age group of patients. Removal of the distal part of a well-fixed broken cemented stem is a challenging procedure. Many techniques have been described, such as femoral bone window distal to the tip of the stem, extended trochanteric osteotomy, knee arthrotomy to push the distal part, and minimally invasive technique through the drilling of the proximal surface of the retained part of the stem and attachment of a threaded extraction device and a proximal femoral cortical window [6, 7]. In this series, we analyzed revision of the well-fixed broken stem of cemented Thompson hemiarthroplasty using anterolateral proximal femoral window without the need of extended trochanteric osteotomy.

2. Patients and Methods

This retrospective study was approved by our Institutional Ethics Committee. From January 2017 till April 2019, eight revisions of hemiarthroplasty in eight patients have been done. The preoperative diagnosis of all cases was a broken stem of cemented (Thompson) hemiarthroplasty. The main indication for surgery was severe hip pain together with the inability to full weight bearing on the affected limb. The mean age of patients was 72 years old (range 65–76), and they were divided into two females and six males. The primary surgeries in all cases were done outside our hospital. Fracture of the stem in all cases occurred after minimal trauma. Stem fracture happened after a period of 1–5 years from the primary surgery. Preoperative ESR and CRP were done for all patients to exclude infection. There were no preoperative signs of infection in all cases. All cases underwent single-stage revision. Surgical technique (Figures 1(a)–1(e)): first, preoperative manual templating was done; lateral approach to the hip with patients on lateral decubitus position was done for all patients; removal of the proximal part of the prosthesis; and then removal of the superficial part of the cement mantle in the lateral aspect of the metaphyseal area of the femur. Then, a rectangular bone window (1.5 cm width and 2.5 cm length) had been done in the anterolateral aspect of the femoral shaft just distal to the lesser trochanter by an electric saw. This window was enough to expose the proximal end of the retained part of the stem. Then, small osteotome was settled on the surface of the stem in an angle about 45° with the stem. In two cases, we did two depressions on the surface of the stem by a carbide drill, connecting them to each other to make the osteotome settle on the stem. Hammering on the osteotome led to pushing of the distal part of the stem proximally until it was delivered from the femur upward. After that, the bone window was closed and secured by cerclage wires, and then cup implantation was done first (Figures 2(a)–2(e)). Cemented dual mobility metal cups were used in four patients (Figure 3(a)–3(c)) and cemented polyethylene cups in the other four patients (Figures 4(a) and 4(b)). Then, cement-in-cement conventional stems have been used in all cases except one case, where the stem was broken into three pieces and the window was extended distally, so cementless long stem has been used.

All patients started full weight bearing on the second postoperative day. Clinical assessment has been done by Harries hip score (HHS) after 3 months, 6 months, and then every year. A radiological examination was done in the postoperative day, 3 months, 6 months, and then every year. No intraoperative or postoperative complications have been detected.

3. Results

The mean follow-up period was about 1.5 years (from 1 year to 3 years). Functional outcome was markedly improved after surgery where the mean preoperative HHS was about 26 (25–30) and became 80 (65–85) postoperatively. Seven cases have good outcome, and one case has fair outcome. No signs of loosening in the cup or stem in the follow-up X-ray were seen. Union of the bone window has been detected in all cases. There were no intraoperative or postoperative complications.

4. Discussion

In this case series, we presented eight cases of revision cemented unipolar (Thompson) hemiarthroplasty after broken cemented stems of Thompson hemiarthroplasty, in which we used the anterolateral bone window techniques for extraction of the distal portion of stem. Most of the cases have good outcome. No signs of loosening in the cup or stem in the follow-up X-ray were seen. Union of the bone window has been detected in all cases. There were no intraoperative or postoperative complications. Mechanical failure of the prosthesis is one of the indications for revision THR. However, nowadays, it is of less common occurrence due to the development of more resistant metal alloys and the evolution of cementing techniques. The fractures of femoral stems have been previously described [8–12], and this type of failure may be due to excessive patient weight, high levels of physical activity, deficient bone support, malposition or loosening of the stem, the presence of a stress riser, and a reduced cross-sectional area within the stem [13–16]. In a study which included 122 patients using an extensively coated cobalt-chrome femoral component, Sotereanos et al. found two fractures of the stem (1.6 percent) [9]. Although Lakstein et al., in his study which included 72 hips at five to ten years of follow-up, reported only one stem fracture at the modular junction [12], Paprosky et al. found relatively high incidence which is six percent of femoral component fractures after revision hip arthroplasty. This may be due to reduction in the proximal support as a result of extended trochanteric osteotomy (ETO) against a distally well-fixed stem [8]. Collis used a technique in which he used a trephine for penetration of the cement-stem interface prior to extraction [5, 8]. Moreland et al. [17]. have described a technique that requires a femoral window through posterior cortex to expose the distal part of the broken femoral stem to perform retrograde impaction. Akwari et al. [7] described a modification of this technique in two patients, but performing reconstructions with standard stems and a cement-in-cement technique. The use of intramedullary nail for the retrograde impaction of the distal part of the stem through knee arthrotomy has also been described for selected cases [18]. The anterolateral bone window technique is easy applicable, less time-consuming than metal drilling, and better bone preservation compared to greater trochanter osteotomy. Although proximal femoral bone window technique has been previously published methods by Akwari et al. and Moreland et al. [7, 17], we did some modifications by making the bone window in the anterolateral aspect of the femur instead of posterior aspect because we did all cases by lateral approach and the anterolateral surface is more accessible than posterior, as we used the lateral approach to the hip in THA, we also used the electric saw instead of osteotome because it is much safer with less possibility in producing femoral fracture, and lastly, we used the cerclage wires instead of a metal cable which is cheaper. This technique is preferable to the distal window technique, where the bone window is done distal to the tip of the stem. Hence, a long-stem THR should be used to avoid stress rising and fracture of femur distal to the stem [17, 19]. But in the proximal window technique, we used a standard stem, which is less invasive, requires limited surgical time, and is cheap. In all of our cases, we did not use long-stem THA except in one patient, where the stem was broken to three pieces, so the window was slightly bigger and we have to remove the

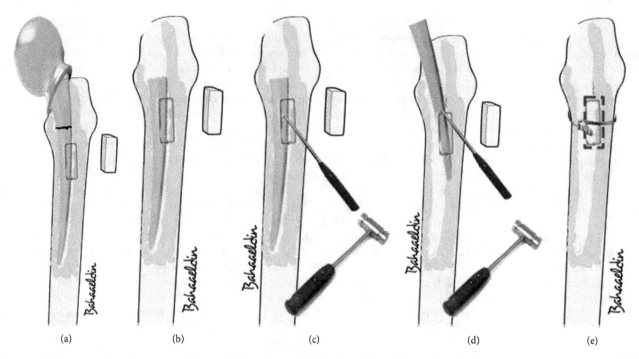

(a)   (b)   (c)   (d)   (e)

FIGURE 1: Sequence of events to extract fractured femoral stem. (a) Broken stem of Thompson prosthesis (b) rectangular bone window (1.5 cm width and 2.5 cm length) at the lateral aspect of the femoral shaft just distal to the lesser trochanter. (c) Small osteotome settled on the surface of the stem in an angle about 45° with the stem. (d) Hammering process to extract the distal part of the stem. (e) Cortical bone window is closed and secured with cerclage (diagrams were designed by Dr. Bahaaeldin Ibrahim).

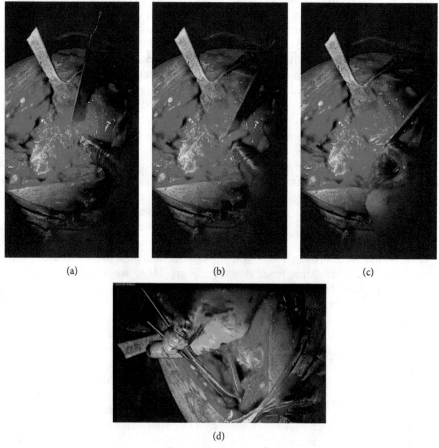

(a)   (b)   (c)

(d)

FIGURE 2: Continued.

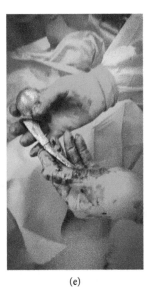

(e)

FIGURE 2: Intraoperative photos of window technique for stem removal. (a) A rectangular bone window done by saw at the lateral surface of proximal femur. (b) Elevation of the bone window to reveal the retained part of the stem. (c) Pushing the stem by an osteotome and hammer. (d) Delivery of the stem from the upper part of the femur. (e) Two parts of the Thompson prosthesis after removal.

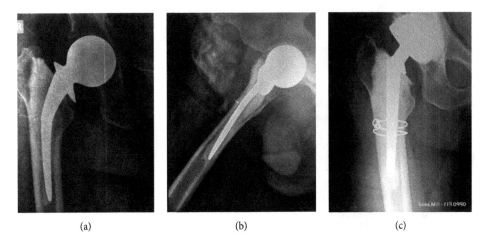

(a)   (b)   (c)

FIGURE 3: Preoperative and postoperative plane X-ray of a case with broken Thompson prosthesis. Removal of the broken stem by lateral bone window and revision by cemented dual mobility cup and DDH cemented stem.

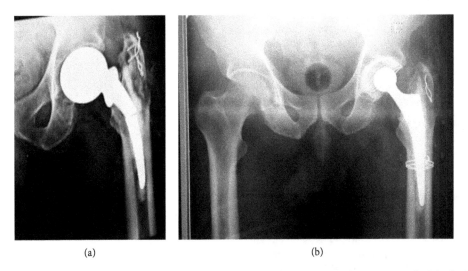

(a)   (b)

FIGURE 4: Preoperative and postoperative plane X-ray of a case with broken Thompson prosthesis. Removal of the broken stem by lateral bone window and revision by cemented polyethylene cup and cemented stem.

whole cement mantle and use cementless long-stem THA to gain better fixation distally and avoid fracture of the femur. The limitation of this study is the limited number of patients, but this is due to the rarity of incidence of fractured stem.

5. Conclusion

Extraction of broken stem is a challenging procedure, and many techniques have been described for revision of cases with fractured stem of hip prosthesis, but we think that the anterolateral femoral bone window is a reproducible technique due to the characteristics of simplicity, time sparing, less invasive, not requiring extra instruments, and can be successful for most patients.

References

[1] J. Charnley, "Fracture of femoral prostheses in total hip replacement: a clinical study," Clinical Orthopaedics and Related Research, vol. 111, pp. 105–120, 1975.

[2] D. A. Heck, C. M. Partridge, J. D. Reuben, W. L. Lanzer, C. G. Lewis, and E. M. Keating, "Prosthetic component failures in hip arthroplasty surgery," The Journal of Arthroplasty, vol. 10, no. 5, pp. 575–580, 1995.

[3] S. J. Hampton, T. P. Andriacchi, and J. O. Galante, "Three dimensional stress analysis of the femoral stem of a total hip prosthesis," Journal of Biomechanics, vol. 13, no. 5, pp. 443–448, 1980.

[4] M. A. Ritter and E. D. Campbell, "An evaluation of Trapezoidal-28 femoral stem fractures," Clinical Orthopaedics and Related Research, vol. 212, pp. 237–244, 1986.

[5] D. K. Collis, "Femoral stem failure in total hip replacement," The Journal of Bone and Joint Surgery, vol. 59, no. 8, pp. 1033–1041, 1977.

[6] F. J. Burgo, D. E. Mengelle, M. Feijoo, and C. M. Autorino, "A minimally invasive technique to remove broken cemented stems and its reconstruction with cement-in-cement," HIP International, vol. 29, no. 1, pp. NP1–NP5, 2019.

[7] H. Akrawi, M. Magra, A. Shetty, and A. Ng, "A modified technique to extract fractured femoral stem in revision total hip arthroplasty: a report of two cases," International Journal of Surgery Case Reports, vol. 5, no. 7, pp. 361–364, 2014.

[8] W. G. Paprosky, S. H. Weeden, and J. W. Bowling Jr., "Component removal in revision total hip arthroplasty," Clinical Orthopaedics and Related Research, vol. 393, pp. 181–193, 2001.

[9] N. G. Sotereanos, C. A. Engh, A. H. Glassman, G. E. Macalino, and C. A. Engh Jr., "Cementless femoral components should be made from cobalt chrome," Clinical Orthopaedics and Related Research, vol. 313, pp. 146–153, 1995.

[10] D. Lakstein, N. Eliaz, O. Levi et al., "Fracture of cementless femoral stems at the mid-stem junction in modular revision hip arthroplasty systems," The Journal of Bone and Joint Surgery, vol. 93, no. 1, pp. 57–65, 2011.

[11] C. A. Busch, M. N. Charles, C. M. Haydon et al., "Fractures of distally-fixed femoral stems after revision arthroplasty," The Journal of Bone and Joint Surgery, vol. 87, no. 10, pp. 1333–1336, 2005.

[12] D. Lakstein, D. Backstein, O. Safir, Y. Kosashvili, and A. E. Gross, "Revision total hip arthroplasty with a porous-coated modular stem: 5 to 10 years follow-up," Clinical Orthopaedics and Related Research, vol. 468, no. 5, pp. 1310–1315, 2010.

[13] T. P. Andriacchi, J. O. Galante, T. B. Belytschko, and S. Hampton, "A stress analysis of the femoral stem in total hip prostheses," The Journal of Bone and Joint Surgery, vol. 58, no. 5, pp. 618–624, 1976.

[14] M. A. Buttaro, M. B. Mayor, D. Van Citters, and F. Piccaluga, "Fatigue fracture of a proximally modular, distally tapered fluted implant with diaphyseal fixation," The Journal of Arthroplasty, vol. 22, no. 5, pp. 780–783, 2007.

[15] E. H. Miller, R. Shastri, and C. I. Shih, "Fracture failure of a forged vitallium prosthesis: a case report," The Journal of Bone and Joint Surgery: American Volume, vol. 64, no. 9, pp. 1359–1363, 1982.

[16] B. A. Ishaque, H. Stürz, and E. Basad, "Fatigue fracture of a short stem hip replacement: a failure analysis with electron microscopy and review of the literature," The Journal of Arthroplasty, vol. 26, no. 4, pp. 665.e17–665.e20, 2011.

[17] J. R. Moreland, R. Marder, and W. E. Anspach Jr., "The window technique for the removal of broken femoral stems in total hip replacement," Clinical Orthopaedics and Related Research, vol. 212, pp. 245–249, 1986.

[18] M. Szendroi, K. Tóth, J. Kiss, I. Antal, and G. Skaliczki, "Retrograde genocephalic removal of fractured or immovable femoral stems in revision hip surgery," HIP International, vol. 20, no. 1, pp. 34–37, 2010.

[19] P. M. Pellicci, E. A. Salvati, and H. J. Robinson, "Mechanical failures in total hip replacement requiring reoperation," The Journal of Bone and Joint Surgery, vol. 61, no. 1, pp. 28–36, 1979.

27

A Knee Size-Independent Parameter for Malalignment of the Distal Patellofemoral Joint in Children

Ferdinand Wagner ⓘ,[1,2,3] Günther Maderbacher,[4] Jan Matussek,[4] Boris M. Holzapfel,[1,5] Birgit Kammer,[6] Jochen Hubertus,[3] Sven Anders,[4] Sebastian Winkler,[4] Joachim Grifka,[4] and Armin Keshmiri[4]

[1]Institute of Health and Biomedical Innovation, Queensland University of Technology, 60 Musk Ave, QLD 4059, Brisbane, Australia
[2]Department of Orthopaedic Surgery, Ludwig-Maximilians-University, Marchioninistrasse 15, 81337 Munich, Germany
[3]Dr. von Hauner Children's Hospital, Ludwig-Maximilians University of Munich, Lindwurmstrasse 4, 80337 Munich, Germany
[4]Department of Orthopaedic Surgery for the University of Regensburg at the Asklepios Clinic Bad Abbach, Kaiser-Karl-V. Allee 3, 93077 Bad Abbach, Germany
[5]Orthopedic Center for Musculoskeletal Research, University of Wuerzburg, Koenig-Ludwig-Haus, Brettreichstr. 11, 97074 Wuerzburg, Germany
[6]Pediatric Radiology, Department of Radiology, Dr. von Hauner Children's Hospital, Ludwig-Maximilians-University, Lindwurmstrasse 4, 80337 Munich, Germany

Correspondence should be addressed to Ferdinand Wagner; dr.med.ferdinand.wagner@gmail.com

Academic Editor: Allen L. Carl

Introduction. Patellar instability (PI) is a common finding in children. Current parameters describing patellofemoral joint alignment do not account for knee size. Additionally, most parameters utilize joint-crossing tibiofemoral landmarks and are prone to errors. The aim of the present study was to develop a knee size-independent parameter that is suitable for pediatric or small knees and determines the malpositioning of the distal patellar tendon insertion solely utilizing tibial landmarks. *Methods.* Sixty-one pediatric knees were included in the study. The tibial tubercle posterior cruciate ligament distance (TTPCL) was measured via magnetic resonance imaging (MRI). The tibial head diameter (THD) was utilized as a parameter for knee size. An index was calculated for the TTPCL and THD (TTPCL/THD). One-hundred adult knees were analyzed to correlate the data with a normalized cohort. *Results.* The THD was significantly lower in healthy females than in males (69.3 mm ± 0.8 mm vs. 79.1 mm ± 0.7 mm; $p < 0.001$) and therefore was chosen to serve as a knee size parameter. However, no gender differences were found for the TTPCL/THD index in the healthy adult study cohort. The TTPCL/THD was significantly higher in adult PI patients than in the control group (0.301 ± 0.007 vs. 0.270 ± 0.007; $p = 0.005$). This finding was repeated in the PI group when the pediatric cohort was analyzed (0.316 ± 0.008 vs. 0.288 ± 0.010; $p = 0.033$). *Conclusion.* The TTPCL/THD index represents a novel knee size-independent measure describing malpositioning of the distal patellar tendon insertion determined solely by tibial landmarks.

1. Introduction

Symptoms of patellar instability (PI) usually occur in childhood and adolescence and therefore pose a common problem in the pediatric population [1]. Extensive clinical experience and detailed stepwise analysis of multiple factors, such as dysplasia of the trochlea and patella, leg axis, and rotational alignment, are crucial to understand the pathology of individual patients. A critical point for therapeutic decision making in PI is the location of the distal insertion of the patellar ligament [2, 3].

A pathologic lateralized tibial tubercle often causes PI and patellar dislocation and is commonly addressed by medializing osteotomies, as described by Elmslie–Trillat, in the mature skeletal system and by soft tissue reconstruction, such as medial patellofemoral ligament (MPFL) plasty and the Roux–Goldthwait procedure, in children [4–7].

A frequently utilized parameter indicating the need for distal realignment is the tibial tubercle-trochlear groove distance (TTTG) [8]. This value indicates a mediolateral mismatch of the center of the femoral trochlear groove and the insertion of the distal patellar tendon as determined in the transversal plane generated via computed tomography (CT) or magnetic resonance imaging (MRI) [8–13]. A value of more than 20 mm is usually considered pathological in CT scans. Regularly, smaller values were described for MRI measurements. In recent studies, three major problems have been raised concerning this parameter. First, different positioning of the joint during imaging results in inconsistent values because the landmarks used to measure the TTTG are located across the joint line at the femur and the tibia [14]. Second, the TTTG reflects the absolute value and therefore does not consider differences in overall knee size [10]. Knee size has been shown not only to be different between men and women but also to vary with age [10, 15]. Third, only 56% of the patients with PI present with a pathological TTTG [16]. Recently, Hingelbaum et al. described a knee size-adjusted TTTG index that includes the tibial tubercle-femoral trochlear entrance (TTTE) distance as a knee size-independent parameter measured in the longitudinal plane by MRI [10]. However, the concern of incorrect joint positioning during imaging is also relevant for this parameter.

Seitlinger et al. recently introduced a novel parameter solely utilizing tibial landmarks [17]. The mediolateral distance between the tibial tubercle (TT) and the medial border of the posterior cruciate ligament (PCL) describes the true lateralization of the distal insertion of the patellar tendon [14]. Other authors evaluated this new measure (TTPCL) and proposed pathological values as indicators for the Elmslie–Trillat procedure in the case of adult PI patients [14, 18].

However, the TTPCL does not consider the knee size, and therefore its applicability for children or small knees is questionable. The aim of the presented study was to describe a knee size-independent measure for pathologic lateral malpositioning of the tibial tubercle by determining the ratio between the TTPCL and the maximal tibial head diameter (THD). This TTPCL/THD index might be used as an additional tool in surgical decision-making.

2. Methods

2.1. Patients. One-hundred MRI scans of knees from adults and 61 knee MRI scans from children were analyzed retrospectively. The presence of open epiphyseal growth plates, and thus the inclusion of each individual patient in the pediatric study cohort, was verified by X-ray examinations. Patients with a history of chronic knee pain without trauma who presented PI in the subsequent clinical examination were included in the PI group. PI was defined as one or more events of patellar dislocation and/or a positive apprehension sign from 0° to 90° of flexion. Patients undergoing MRI because of acute knee pain due to trauma served as a control

cohort [15]. These patients had no history of chronic knee pain, retropatellar cartilage defects, or surgery addressing the patellofemoral joint. Standard MRI scans were acquired as a routine procedure in several outpatient radiology clinics.

2.2. Measurements. MRI scans were blinded, and three different parameters were assessed by two independent orthopedic surgeons (F. W. and G. M.) utilizing the transversal planes of the T2 sequence. IMPAX Xerox 2014 software (Agfa Health Care, Mortsel, Belgium) was used for the measurements.

The TTTG was defined as the mediolateral distance between the midpoint of the insertion of the patellar tendon and the trochlear groove as described by Goutallier et al. [8]. This distance was measured parallel to the dorsal femoral condylar line.

The mediolateral TTPCL distance was measured from the midpoint of the tibial tubercle and the medial border of the posterior cruciate ligament (PCL) as proposed by Seitlinger et al. [17]. The distance was measured parallel to the dorsal tibia condylar line (Figures 1(a) and 1(b)).

For all the measurements, the bony margins in the MRI scans were used, except when measuring the maximal THD. The THD was defined as the proximal part of the tibia with maximal diameter (Figure 1(c)). To determine the THD, the transverse plane with the maximum diameter of the proximal tibial head was identified by the examiner. The outer cartilaginous margin of the tibial head was used when analyzing MRI scans of children as they can be easily determined in the T2 MRI sequence.

2.3. Statistical Analysis. Retrospective data acquisition and analysis were approved by the ethics committee of the University of Regensburg (Approval No.: 6-104-0131) and performed according to the Declaration of Helsinki. Inter- and intraobserver variabilities were assessed via intraclass coefficient (ICC) analysis for TTPCL, TTTG, THD, and TTPCL/THD. All parameters were measured twice by both orthopedic surgeons on two separate days. The mean of these parameters for every patient was utilized for consecutive calculations in order to determine significant differences between groups. The results were expressed as the mean per group ± the standard error of the mean (±SEM). The Mann–Whitney U test was performed using SPSS (IBM, Ver. 20) to determine statistical significance between groups.

3. Results

3.1. Patient Characteristics. Forty-two of 100 adult patients suffered from PI, while 58 patients were included in the healthy control group (see Table 1 for detailed patient characteristics). In the second step, 61 knee MRI scans from patients with open epiphyseal growth plates were analyzed. Of the 61 pediatric patients, 32 knees exhibited PI and the remaining knees were assessed as control knees. The mean ages were 12.3 years old (±0.4) in the pediatric PI group and 13.3 years old (±0.3) in the control group ($p = 0.230$).

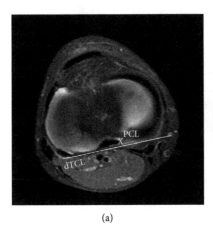
(a)

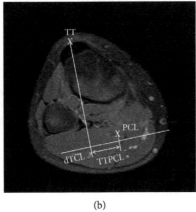
(b)

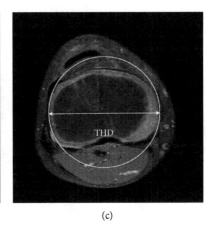
(c)

FIGURE 1: Measurement technique for the TTPCL/THD. Representative T2 MRI sequences acquired from a healthy 9-year-old boy. The mediolateral tibial tubercle-posterior cruciate ligament (TTPCL) distance was measured from (a) the medial border of the tibial insertion of the posterior cruciate ligament (PCL) and (b) the midpoint of the tibial tubercle (TT). The distance was measured parallel to the dorsal tibial condylar line (dTCL). The bony margins in the MRI scans were utilized except when measuring the tibial head diameter (THD). To determine the THD, the transversal plane with the maximum diameter of the tibial head was identified by the examiner (c).

TABLE 1: Patients' characteristics.

	PI	Control
Adults		
n	58	42
Age	28.7 years ± 1.8 SEM	21.2 years ± 1.1 SEM
Sex (male/female)	32/26	20/22
Side (right/left)	27/31	23/19
Children		
n	32	29
Age	12.3 years ± 0.4 SEM	13.3 years ± 0.3 SEM
Min/max	9/16 years	9/16 years
Sex (male/female)	22/10	16/13
Side (right/left)	13/19	15/14

3.2. TTPCL, TTTG, and TTPCL/THD. In adult patients, the TTTG and TTPCL were significantly higher in the PI group (TTTG: 13.4 mm ± 0.94 mm vs. 9.3 mm ± 0.50 mm; $p \leq 0.001$; TTPCL: 22.1 mm ± 0.57 mm vs. 20.2 mm ± 0.60 mm; $p = 0.031$; Table 2 and Figure 2(a)). No difference was observed between the PI and controls for the mean THD when all adult knees were compared. However, our analysis found that the TTPCL/THD index was significantly higher in the adult PI group than in the adult control group (0.301 ± 0.007 vs. 0.270 ± 0.007; $p = 0.005$). Accordingly, similar results were found in the pediatric patient population (Table 2 and Figure 2(b)).

3.3. Knee Size-Dependent Differences. The TTPCL differed significantly between healthy male and female participants ($p < 0.001$; Table 3). As the mean THD was also approximately 10 mm smaller in adult women than in men (69.3 mm ± 0.8 mm vs. 79.1 mm ± 0.7 mm; $p < 0.001$; Table 3 and Figure 3), we regarded both parameters to be knee size-dependent. Therefore, we divided our healthy adult patient cohort into male and female groups to determine whether the TTPCL/THD index is gender- independent and

therefore knee size-independent. Consequently, no difference in the TTPCL/THD index was found between the sexes in the healthy adult population (Table 3 and Figure 3).

3.4. TTPCL/THD in Children. Because no difference was found in the TTPCL/THD between sexes in adults and, more specifically between knee sizes, we regarded this value as knee size-independent. Therefore, we calculated the TTPCL/THD index for the pediatric study population. We found significantly higher values again in the PI group than that in the pediatric control group (0.316 ± 0.008 vs. 0.288 ± 0.010; $p = 0.033$; Table 2 and Figure 2(b)).

3.5. Inter- and Intraobserver Correlation. Good to excellent inter- and intraobserver correlations were found between the measurements. The ICC was >0.900 for all parameters when the intraobserver variability was analyzed. The interobserver variability values were ≥0.950 for both the TTPCL/THD and THD. We calculated an interobserver variability of 0.888 for the TTTG and 0.711 for the TTPCL.

4. Discussion

Pathologies of the patellofemoral joint leading to PI with consecutive anterior knee pain or patellar dislocation are multifactorial and therefore complex [2]. Although a broad variety of clinical and radiological measures seem to assist in clinical decision-making, safe algorithms have not been established [1, 14, 15]. A major concern in pediatric orthopedics is that many parameters are established in the adult patient population but are not normalized for different joint sizes and consequently are not suitable for immature patients [10, 15]. The TTTG, which is expressed as an absolute value in millimeters, does not consider the fact that a lower TTTG value in a smaller knee is considered abnormal [10]. For that purpose, Hingelbaum et al. have recently described a TTTG Index, measuring the TTTG as well as the

TABLE 2: Measurements of the TTTG, TTPCL, THD, and TTPCL/THD for the control and patellar instability (PI) groups for adults and children.

	Adults			Children		
	Control	PI	p value	Control	PI	p value
TTTG (mm)	9.3 ± 0.50	13.4 ± 0.94	<0.001	8.2 ± 0.55	13.2 ± 1.10	<0.001
TTPCL (mm)	20.2 ± 0.60	22.1 ± 0.57	0.031	20.6 ± 0.64	22.6 ± 0.62	0.031
THD (mm)	74.7 ± 0.82	73.5 ± 0.82	0.247	71.8 ± 1.03	71.6 ± 1.00	0.902
TTPCL/THD	0.270 ± 0.007	0.301 ± 0.007	0.005	0.288 ± 0.010	0.316 ± 0.008	0.033

The results are expressed as the mean values of the group ± SEM.

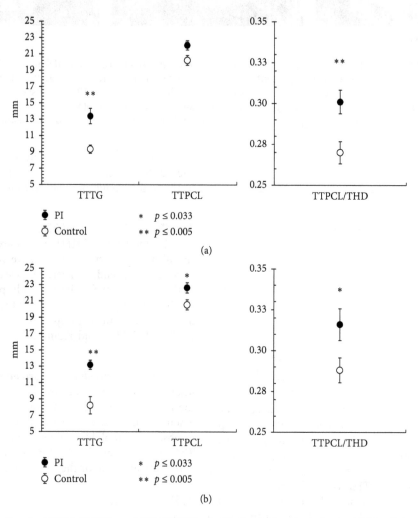

(a)

(b)

FIGURE 2: Graphs illustrating the TTTG, TTPCL, and TTPCL/THD for the control and patellar instability (PI) groups for adults (a) and children (b). The results are expressed as the mean values of the group ± the standard error of the mean (SEM).

TABLE 3: Gender-specific results for the TTTG, TTPCL, THD and TTPCL/THD in the healthy study population.

	Healthy adults			Healthy children		
	Male	Female	p value	Male	Female	p value
n	32	26		22	10	
TTTG (mm)	9.7 ± 0.8	8.8 ± 0.6	0.070	8.7 ± 0.72	7.3 ± 0.76	0.100
TTPCL (mm)	22.1 ± 0.7	17.9 ± 0.8	<0.001	20.9 ± 0.76	19.9 ± 1.20	0.562
THD (mm)	79.1 ± 0.7	69.3 ± 0.8	<0.001	73.2 ± 1.32	68.7 ± 1.16	0.039
TTPCL/THD	0.279 ± 0.009	0.259 ± 0.010	0.231	0.287 ± 0.012	0.290 ± 0.018	0.862

The results are expressed as the mean values of the group ± SEM.

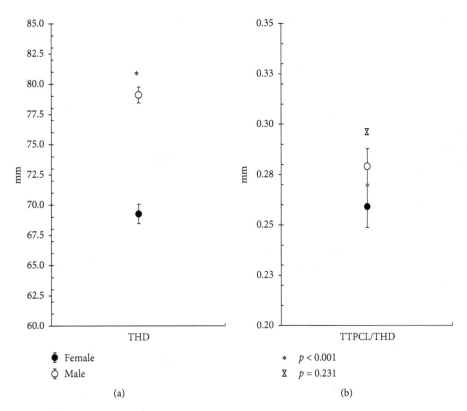

FIGURE 3: Graphs illustrating the THD and TTPCL/THD for healthy male and female adults. The results are expressed as the mean values of the group ± SEM.

distance from the tibial tubercle to the deepest point of the chondral entrance of the trochlea (TTTE) as a parameter for knee size [10]. Studies confirming the reliability of this parameter are missing to date. Others like Graf et al. recently highlighted the quantification of the q vector and the TTTG angle in order to appropriately address TTTG in surgical decision-making [19, 20]. To our knowledge, no attempts have been made to implement age-dependent percentiles for the TTTG.

Recently, a novel parameter was described by Seitlinger et al. that eliminated the limitation of joint line-crossing landmarks as is reported for the TTTG [17, 21]. The TTPCL solely utilizes tibial landmarks and describes the pathological lateralization of the distal insertion of the patellar tendon at the tibial tubercle [17]. However, joint size is still not considered with this measure [14].

Therefore, we designed our study to include a measure of joint size, such as the THD, when analyzing the TTPCL [22]. In analogy to Hingelbaum et al., we performed a stepwise analysis in order to determine, if our parameter is size independent [10]. In a first step, we found that the TTPCL/THD ratio is significantly higher in adult PI patients than in the healthy study population, and we regarded this parameter as a valuable measure for the lateralization of the tibial tubercle. The fact that previously established parameters such as the TTTG and TTPCL were also higher in the PI group confirmed that we analyzed adequate study cohorts that reflect the disease. In a second step, we showed that the THD is a measure of knee size, as it was significantly smaller in women than in men. The TTPCL was also significantly

smaller in women than in men. However, no difference was found in the TTPCL/THD index between healthy male and female study participants, indicating that including the THD into the TTPCL parameter eliminates knee size-dependent differences. We also found no difference in the TTPCL/THD index between healthy boys and girls. Nevertheless, a significant difference was found between children with and without PI. Therefore, we also concluded that this measure is a novel knee size-independent parameter for the true lateralization of the tibial tubercle that is applicable in the growing and maturing musculoskeletal system. The finding that healthy adult women have a significantly smaller TTPCL and a smaller THD than men also reflects the importance of the knee size component in adults for this specific parameter.

The mean TTTG was 13.2 mm in our pediatric PI group and only 13.4 mm in the adult group. Both are near the recommended normal position of the tibial tubercle as proposed by Dejour et al. [16] and lower than the pathologic values, which are generally described in the literature to be higher than 15 or 20 mm in CT scans [3, 16]. A study by Camp et al. showed that measuring TTTG by MRI modalities is generally lower than when determined via CT scans (16.9 mm in CT scans versus 14.7 mm in MRI scans in a PI group of 59 knees) [23]. In a subgroup of their patients presenting with a TTTG >20 mm in CT scans (mean 22.5 mm), the mean TTTG distance was only 18.7 mm in MRIs. This resulted in a mean difference of 3.8 mm between both imaging modalities ($p < 0.001$).

The described TTPCL/THD index utilizes only tibial landmarks and therefore is independent of certain modalities during imaging such as joint positioning. This is of particular value as significant variations in the current standard parameter, namely, the TTTG, can be generated by variations in positioning of the joint during MRI or CT examinations [14]. Dietrich et al. described a high variability in TTTG values in healthy volunteers depending on the knee positioning during MRI (ranging from 15.1 mm in full knee extension and 8.1 mm in 30° flexion) [24, 25]. Nevertheless, our TTTG values measured for the pediatric and adult PI cohort are out of the usually recommended cutoff for surgical intervention [26]. As we found no significant difference in TTTG between pediatric and adult patients, our results cannot fully refute TTTG as a non-applicable parameter for pediatric PI patients. Additionally, our data found differences in value ranges (SEM and min-max) between groups opening up the question if our cohorts are representative for the investigated question. However, we did not want to specify our PI cohort on single radiological parameters and used clinical measures as PI is a multifactorial condition [3]. PI was defined as one or more events of patellar dislocation and/or chronic anterior knee pain with a positive apprehension sign from 0° to 90° of flexion. Patients undergoing MRI because of acute knee pain due to trauma served as a control cohort [15]. Another limitation of our retrospective study is that the pediatric patient cohort was rather small.

We used MRI to evaluate our novel index for two reasons. In contrast to CT, this imaging modality is free of radiation and is therefore favorable for children [27]. Additionally, cartilaginous landmarks can be determined easily by MRI [9, 28], which is especially helpful when measuring the true maximal THD in children.

We found good to excellent intra- and interobserver correlation for all parameters. This corresponds with other reports [14, 17]. Although the ICC for the TTPCL was only fair—with a value of 0.711—the results were comparable to those published by Seitlinger et al. [17]. Additionally, other authors have previously reported values >0.900 for the TTPCL. More importantly, we found excellent values when calculating the TTPCL/THD index consecutively [14].

5. Conclusion

At this stage, we propose TTPCL/THD >0.30 as a possible pathologic value because the mean TTPCL/THD index was >0.300 in all PI groups and ≤0.290 in all the controls. However, further prospective studies with larger study cohorts, a broader age distribution, and the inclusion of additional parameters like rotational analysis of the limb are needed to evaluate the significance of this novel index and its potential in clinical practice. The described TTPCL/THD index might circumvent the need for the impractical age- and gender-adjusted percentiles required when applying the TTPCL.

Disclosure

F. W. participated in a Research Fellowship funded by the Deutsche Forschungsgemeinschaft (DFG WA 3606/1-1) during the time this study was performed. The Fellowship was not related to this work. No other funding for the reported research has been applied.

References

[1] D. M. Atkin, D. C. Fithian, K. S. Marangi, M. L. Stone, B. E. Dobson, and C. Mendelsohn, "Characteristics of patients with primary acute lateral patellar dislocation and their recovery within the first 6 months of injury," *The American Journal of Sports Medicine*, vol. 28, no. 4, pp. 472–479, 2000.

[2] S. Frosch, P. Balcarek, T. Walde et al., "Die therapie der patellaluxation: eine systematische literaturanalyse," *Zeitschrift für Orthopädie und Unfallchirurgie*, vol. 149, no. 6, pp. 630–645, 2011.

[3] A. E. Weber, A. Nathani, J. S. Dines et al., "An algorithmic approach to the management of recurrent lateral patellar dislocation," *The Journal of Bone and Joint Surgery*, vol. 98, no. 5, pp. 417–427, 2016.

[4] J. E. Goldthwait, "Slipping or recurrent dislocation of the patella: with the report of eleven cases. American journal of orthopedic surgery, vol. 1, pp. 293–308, 1903," *Journal of Bone and Joint Surgery*, vol. 85-A, no. 12, p. 2489, 2003.

[5] D. E. Brown, A. H. Alexander, and D. M. Lichtman, "The Elmslie-Trillat procedure: evaluation in patellar dislocation and subluxation," *The American Journal of Sports Medicine*, vol. 12, no. 2, pp. 104–109, 1984.

[6] K. L. Huston, U. C. Okoroafor, S. G. Kaar, C. L. Wentt, P. Saluan, and L. D. Farrow, "Evaluation of the schottle technique in the pediatric knee," *Orthopaedic Journal of Sports Medicine*, vol. 5, no. 11, Article ID 2325967117740078, 2017.

[7] M. Nelitz and S. R. M. Williams, "Anatomic reconstruction of the medial patellofemoral ligament in children and adolescents using a pedicled quadriceps tendon graft," *Arthroscopy Techniques*, vol. 3, no. 2, pp. e303–e308, 2014.

[8] D. Goutallier, J. Bernageau, and B. Lecudonnec, "The measurement of the tibial tuberosity: patella groove distanced technique and results (author's transl)," *Revue de Chirurgie Orthopedique et Reparatrice de l'Appareil Moteur*, vol. 64, no. 5, pp. 423–428, 1978.

[9] P. B. Schoettle, M. Zanetti, B. Seifert, C. W. A. Pfirrmann, S. F. Fucentese, and J. Romero, "The tibial tuberosity-trochlear groove distance; a comparative study between CT and MRI scanning," *The Knee*, vol. 13, no. 1, pp. 26–31, 2006.

[10] S. Hingelbaum, R. Best, J. Huth, D. Wagner, G. Bauer, and F. Mauch, "The TT-TG index: a new knee size adjusted measure method to determine the TT-TG distance," *Knee Surgery, Sports Traumatology, Arthroscopy*, vol. 22, no. 10, pp. 2388–2395, 2014.

[11] A. Aarvold, A. Pope, V. K. Sakthivel, and R. V. Ayer, "MRI performed on dedicated knee coils is inaccurate for the measurement of tibial tubercle trochlear groove distance," *Skeletal Radiology*, vol. 43, no. 3, pp. 345–349, 2014.

[12] K. Izadpanah, E. Weitzel, M. Vicari et al., "Influence of knee flexion angle and weight bearing on the tibial tuberosity-trochlear groove (TTTG) distance for evaluation of patellofemoral alignment," *Knee Surgery, Sports Traumatology, Arthroscopy*, vol. 22, no. 11, pp. 2655–2661, 2014.

[13] G. Seitlinger, G. Scheurecker, R. Högler, L. Labey, B. Innocenti, and S. Hofmann, "The position of the tibia tubercle in 0°–90° flexion: comparing patients with patella dislocation to healthy volunteers," *Knee Surgery, Sports Traumatology, Arthroscopy*, vol. 22, no. 10, pp. 2396–2400, 2014.

[14] C. M. Anley, G. V. Morris, A. Saithna, S. L. James, and M. Snow, "Defining the role of the tibial tubercle-trochlear groove and tibial tubercle-posterior cruciate ligament distances in the work-up of patients with patellofemoral disorders," *The American Journal of Sports Medicine*, vol. 43, no. 6, pp. 1348–1353, 2015.

[15] P. Balcarek, K. Jung, K.-H. Frosch, and K. M. Stürmer, "Value of the tibial tuberosity-trochlear groove distance in patellar instability in the young athlete," *The American Journal of Sports Medicine*, vol. 39, no. 8, pp. 1756–1762, 2011.

[16] H. Dejour, G. Walch, L. Nove-Josserand, and C. Guier, "Factors of patellar instability: an anatomic radiographic study," *Knee Surgery, Sports Traumatology, Arthroscopy*, vol. 2, no. 1, pp. 19–26, 1994.

[17] G. Seitlinger, G. Scheurecker, R. Högler, L. Labey, B. Innocenti, and S. Hofmann, "Tibial tubercle-posterior cruciate ligament distance," *The American Journal of Sports Medicine*, vol. 40, no. 5, pp. 1119–1125, 2012.

[18] J. Daynes, B. B. Hinckel, and J. Farr, "Tibial tuberosity-posterior cruciate ligament distance," *The Journal of Knee Surgery*, vol. 29, no. 6, pp. 471–477, 2015.

[19] K. H. Graf, M. A. Tompkins, J. Agel, and E. A. Arendt, "Q-vector measurements: physical examination versus magnetic resonance imaging measurements and their relationship with tibial tubercle-trochlear groove distance," *Knee Surgery, Sports Traumatology, Arthroscopy*, vol. 26, no. 3, pp. 697–704, 2018.

[20] B. B. Hinckel, R. G. Gobbi, C. C. Kaleka, G. L. Camanho, and E. A. Arendt, "Medial patellotibial ligament and medial patellomeniscal ligament: anatomy, imaging, biomechanics, and clinical review," *Knee Surgery, Sports Traumatology, Arthroscopy*, vol. 26, no. 3, pp. 685–696, 2018.

[21] M. J. Heidenreich, C. L. Camp, D. L. Dahm, M. J. Stuart, B. A. Levy, and A. J. Krych, "The contribution of the tibial tubercle to patellar instability: analysis of tibial tubercle-trochlear groove (TT-TG) and tibial tubercle-posterior cruciate ligament (TT-PCL) distances," *Knee Surgery, Sports Traumatology, Arthroscopy*, vol. 25, no. 8, pp. 2347–2351, 2015.

[22] G. Maderbacher, A. Keshmiri, J. Schaumburger et al., "Accuracy of bony landmarks for restoring the natural joint line in revision knee surgery: an MRI study," *International Orthopaedics*, vol. 38, no. 6, pp. 1173–1181, 2014.

[23] C. L. Camp, M. J. Stuart, A. J. Krych et al., "CT and MRI measurements of tibial tubercle-trochlear groove distances are not equivalent in patients with patellar instability," *The American Journal of Sports Medicine*, vol. 41, no. 8, pp. 1835–1840, 2013.

[24] T. J. Dietrich, M. Betz, C. W. A. Pfirrmann, P. P. Koch, and S. F. Fucentese, "End-stage extension of the knee and its influence on tibial tuberosity-trochlear groove distance (TTTG) in asymptomatic volunteers," *Knee Surgery, Sports Traumatology, Arthroscopy*, vol. 22, no. 1, pp. 214–218, 2014.

[25] T. J. Dietrich, S. F. Fucentese, and C. W. Pfirrmann, "Imaging of individual anatomical risk factors for patellar instability," *Seminars in Musculoskeletal Radiology*, vol. 20, no. 1, pp. 65–73, 2016.

[26] J. M. Brady, A. S. Rosencrans, and B. E. Shubin Stein, "Use of TT-PCL versus TT-TG," *Current Reviews in Musculoskeletal Medicine*, vol. 11, no. 2, pp. 261–265, 2018.

[27] R. R. Jimenez, M. A. Deguzman, S. Shiran, A. Karrellas, and R. L. Lorenzo, "CT versus plain radiographs for evaluation of c-spine injury in young children: do benefits outweigh risks?," *Pediatric Radiology*, vol. 38, no. 6, pp. 635–644, 2008.

[28] J. W. Xerogeanes, K. E. Hammond, and D. C. Todd, "Anatomic landmarks utilized for physeal-sparing, anatomic anterior cruciate ligament reconstruction," *The Journal of Bone and Joint Surgery-American Volume*, vol. 94, no. 3, pp. 268–276, 2012.

28

Diagnosis and Treatment of Peritalar Injuries in the Acute Trauma Setting

Abdul R. Arain (ID), **Curtis T. Adams, Stefanos F. Haddad, Muhammad Moral, Joseph Young, Khusboo Desai, and Andrew J. Rosenbaum** (ID)

Albany Medical Center, Albany, NY, USA

Correspondence should be addressed to Abdul R. Arain; mrbonelover@gmail.com

Academic Editor: Benjamin Blondel

The bony and ligamentous structure of the foot is a complex kinematic interaction, designed to transmit force and motion in an energy-efficient and stable manner. Visible deformity of the foot or atypical patterns of swelling should raise significant concern for foot trauma. In some instances, disruption of either bony structure or supporting ligaments is identified years after injury due to chronic pain in the hindfoot or midfoot. This article will focus on injuries relating to the peritalar complex, the bony articulation between the tibia, talus, calcaneus, and navicular bones, supplemented with multiple ligamentous structures. Attention will be given to the five most common peritalar injuries to illustrate the nature of each and briefly describe methods for achieving the correct diagnosis in the context of acute trauma. This includes subtalar dislocations, chopart joint injuries, talar fractures, navicular fractures, and occult calcaneal fractures.

1. Introduction

Fractures and ligamentous injuries of the foot are significant and challenging entities in the context of orthopaedic trauma [1]. Foot fractures are regarded as the most frequently missed extremity fracture [2]. Similarly, ligamentous injuries and related dislocations present many diagnostic challenges. There are multiple potential causalities underlying these missed injuries, which will be discussed in detail.

In the acute trauma patient, priority is given to executing ATLS protocol and emergent resuscitation. Hemodynamically unstable patients necessitate immediate life-saving measures while stable patients can undergo full clinical and radiologic workup to identify less obvious injuries.

In the resuscitated patient, priority is initially directed toward open injuries, fractures causing neurologic impairment, or injuries at high risk for compartment syndrome. Beyond this, a thorough primary survey with direct examination and palpation of every joint and extremity is critically important, and its importance cannot be overstated. The physical exam should further be correlated with radiographic evaluation of any site of suspected fracture, utilizing stress tests where appropriate and maintaining high clinical suspicion for particular fracture patterns based on the mechanism of injury.

In recent years, lisfranc injuries have been discussed extensively due to the frequency with which they are missed and the high probability for requiring operative treatment [3, 4]. In contrast, hindfoot injuries, particularly peritalar fractures and dislocations, have received significantly less attention. Both are relatively rare in the context of orthopaedic trauma; however, the previous literature has demonstrated a significant increase in morbidity of polytraumatized patients with an untreated foot injury [5]. Within the category of peritalar injuries, the most common missed injury is a fracture of the talus. Together with occult fractures of the calcaneus and navicular, these form roughly 70% of all missed foot injuries in high and low energy trauma [3].

Previous research has identified several signs useful in identifying occult foot fractures [4]. These include pain out of proportion to provisional diagnosis, which suggests a radiographically invisible fracture or ligamentous injury. Visible deformity of the foot or atypical patterns of swelling also raise significant concern. In the long-term, one should suspect missed foot injury when there is failure of symptoms to improve in the days and weeks following the initial trauma. Finally, a high-energy or classically described mechanism, such as an axial load on a plantar-flexed foot, should raise serious concern for an occult injury.

2. Peritalar Complex

The peritalar complex is a bony articulation between the tibia, talus, calcaneus, and navicular bones, supplemented with multiple ligamentous structures. Within this complex, the talar-navicular interaction, coupled with the spring ligament, is most important for maintaining integrity of the medial column [6]. The peritalar joints have been described to consist of two separate, independently functioning capsules involving the subtalar and talocalcaneonavicular joints, respectively [7]. Recent studies have emphasized the complex anatomic and kinematic relationship between the talocalcaneal and talonavicular joints and their contributions to hindfoot function [8].

In its uninjured state, the peritalar complex carries out several critical functions. The talus, in its relation between the calcaneus and tibia, acts to transmit a valgus force upon heel strike from the laterally-oriented calcaneus through the talus to the mid- and forefoot. This thrust unlocks the transverse tarsal joints and enables the talus to transmit directional torque away from the tibiotalar joint, thereby decreasing tibiotalar tilt stress. Hence, the subtalar joint functions to convert the foot from a mobile structure at heel strike to a rigid structure at toe off [7]. The talonavicular joint, supported by the plantar spring ligament complex of the calcaneonavicular ligaments, is the most important contributor of medial column stability. Additionally, the spring ligament supports the head of the talus and acts as a primary static restraint at the talonavicular joint to prevent excursion [9].

Peritalar injuries have been defined as fractures or ligamentous disruption resulting in instability of one or more peritalar joints: tibiotalar, subtalar, calcaneocuboid, and talonavicular [3]. As discussed, the bony and ligamentous structure of the foot is a complex kinematic interaction, designed to transmit force and motion in an energy-efficient and stable manner. Disruption of either bony structure or supporting ligaments results in long-term functional deficits, sometimes only identified years after injury by chronic pain in the hindfoot or midfoot due to progressive wear and strain.

The following sections will review the five most common peritalar injuries in order to illustrate the nature each and briefly describe methods for achieving the correct diagnosis in the context of acute trauma.

3. Subtalar Dislocation

Subtalar joint stability is primarily dependent on ligamentous structures, as described above. Forceful inversion, eversion, or extreme plantar flexion may cause ligamentous failure resulting in traumatic displacement of the calcaneus and navicular. Isolated subtalar dislocations are rare and more often present with associated fractures of the malleoli, fifth metatarsal, or talus (Figure 1). Patients with ligamentous insufficiency, malleolar hypoplasia, or other peritalar deformity are at increased risk of sustaining subtalar dislocation [4].

Subtalar dislocations almost invariably present as either grossly dislocated or spontaneously reduced. In the case of gross dislocation, there is visible deformity with skin tension on the opposing side. The amount of force required frequently results in a substantial skin defect on the tension side of the wound, creating an open subtalar dislocation. Conversely, many subtalar dislocations spontaneously reduce, leaving no radiographic sign of associated fractures. These patients present with significant soft tissue swelling and ecchymosis of the mid- and hindfoot, often similar to an ankle sprain. MRI studies may be helpful in cases of high clinical suspicion for a spontaneously reduced subtalar dislocation.

Broca was among the first to suggest a classification scheme for subtalar dislocations, describing medial, lateral, and posterior dislocations of the calcaneus and foot from beneath the talus [10]. Later, it was noted that anterior dislocations can occur; however, these are exceedingly rare. Medial dislocations are most common in the context of lower extremity trauma. Forceful inversion of the forefoot in a plantarflexed position loads the lateral collateral ligaments, resulting in rupture of the talocalcaneal and talonavicular ligaments and pivot of the talus on the sustentaculum tali. Conversely, lateral dislocations are caused by traumatic eversion of the foot and posterior dislocation by forceful plantar flexion alone [11].

Treatment of subtalar dislocations is highly dependent on skin integrity and associated fracture patterns. In cases of isolated ligamentous injury with intact skin, closed reduction and immobilization is almost universally recommended. Previously literature supports both immobilization for greater than 4 weeks, and early protected range of motion exercises with the goal of avoiding subtalar stiffness [11]. Lateral dislocations carry a poorer prognosis overall, in part due to the higher energy force necessary to cause sufficient eversion of the foot and dislocation of the calcaneus and navicular [12]. Significant soft tissue injury and skin defects overlying the site of dislocation should be treated as an open injury, requiring formal debridement, irrigation, reduction, closure, and course of parenteral antibiotics.

Complications following subtalar dislocation are well described in the literature. Posttraumatic arthritis is noted in up to 80% of patients and may present in the talonavicular, tibiotalar, or talocalcaneal joints. Osteonecrosis of the talus has also been described as a late complication of subtalar dislocation. Finally, subtalar joint stiffness is commonly observed as a result of fibrosis of the joint capsule following injury [3]. Newer evidence supports shorter-term immobilization followed by early range of motion after the initial injury in order to prevent stiffness [11].

4. Chopart Joint Injury

The chopart joint consists of the combined talonavicular and calcaneocuboid joints. The talonavicular joint allows for

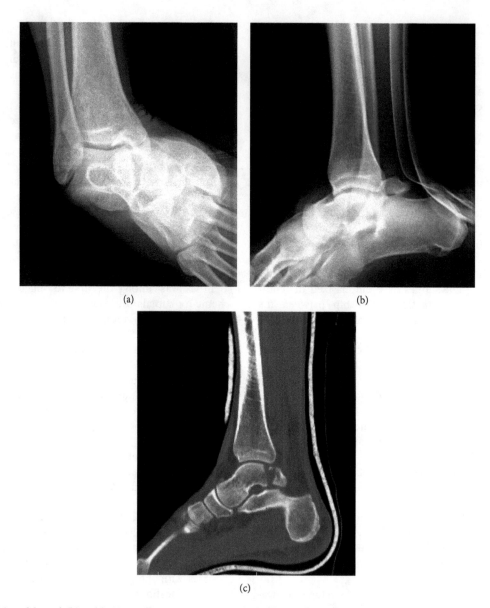

FIGURE 1: AP (a) and lateral (b) ankle X-rays demonstrating a medial subtalar fracture dislocation. The talar dome remains in normal articulation with the ankle joint, with the ankle mortise intact. Postreduction CT (c) reveals a coronally oriented, comminuted, and displaced fracture of the posterior talar dome and posterior talar process, with intraarticular extension into the subtalar joint.

pronation and supination of the foot as part of the talocalcaneonavicular joint. The calcaneocuboid joint lies in the lateral column and provides both flexibility and suspension to the foot.

Chopart joint injuries may be purely ligamentous or combined fracture and ligamentous injury. In both cases, there is loss of stability across the transverse tarsal joints. These injuries may occur in conjunction with a talar head, navicular, or cuboid fracture, which should raise suspicion for an associated ligamentous injury [8].

Chopart joint injuries are uncommon and may be difficult to detect clinically. Kou and Fortin recommend evaluating joint space asymmetry across the transverse tarsal joints on foot radiographs [3]. This may reveal a ligamentous disruption, especially in the setting of soft tissue swelling and midfoot pain. We recommend manual stress or weightbearing films with

contralateral comparison in order to highlight ligamentous insufficiency of the talonavicular or calcaneocuboid joints.

The treatment of Chopart joint injuries is largely based on case reports and individual surgeon preference, given the relative paucity of the literature. Initial management begins with immobilization of the joint. In cases of refractory pain or continued tarsal instability, transverse tarsal fusion may be necessary [13]. The use of bilateral stress films is helpful in identifying instability and guiding surgical management. In cases of minimal instability identified on stress views, temporary percutaneous fixation is often sufficient to stabilize the anatomic joint. Malreduction or gross deformity may require open reduction and internal fixation. As a last resort, salvage arthrodesis may prevent midfoot collapse and resultant loss of function. A previous literature has demonstrated that fusion of the calcaneocuboid joint may provide indirect stability of the talonavicular joint, and results in less functional impairment given the inherent flexibility of the lateral column [14]. Following reduction and/or fixation of Chopart joint injuries, weight bearing is generally restricted for 8–10 weeks following injury, with graduated range of motion exercises and slow return to activity thereafter.

5. Talar Fracture

Multiple fracture patterns of the talus have been described in their relation to peritalar injuries (Figures 2 and 3). These include fractures of the talar head and neck as well as of the lateral and posterior processes [15]. In addition, occult talar dome injury may be present. In each case, as with all peritalar injuries, findings range from radiologically benign to grossly displaced fragments. Pain out of proportion to provisional diagnosis can be key to further investigating a possible talar fracture.

Fracture of the talar head is relatively rare, with a described incidence of <10% of talar fractures. This pattern is caused by a combined dorsiflexion and inversion force that longitudinally loads the talus, resulting in a shear fracture across the talar head [16]. As a result, the medial column is functionally shortened, often resulting in a cavovarus foot with abnormal loading of the lateral column. Patients often present after a high-energy motor vehicle accident or fall. Clinically they demonstrate soft tissue swelling at the midfoot, variable gross deformity, ecchymosis, and significant pain on palpation or range of motion. Gross ecchymosis often signifies injury beyond a simple sprain. Radiographic findings are variable; therefore, CT scans of the foot are most helpful in diagnosis and treatment planning.

Treatment of talar head fractures varies from conservative immobilization to percutaneous pinning and to open reduction and internal fixation of displaced fragments [16]. In cases of late or missed diagnosis, salvage arthrodesis may be an additional option. Medial column shortening may also require distraction and bone block fusion. Avascular necrosis, although commonly described in talar neck fractures, is rare in the setting of talar head fracture due to adequate blood supply and multiple ligamentous attachments.

Similar to the talar head, lateral process fractures are often missed due to subtle or absent radiographic findings. Commonly referred to as "snowboarder's ankle," the lateral process comprises up to 24% of talar body fractures [17]. The mechanism of injury involves a dorsiflexed, inverted foot subjected to an external rotatory force, commonly due to high energy forces. Clinically, lateral process fractures can be misdiagnosed as ankle sprains of the anterior tibiofibular ligament, given the similarity of presentation and site of localized pain [17]. Radiographically, ankle mortise views provide a profile of the lateral process. CT scan remains the imaging modality of choice and frequently reveals more extensive comminution and displacement than originally evident on radiographs.

Unlike the talar head, lateral process fractures are typically classified as intraarticular injuries. These fractures extend to the facets that articulate with the distal fibula and the anterolateral subtalar joint. As a result, missed diagnoses pose increased risk of significant subtalar arthritis [5]. Similar to talar head fractures, nondisplaced lateral process fractures may be treated with immobilization and graduated weight bearing, while open reduction and internal fixation is appropriate where there is articular comminution or displacement. Chronic pain after a missed, remote injury may necessitate subtalar fusion if significant joint arthrosis is present.

Fractures of the posterior process of the talus involve a larger portion of the talar body, roughly 25% of the articulating subtalar surface [3]. Like other talar fractures, these typically involve high energy mechanisms. Avulsion of the lateral tubercle can occur through forceful inversion, whereas extreme plantar flexion crushes the posterior malleolus against the posterior process of the talus. Similarly, the medial tubercle of the posterior process may avulse through tension of the deltoid ligament in forceful dorsiflexion with pronation. Clinically, patients experience pain with forced plantar flexion as the posterior process of the talus is compressed. Location of pain is dependent on the location of the fracture within the posterior process; fragments that disrupt the groove for the flexor hallucis longus often elicit pain with great toe flexion and extension. Fractures that involve the posteromedial tubercle are universally accompanied by medial subtalar joint dislocation and frequent tenderness to palpation over the medial posterior ankle [11].

On radiographs, posterior process fractures must be distinguished from an intact os trigonum, a secondary talar ossification center. If present, the os trigonum is located posterior to the lateral tubercle and may resemble a fracture fragment. As with other talar fractures, a CT scan remains the most reliable method of identifying subtle fractures, especially in the presence of suggestive clinical symptoms.

Displaced posterior process fractures are treated via open reduction and internal fixation, while nonsurgical treatment may be judiciously employed for nondisplaced, minimally comminuted fractures. In the presence of significant displaced comminution, surgical removal of fragments may improve long-term outcomes. As with other talar fractures, subtalar arthrodesis may be required for posttraumatic subtalar arthrosis.

6. Navicular Fracture

Fractures of the tarsal navicular occur when the talus and the cuneiforms of the midfoot compress the navicular (Figure 4). This combination of forces most often results in transverse fractures towards the plantar aspect of the navicular, resulting in superior displacement of the dorsal navicular fragment [9]. As a result, the medial column is fundamentally damaged and frequently demonstrates gross instability. Clinically, navicular fractures may present with gross deformity, such as tenting of the skin overlying a displaced navicular fragment, or patients may only endorse midfoot pain and swelling. Plain films should be taken to evaluate the continuity between the dorsal and plantar aspects of the navicular and associated cuneiforms; displacement is indicative of fracture. CT scans are most useful in determining whether there is plantar comminution.

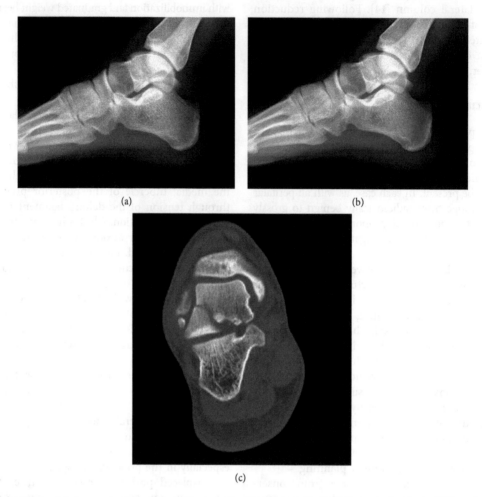

(a)

(b)

(c)

FIGURE 2: Lateral foot X-ray (a) demonstrating subtle fracture, vertically oriented across the talar body. Sagittal (b) and coronal (CT) cuts better elucidating fracture pattern. Primary fracture line extends posterior to the lateral process of the talus. There is intraarticular extension into the middle and posterior subtalar joints. Fracture extends into the anterior talar dome with articular step-off.

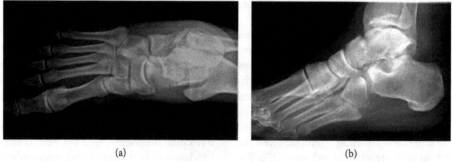

(a)

(b)

FIGURE 3: Continued.

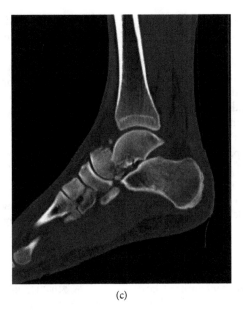

(c)

FIGURE 3: AP (a) and lateral (b) foot X-rays demonstrating a displaced talar neck fracture. CT scan (c) better elucidates the comminution and fracture pattern.

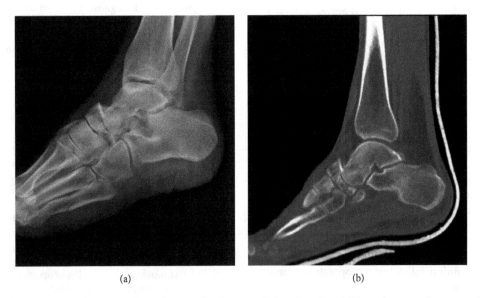

(a)   (b)

FIGURE 4: Lateral foot X-ray (a) demonstrating talonavicular fracture dislocation. In addition, there are fractures of the 4th and 5th metatarsal shafts. CT scan (b) better elucidates the fracture pattern. The talus was driven into the lateral aspect of the navicular producing a comminuted fracture.

Treatment in the acute setting consists of immobilization and protected weight bearing for nondisplaced fractures, with open reduction and internal fixation if displacement is present. Consideration in either case must be given to the propensity of the navicular for nonunion or avascular necrosis, given its limited blood supply. As with talar fractures, chronic pain after remote navicular fracture can be treated with talonavicular arthrodesis.

7. Occult Calcaneal Fracture

The calcaneus is the largest tarsal bone in the foot and the most commonly fractured. There are several major fracture variants which present with obvious clinical or radiographic findings; however, in the context of traumatic peritalar injuries, two important subtler fracture patterns can be difficult to identify [3]. A Sanders Type II fracture with a lateral calcaneal fragment involving the calcaneal tuberosity displaced laterally and proximally may result in lateral dislocation of the subtalar joint. Unlike the majority of high energy calcaneal fractures, this variant has been shown to result from lower energy axial, twisting forces. This lateral calcaneal displacement is often difficult to distinguish on AP and lateral radiographs but may be visible on a mortise view of the ankle, where the displaced lateral calcaneal facet appears beneath the distal fibula. Open reduction and internal fixation provides definitive treatment, with subtalar fusion for posttraumatic subtalar arthrosis [18].

A rare calcaneal variant is an isolated sustentaculum tali fracture, where the Bohler angle is again preserved [3]. In contrast to a Sanders Type II fracture, this variant involves high energy axial forces with varus loading and rotation, a mechanism which can produce concomitant talus fractures. Clinical suspicion in the presence of hind or midfoot swelling, ecchymosis, or unexplained pain should prompt thorough evaluation, with CT imaging if there is concern for fracture not apparent on plain films. As with the majority of calcaneal fractures, open reduction and internal fixation is the treatment of choice for sustentacular fractures.

8. Summary

In the context of trauma, with frequent concomitant large bone injury, neurologic deficit, or hemodynamic instability, injuries of the foot can prove both less urgent and more difficult to treat. Once a patient is stabilized and, however, other injuries have been addressed, appropriate orthopaedic care should be undertaken of all extremities. Given the frequency of tarsal bone injury in the context of high energy trauma, attention must be given to identifying possible fractures, ligamentous injuries, and dislocations of the hind and midfoot.

A high degree of clinical acumen and suspicion for injury must be employed in the presence of significant soft tissue swelling, hind or midfoot ecchymosis, gross deformity, crepitus, instability, or pain out of proportion to the provisional diagnosis. Standard foot X-rays along with oblique views should be obtained to evaluate for fractures. We also recommend obtaining contralateral foot films to thoroughly assess for occult injuries and posttraumatic changes. When initial films are unrevealing, CT scanning is invaluable in evaluating the degree of comminution and displacement of known fractures. It can also help with operative planning and assessment of union following nonoperative management of known injuries.

A thorough understanding of peritalar injuries is important as a high degree of morbidity results if the injury is missed. The most common consequence is chronic pain and progressive arthrosis, often necessitating salvage arthrodesis. As we have noted above, several fracture variants, including chopart joint injury and occult calcaneal fractures, are mentioned primarily in case reports. Further research of peritalar injuries should include more thorough retrospective reviews of these fractures.

Authors' Contributions

All authors contributed extensively to the construction of this manuscript and were involved with final edits. All authors approve the submission of this manuscript. ARA conceived the idea, edited the manuscript, and completed the abstract, introduction, and conclusion sections. CTA also helped conceive the idea, recruited authors, helped with editing the document, and completed the subtalar dislocations section. SFH and JY wrote the chopart joint injury and talar fracture section. MM and KD helped with final edits and wrote the navicular fractures and occult calcaneal fractures sections. AR wrote remaining sections, helped with final edits, and oversaw the entire project.

References

[1] S. Lau, M. Bozin, and T. Thillainadesan, "Lisfranc fracture dislocation: a review of a commonly missed injury of the midfoot," *Emergency Medicine Journal*, vol. 34, no. 1, pp. 52–56, 2017.

[2] C.-J. Wei, W.-C. Tsai, C.-M. Tiu, H.-T. Wu, H.-J. Chiou, and C.-Y. Chang, "Systematic analysis of missed extremity fractures in emergency radiology," *Acta Radiologica*, vol. 47, no. 7, pp. 710–717, 2006.

[3] J. X. Kou and P. T. Fortin, "Commonly missed peritalar injuries," *JAAOS*, vol. 17, pp. 775–786, 2019.

[4] S. A. Matuszak, E. A. Baker, C. M. Stewart, and P. T. Fortin, "Missed peritalar injuries an analysis of factors in cases of known delayed diagnosis and methods for improving identification," *Foot and Ankle Specialists*, vol. 7, no. 5, pp. 863–871, 2014.

[5] T. Schepers and S. Rammelt, "Complex foot injury," *Foot and Ankle Clinics*, vol. 22, no. 1, pp. 193–213, 2017.

[6] R. Sanders and S. Papp, "Fractures of the midfoot and forefoot," *Surgery of the Foot and Ankle*, vol. 8, pp. 2204–2211, 2007.

[7] A. Sangeorzan and B. Sangeorzan, "Subtalar joint biomechanics," *Foot and Ankle Clinics*, vol. 23, no. 3, pp. 341–352, 2018.

[8] J. B. Arnold, P. Caravaggi, F. Fraysse, D. Thewlis, and A. Leardini, "Movement coordination patterns between the foot joints during walking," *Journal of Foot and Ankle Research*, vol. 10, no. 1, pp. 1–7, 2017.

[9] S. G. Burne, C. M. Mahoney, B. B. Forster, M. S. Koehle, J. E. Taunton, and K. M. Khan, "Tarsal navicular stress injury," *The American Journal of Sports Medicine*, vol. 33, no. 12, pp. 1875–1881, 2005.

[10] D. Giannoulis, D. V. Papadopoulos, M. G. Lykissas, P. Koulouvaris, I. Gkiatas, and A. Mavrodontidis, "Subtalar dislocation without associated fractures: case report and review of literature," *World Journal of Orthopedics*, vol. 6, no. 3, pp. 374–379, 2015.

[11] B. J. Grear, "Review of talus fractures and surgical timing," *Orthopedic Clinics of North America*, vol. 47, no. 3, pp. 625–637, 2016.

[12] A. Prada-Cañizares, I. Auñón-Martín, J. Vilá y Rico, and J. Pretell-Mazzini, "Subtalar dislocation: management and prognosis for an uncommon orthopaedic condition," *International Orthopaedics*, vol. 40, no. 5, pp. 999–1007, 2016.

[13] K. Zhang, Y. Chen, M. Qiang, and Y. Hao, "Effects of five hindfoot arthrodeses on foot and ankle motion: measurements in cadaver specimens," *Scientific Reports*, vol. 6, no. 1, pp. 1–8, 2016.

[14] J. A. Cross, B. D. McHenry, R. Molthen, E. Exten, T. G. Schmidt, and G. F. Harris, "Biplane fluoroscopy for hindfoot motion analysis during gait: a model-based evaluation," *Medical Engineering and Physics*, vol. 43, pp. 118–123, 2017.

[15] J. R. Shank, S. K. Benirschke, and M. P. Swords, "Treatment of peripheral talus fractures," *Foot and Ankle Clinics*, vol. 22, no. 1, pp. 181–192, 2017.

[16] S. Sundararajan, A. Badurudeen, R. Ramakanth, and S. Rajasekaran, "Management of talar body fractures," *Indian Journal of Orthopaedics*, vol. 52, no. 3, pp. 258–268, 2018.

[17] P. McCrory and C. Bladin, "Fractures of the lateral process of the talus," *Clinical Journal of Sport Medicine*, vol. 6, no. 2, pp. 124–128, 1996.

[18] A. Razik, M. Harris, and A. Trompeter, "Calcaneal fractures: where are we now?," *Strategies Trauma Limb Reconstr*, vol. 13, no. 1, pp. 1–11, 2018.

The Ischial Spine in Developmental Hip Dysplasia: Unraveling the Role of Acetabular Retroversion in Periacetabular Osteotomy

Gerard El-Hajj[1] **Hicham Abdel-Nour,**[2] **Rami Ayoubi,**[2] **Joseph Maalouly,**[2] **Fouad Jabbour,**[2] **Raja Ashou,**[1] **and Alexandre Nehme**[2]

[1]*Department of Radiology, Saint George Hospital University Medical Center, University of Balamand, P.O. Box 166378, Achrafieh, Beirut 1100 2807, Lebanon*
[2]*Department of Orthopedic Surgery and Traumatology, Saint George Hospital University Medical Center, University of Balamand, P.O. Box 166378, Achrafieh, Beirut 1100 2807, Lebanon*

Correspondence should be addressed to Gerard El-Hajj; gerard.hajj@gmail.com

Academic Editor: Allen L. Carl

Purpose. Radiological diagnosis of acetabular retroversion (AR) is based on the presence of the crossover sign (COS), the posterior wall sign (PWS), and the prominence of the ischial spine sign (PRISS). The primary purpose of the study is to analyze the clinical significance of the PRISS in a sample of dysplastic hips requiring periacetabular osteotomy (PAO) and evaluate retroversion in symptomatic hip dysplasia. *Methods.* In a previous paper, we reported the classic coxometric measurements of 178 patients with symptomatic hip dysplasia undergoing PAO where retroversion was noted in 42% of the cases and was not found to be a major factor in the appearance of symptoms. In the current study, we have added the retroversion signs PRISS and PWS to our analysis. Among the retroverted dysplastic hips, we studied the association of the PRISS with the hips requiring PAO. We also defined the ischial spine index (ISI) and studied its relationship to the coxometric measurements and AR. *Results.* In hips with AR, the operated hips were significantly associated with the PRISS compared to the nonoperated ones ($\chi^2 = 4.847$). Additionally, the ISI was able to classify acetabular version (anteverted, neutral, and retroverted acetabula). A direct correlation between the ISI and the retroversion index (RI) was found, and the highest degree of retroversion was found when the 3 signs of acetabular retroversion were concomitantly present (RI = 33.6%). *Conclusion.* The PRISS, a radiographic sign reflecting AR, was found to be significantly associated with dysplastic hips requiring PAO where AR was previously not considered a factor in the manifestation of symptoms and subsequent requirement for surgery. Moreover, the PRISS can also serve as an adequate radiographic sign for estimating acetabular version on pelvic radiographs.

1. Introduction

Subtle variations in normal anatomy of the hip joint labeled by Ganz et al. as CAM and pincer-type impingement can cause a premature contact between the head-neck junction and the anterior wall of the acetabulum leading to early hip osteoarthritis (OA). This was later confirmed by Tanzer et al., and a clear relationship between FAI and early OA was established [1–3]. Reynold defined the crossover sign (COS) and the posterior wall sign (PWS) as the radiological parameters to detect acetabular retroversion on a typical AP pelvic radiograph [4]. The COS is positive in all retroversion

cases, whereas the PWS is positive only in hips with deficient posterior wall. Jamali et al. confirmed that the presence of a positive crossover sign is a highly reliable indicator of acetabular retroversion with anatomic correlations performed on 43 cadavers [5]. However, despite being good radiological indicators, the COS and PWS both rely on difficult visualization of the acetabular walls [6–8].

As a result, the prominence of the ischial spine (PRIS) inside the pelvic brim emerged as a more reproducible sign reflecting acetabular retroversion because it is easier to detect. It was first described by Kalberer et al. in 2008, with excellent sensitivity and a positive predictive value [9]. It has been shown to have high interobserver and intraobserver reliability among orthopedic surgeons and radiologists [10]. This sign has been studied in a series of retroverted hips including mostly normally covered hips but never on a series including only patients operated for unilateral or bilateral hip dysplasia.

In fact, in patients with hip dysplasia, whether unilateral or bilateral, the dysplastic retroverted sockets constitute a specific subgroup (42%) [11]. The surgical decision of performing a periacetabular osteotomy (PAO) in this subgroup is dictated by the amount of dysplasia and not by retroversion [12].

However, at the time of the study, the ischial spine was not a well-established sign of retroversion. In our study, we found that the addition of the sign can be used to uncover potential morphological associations reflected by the ischial spine.

Retroversion in the setting of dysplasia does not seem to produce impingement even though a COS is present. In fact, there is global insufficient development of the anterior and posterior walls associated with a steeper inclination of the neck in the setting of increased valgus, which makes a premature contact between both nearly inexistent.

Moreover, it is paramount to diagnose retroversion in those hips in order to be able to correctly orient the osteotomized fragment and thus avoid postoperative impingement. Because when corrected, those hips becoming normally covered but still retroverted, will have the distance of the anterior wall to the head-neck junction shortened, and hence will become symptomatic [13–15].

Therefore, our aim is to study the variation of the PRIS sign (PRISS) in a series of patients undergoing PAOs to correct unilateral or bilateral dysplasia, according to acetabular version, and to the presence (requiring PAO) or absence (conservative treatment) of symptoms in dysplasia.

2. Materials and Methods

A total of 227 patients underwent PAO between 1995 and December 2003. Patients who were asymptomatic, even when presenting with radiological signs of congenital dysplasia, were treated conservatively. Only symptomatic patients who were experiencing pain secondary to their congenital hip dysplasia underwent surgeries; 204 patients underwent unilateral PAO, and 23 patients underwent bilateral two-staged PAO.

The following inclusion criteria were used for reviewing the preoperative radiographs:

(1) The anterior and posterior walls, the bearing surface, as well as the external edge of the acetabulum were well defined on the radiographs.

(2) The symmetries of the iliac wings and the obturator foramens were used to check for neutral rotation.

(3) Coccyx to pubic symphysis distance of less than 2 cm was measured to have neutral tilts of the pelvis.

(4) Percentage of femoral head coverage was measured on hips in neutral abduction.

(5) A Lequesne false profile radiograph was obtained for each patient.

Radiographs that did not meet the inclusion criteria were excluded from this study. Patients with a diagnosis of neuromuscular dysplasia or Legg-Perthes-Calvé disease were also omitted. The remaining number of patients was 174 (348 hips), with a mean age of 30 years (range, 15–56 years; SD = 10.5), 137 were females (79%) and 37 were males (21%). The selection and total patients are shown in Figure 1.

2.1. Radiographic Hip Parameters

(1) Prominence of the ischial spine (PRIS) is an alternate radiographic sign for acetabular retroversion because in these hips, the whole hemipelvis is rotated. PRIS 1 measured the ischial spine protruding into pelvic inlet, and PRIS 2 measured the entire ischial spine extending to the ilioischial line (Figure 2). If the ischial spine extends beyond the pelvic brim, it is considered a positive sign (PRIS 1 > 0).

(2) Ischial spine index (ISI), newly described ratio of PRIS 1 over PRIS 2, which accounts for the percentage of the ischial spine protruding into the pelvic inlet.

(3) Lateral center-edge (Wiberg's) angle, measured by a vertical line and a line connecting the femoral head center with the lateral edge of the acetabulum. Normal LCE angles ranges from 20° to 40°. Angles below 20° indicate hip dysplasia.

(4) Vertical-center-anterior edge (VCA) angle, formed by intersection of a vertical line through the center of the femoral head and a line extending through the center of the femoral head to the anterior sourcil. It measures anterior dysplasia on the false profile view and is an indicator of the degree of femoral head anterior coverage. Normal values range from 20 to 50 degrees.

(5) Tönnis angle, formed between a horizontal line and a line extending from the medial to lateral edges of the sourcil. Acetabula having a Tönnis angle of 0°–10° are considered normal, whereas those having an angle of >10° or <0° are considered to have increased and decreased inclination, respectively. Acetabula with increased Tönnis angles are subject to structural instability, whereas those with decreased Tönnis angles are at risk for pincer-type femoroacetabular impingement.

(6) The index of extrusion of the femoral head measured as the lateral part of the femoral head not covered by the acetabulum divided by the total width of the head. Values under 25% are usually indicators of an adequately covered femoral head.

(7) Acetabular index depth to width: it is the depth of central portion of acetabulum divided by the width of acetabular opening.

(8) Acetabular orientation was assessed using the crossover sign.

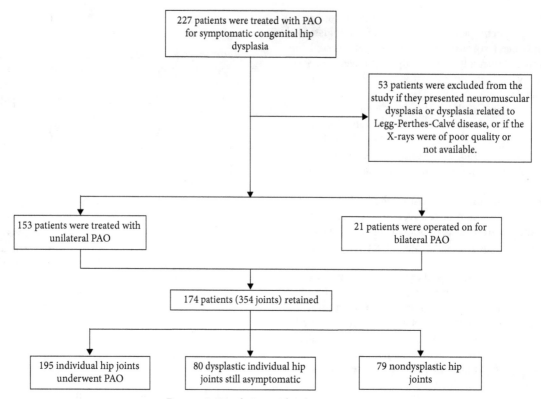

FIGURE 1: Population with selection criteria.

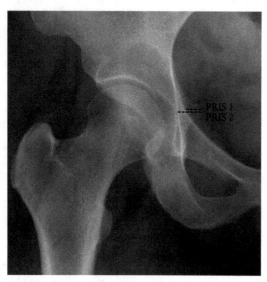

FIGURE 2: Pelvic AP radiograph showing PRIS 1 and PRIS 2 measurements.

(9) Crossover distance, distance between the supero-lateral edge of the acetabulum and the crossover sign.

2.2. Statistical Analysis. To compare the coxometric measurements according to the presence or absence of the ischial spine, a *t*-test was used to analyze the difference between the 2 groups. A Pearson product-moment correlation coefficient was computed to assess the relationship between length of the ischial spine and the following parameters: retroversion

index and crossover distance. The following correlation scale was taken: 0.00–0.19 "very weak," 0.20–0.39 "weak," 0.40–0.59 "moderate," 0.60–0.79 "strong," and 0.80–1.0 "very strong." One-way analysis of variance (ANOVA) was used to compare the 3 acetabular version groups. The chi-square independence test was used to study the association between the signs and the surgical hips.

2.3. Interobserver Reproducibility. Interobserver reproducibility of ischial spine measurements was evaluated by 2 different radiologists in a subset of 100 hips using a two-way, mixed, consistency single-measures intraclass correlation coefficient (ICC). ICC values greater than 0.80 indicate excellent reliability, 0.61–0.80 substantial reliability, 0.41–0.60 moderate reliability, 0.21–0.40 fair reliability, and <0.20 poor reliability [16]. The ICC showed excellent reliability for measurements of PRIS 1 (ICC ¼ 0.823, 95% confidence interval (CI) 0.776–0.876).

3. Results and Discussion

3.1. Analysis of the Length of the Ischial Spine. When classified according to acetabular version (anteverted, neutral, and retroverted), there was a statistically significant difference in the ISI between groups as determined by one-way ANOVA (F (2,183) = 33.665, $P < 0.001$). A Tukey post hoc test revealed that the ISI was statistically significantly lower in the anteverted (5.64 ± 13.08%, $P < 0.001$) and neutral (21.33 ± 24.68%, $P < 0.0001$) acetabula compared to the retroverted group (34.16 ± 24.83%, $P < 0.001$). The

TABLE 1: Comparison of the 3 acetabular version groups where analysis of variance was performed.

Acetabular version	Ischial spine index (%)	PRIS 1 (mm)	PRIS 2 (mm)	Age (years)	CE angle (degrees)	CA angle (degrees)	Tönnis angle
Anteverted	5.64 ± 13.08	0.46 ± 1.17	6.29 ± 2.55	31.32 ± 10.87	5.31 ± 10.39	-0.33 ± 14.44	25.36 ± 6.70
($n = 72$)	(0–63)	(0–6.4)	(2.40–18.1)	(15–56)	(-26–30)	(-44–28)	(7–45)
Neutral	20.30 ± 24.68	1.73 ± 2.19	7.16 ± 2.33	33.06 ± 9.76	8.22 ± 9.30	1.03 ± 14.96	22.16 ± 5.82
($n = 34$)	(0–80)	(0–7)	(3–11.8)	(15–48)	(−17–24)	(−30–32)	(9–35)
Retroverted	34.16 ± 25.48	3.32 ± 3.09	8.47 ± 3.26	28.12 ± 10.04	4.28 ± 12.54	-0.11 ± 19.52	24.11 ± 8.04
($n = 78$)	(0–80)	(0–13.80)	(3–17.8)	(15–48)	(−50–26)	(−46–47)	(0–44)
Total ($n = 184$)	21.33 ± 24.83	1.90 ± 2.66	7.38 ± 2.99	30.29 ± 10.45	5.42 ± 11.21	0.02 ± 16.76	24.23 ± 7.21
	(0–80)	(0–13.8)	(2.4–18.1)	(15–56)	(−50–30)	(−46–57)	(0–45)
F	33.665	27.94	11.1	3.44	1.55	0.07	2.43
Mean square	15299.248	153.843	90.380	367.355	194.053	20.993	124.857
P	<0.001	<0.001	<0.001	0.03	0.21	0.92	0.09

All values are described as mean ± SD (range). CE angle = Wiberg lateral coverage angle; Tönnis angle = acetabular bearing surface index; CA angle = Lequesne anterior coverage angle.

TABLE 2: Correlations of coxometric measurements with length of ischial spine.

	PRIS 1		PRIS 2		ISI	
	r coefficient	P	r coefficient	P	r coefficient	P
CD	0.612**	<0.001	0.466**	<0.001	0.556**	<0.001
RI	0.416**	0.003	0.154	0.221	0.294**	0.009

PRIS = prominence of the ischial spine; ISI = ischial spine index; CD = crossover distance; RI = retroversion index.

demographics and other radiographic parameters are shown in Table 1.

Furthermore, we found a good positive correlation with the crossover distance (Pearson's $r = 0.612$, $P < 0.0001$) and a moderate positive correlation with the retroversion index (Pearson's $r = 0.416$, $P = 0.003$). As for the PRISS 2, we only found significant correlations with the crossover distance ($r = 0.466$) (Table 2).

3.2. Coxometric Measurements according to the Presence of the PRISS (Ischial Spine as a Positive or Negative Sign).
When compared according to the PRISS, hips with the positive sign were significantly associated with greater crossover distance compared to those without the PRISS (Table 3).

3.3. Validity of the PRISS in Determining Acetabular Version.
Figure 3 shows the association between the PRISS and acetabular version in hips requiring PAO (χ^2 (2, $N = 184$) = 52.03, Cramer's $V = 0.527$, $P < 0.001$). The proportion of the PRISS in the groups was gradually increasing moving from anteverted, neutral, to retroverted.

Table 4 shows the acetabular retroversion index in different combination of radiographic markers. RI (corresponding to the amount of acetabulum that is retroverted) was found to be highest when all the signs are positive and lowest when all are negative.

We compared the radiographic measurements between operated and nonoperated hips. We found no significant difference in the ISI (Table 5). However, when taken as a binary sign, we found a significant association of the PRISS with the operated hips (Figure 4), whereas when

TABLE 3: Comparison of coxometric measurements according to ischial spine sign.

	Ischial spine		Mean difference (%)	P
	Present (%)	Absent (%)		
RI	33.37	31.60	1.76	0.593
CD	11.45	2.48	8.97	<0.001

RI = retroversion index; CD = crossover distance.

assessed by the COS, there was no significant association (Figure 5).

4. Discussion

Due to the irregular nature of acetabular walls in dysplastic hips, these walls might provide unclear morphological data of acetabular version. We showed that the use of the ischial spine as a surrogate sign for acetabular retroversion is a valid method and that it can reflect general acetabular orientation.

In this study, when PRIS was positive, not only did it show that in hip dysplasia the ischial spine was able to reflect retroversion but its degree of pelvic protrusion (ischial spine index) was able to classify the acetabular version (Table 1 and Figure 3).

Additionally, the simultaneous presence of the COS, PWS, and PRISS signs returned the highest degree of retroversion index (Table 4). Consequently, this reflects a higher degree of acetabular retroversion. These 3 signs may indicate the involvement of the whole midsegment of the pelvis composed of the whole acetabulum and the ischial spine in the setting of retroversion. These hips were associated with an average of 33.6% retroversion index, the most pronounced among all groups tested. No studies were able to

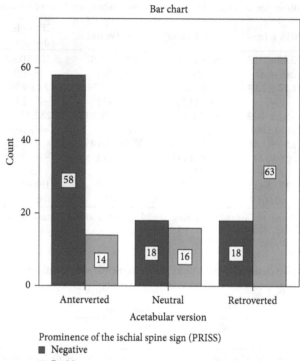

FIGURE 3: Distribution of the PRISS according to acetabular version (χ^2 (2, $N = 184$) = 52.03, Cramer's $V = 0.527$, $P < 0.001$).

TABLE 4: Retroversion index according to radiographic markers (PWS, COS, and ISS).

	Retroversion index	
	PRISS (+) (%)	PRISS (−) (%)
(+) COS, (+) PWS	33.6%	29.9
(+) COS, (−) PWS	25.6%	23.8

TABLE 5: Comparison of the dysplastic PAO vs. dysplastic non-PAO groups.

Dysplastic hips	ISI (%)	PRIS 1 (mm)	PRIS 2 (mm)	RI (%)	Age (years)	CE angle (degrees)	CA angle (degrees)	Tönnis angle (degrees)
Operated hips (n = 192)	20.51 ± 24.77 (0–80)	1.91 ± 2.66 (0–6.4)	7.38 ± 2.99 (2.40–18.1)	32.97 ± 12.25 (10.2–64.3)	30.32 ± 10.87 (15–56)	5.45 ± 11.19 (−50–30)	6.59 ± 16.19 (−46–47)	24.19 ± 7.21 (0–45)
Nonoperated hips (n = 80)	16.05 ± 22.59 (0–81)	1.35 ± 2.01 (0–7)	7.06 ± 2.87 (2.3–20)	28.64 ± 9.24 (17.8–51.2)	30.75 ± 10.43 (15–56)	15.43 ± 8.14 (−10–28)	0.02 ± 16.71 (−25–37)	17.76 ± 5.95 (5–37)
Total (n = 272)	19.18 ± 24.18 (0–81)	1.90 ± 2.66 (0–13.8)	7.38 ± 2.99 (2.3–20)	31.8 ± 11.64 (10.2–64.3)	30.44 ± 10.53 (15–56)	8.39 ± 11.33 (−50–30)	0.02 ± 16.76 (−46–47)	22.30 ± 7.45 (0–45)
P	0.171	0.03	0.449	0.081	0.761	<0.001	0.059	<0.001

All values are described as mean ± SD (range). ISI = ischial spine index; RI = retroversion index.

correlate the length of the ischial spine to measure the degree of acetabular version.

4.1. Ischial Spine Sign in Operated Hips.

It was previously suggested that the presence of acetabular retroversion is probably independent of congenital hip dysplasia and that it appears to be a secondary factor in the appearance of acetabular dysplasia symptoms [12]. In that former study, retroversion was assessed using the retroversion index

derived from the COS. The corresponding hips were tagged as retroverted based solely on the presence of the COS. Consequently, hips that are actually anatomically different (i.e., hips with the COS having a positive (Figure 6(f)) or negative PRISS (Figure 6(e)) were studied as one group, and no significant association was found between the COS and the requirement for PAO (Figure 5).

These seemingly identically retroverted hips (positive COS on AP radiograph) can be further subcategorized according to the PRISS, where in our current study, we

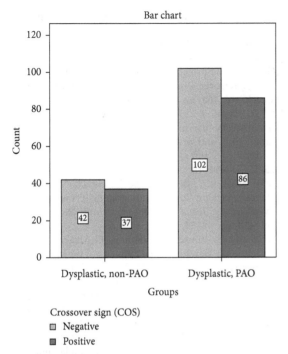

FIGURE 4: The ischial spine sign in retroverted dysplastic hips (PAO vs. non-PAO); $\chi^2 = 4.847$, $P = 0.027$.

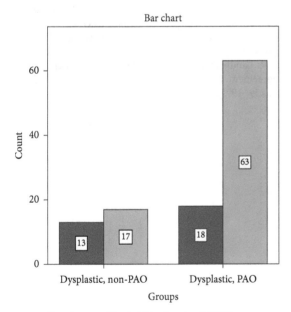

FIGURE 5: The crossover sign in all dysplastic hips (PAO vs. non-PAO); $\chi^2 = .027$, $P = 0.488$.

filtered the retroverted dysplastic group according to this sign and showed that the dysplastic group requiring PAO (i.e. patient with symptomatic hip dysplasia) was, in addition to being more dysplastic, significantly associated with the PRISS (Figure 4). This hints that in the setting of hip

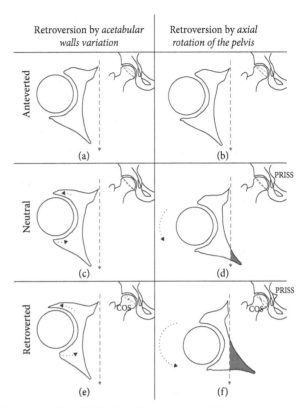

FIGURE 6: Simplified hip illustrations explaining the possible mechanisms of retroversion: acetabular walls variation versus axial rotation of the pelvis. The arrow depicts the direction of AP pelvic radiographs projection. The hip at the top right is a simulation of an AP pelvic X-ray showing the COS and PRISS for each corresponding setting where the anterior and posterior (green and blue dashed lines, respectively) acetabular walls are outlined. COS = crossover sign; PRISS = prominence of the ischial spine sign.

dysplasia, acetabular retroversion might be involved in the manifestation of hip symptoms leading to PAO.

In order to interpret our results, we have to consider the midsegment of the pelvis including both the acetabulum and the ischial spine as a whole unit. In that setting, whenever you have a positive ischial spine sign protruding beyond the pelvic brim in the inner pelvis, it reflects an external rotation of this midsegment (Figure 6(f)).

Therefore, in this setting of a positive PRISS, the presence of a retroverted acetabulum with a positive PRISS could be explained by the concept of "combined retroversion" including first, the classic Reynolds theory where retroversion is caused by an overhang of the anterior wall or an underdeveloped posterior wall both producing a crossover sign on AP X-ray and occasionally causing pincer-type impingement. And second, the associated external rotation of the whole mid-pelvic segment exaggerating the retroversion and protruding the ischial spine internally beyond the pelvic brim.

We can conclude that surgical retroverted dysplastic hips were more dysplastic and had a more pronounced combined retroversion as assessed by the association of a positive PRISS. It suggests that retroversion does contribute to the presence of symptoms but only as long as the retroversion is associated with axial rotation of the hemipelvis.

For the surgeon dealing with PAO surgery, the presence of the positive PRISS should trigger caution that this hip might be more dysplastic and more symptomatic and hence more surgical. And the surgeon should also have the notion of combined retroversion in mind, while reorienting the osteotomized fragment.

To note, the lack of significant association of the length of the ischial spine does not reflect contradicting results when comparing the PAO group to the non-PAO one. Ultimately, the surgeon relies on the presence or absence of the studied ischial spine sign radiographically to aid in the surgical decision making (rather than measuring its corresponding length that was shown here to lack any clinical significance).

5. Conclusions

The PRISS is a valid sign for diagnosing acetabular retroversion in dysplastic hips requiring corrective surgery. The findings in our study are important in guiding corrective osteotomy of the acetabulum. Additionally, ISI, the newly described ischial spine index, allows comprehensive assessment of the ischial spine taking into account variation in hip anatomy and ischial spine patient-specific morphology.

Lastly, the association of the PRISS with hips requiring PAO alludes to a considerable role of retroversion in symptomatic patients. The ischial spine conveys morphological information pertaining to acetabular retroversion that is otherwise lacking with the COS and PWS in the setting of surgical hip dysplasia.

References

[1] R. Ganz, J. Parvizi, M. Beck, M. Leunig, H. Nötzli, and K. A. Siebenrock, "Femoroacetabular impingement: a cause for osteoarthritis of the hip," *Clinical Orthopaedics and Related Research*, vol. 417, pp. 112–120, 2003.

[2] M. Tanzer and N. Noiseux, "Osseous abnormalities and early osteoarthritis: the role of hip impingement," *Clinical Orthopaedics and Related Research*, vol. 429, pp. 170–177, 2004.

[3] M. Beck, "Hip morphology influences the pattern of damage to the acetabular cartilage: femoroacetabular impingement as a cause of early osteoarthritis of the hip," *The Journal of Bone and Joint Surgery. British volume*, vol. 87, no. 7, pp. 1012–1018, 2005.

[4] D. Reynolds, J. Lucas, and K. Klaue, "Retroversion of the acetabulum," *The Journal of Bone and Joint Surgery. British volume*, vol. 81-B, no. 2, pp. 281–288, 1999.

[5] A. A. Jamali, K. Mladenov, D. C. Meyer et al., "Anteroposterior pelvic radiographs to assess acetabular retroversion: high validity of the "cross-over-sign"" *Journal of Orthopaedic Research*, vol. 25, no. 6, pp. 758–765, 2007.

[6] C. Dora, M. Leunig, M. Beck, R. Simovitch, and R. Ganz, "Acetabular dome retroversion: radiological apperance, incidence and relevance," *HIP International*, vol. 16, no. 3, pp. 215–222, 2006.

[7] I. Zaltz, B. T. Kelly, I. Hetsroni, and A. Bedi, "The crossover sign overestimates acetabular retroversion hip," *Clinical Orthopaedics and Related Research*, vol. 471, no. 8, pp. 2463–2470, 2013.

[8] K. A. Siebenrock, D. F. Kalbermatten, and R. Ganz, "Effect of pelvic tilt on acetabular retroversion: a study of pelves from cadavers," *Clinical Orthopaedics and Related Research*, vol. 407, pp. 241–248, 2003.

[9] F. Kalberer, R. J. Sierra, S. S. Madan, R. Ganz, and M. Leunig, "Ischial spine projection into the pelvis: a new sign for acetabular retroversion," *Clinical Orthopaedics and Related Research*, vol. 466, no. 3, pp. 677–683, 2008.

[10] O. R. Ayeni, K. Chan, D. B. Whelan et al., "Diagnosing femoroacetabular impingement from plain radiographs: do radiologists and orthopaedic surgeons differ?" *Orthopaedic Journal of Sports Medicine*, vol. 2, no. 7, Article ID 232596711454141, 2014.

[11] J. W. Mast, R. L. Brunner, and J. Zebrack, "Recognizing acetabular version in the radiographic presentation of hip dysplasia," *Clinical Orthopaedics and Related Research*, vol. 418, pp. 48–53, 2004.

[12] A. Nehme, R. Trousdale, Z. Tannous, G. Maalouf, J. Puget, and N. Telmont, "Developmental dysplasia of the hip: is acetabular retroversion a crucial factor?" *Orthopaedics & Traumatology: Surgery & Research*, vol. 95, no. 7, pp. 511–519, 2009.

[13] S. R. Myers, H. Eijer, and R. Ganz, "Anterior femoroacetabular impingement after periacetabular osteotomy," *Clinical Orthopaedics and Related Research*, vol. 363, pp. 93–99, 1999.

[14] P. Castañeda, C. Vidal-Ruiz, A. Méndez, D. P. Salazar, and A. Torres, "How often does femoroacetabular impingement occur after an innominate osteotomy for acetabular dysplasia?" *Clinical Orthopaedics and Related Research*, vol. 474, no. 5, pp. 1209–1215, 2016.

[15] C. E. Albers, S. D. Steppacher, R. Ganz, M. Tannast, and K. A. Siebenrock, "Impingement adversely affects 10-year survivorship after periacetabular osteotomy for DDH," *Clinical Orthopaedics and Related Research*, vol. 471, no. 5, pp. 1602–1614, 2013.

[16] J. R. Landis and G. G. Koch, "The measurement of observer agreement for categorical data," *Biometrics*, vol. 33, no. 1, p. 159, 1977.

Permissions

List of Contributors

Georgios Gkagkalis, G.-Yves Laflamme, Dominique M. Rouleau, Stéphane Leduc and Benoit Benoit
Orthopedic Surgery, Department of Surgery, Hôpital Sacré-Coeur de Montréal, 5400 Boul. Gouin O., Montréal, Québec H4J 1C5, Canada

Kevin Moerenhout
Orthopedic Surgery, Department of Surgery, Hôpital Sacré-Coeur de Montréal, 5400 Boul. Gouin O., Montréal, Québec H4J 1C5, Canada
Department of Orthopaedics and Traumatology, Lausanne University Hospital, Rue du Bugnon 46, CH 1011 Lausanne, Switzerland

Eric K. Kim and Madeline Tiee
University of California San Francisco, School of Medicine, San Francisco, California, USA

Claire A. Donnelley and Ericka Von Kaeppler
Institute for Global Orthopaedics and Traumatology, Department of Orthopaedics, University of California, San Francisco, California, USA

Heather J. Roberts and David Shearer
University of California San Francisco, Department of Orthopaedic Surgery, San Francisco, California, USA

Saam Morshed
University of California San Francisco, Department of Orthopaedic Surgery, San Francisco, California, USA
University of California San Francisco, Department of Epidemiology and Biostatistics, San Francisco, California, USA

Varah Yuenyongviwat, Chonthawat Jiarasrisatien, Khanin Iamthanaporn, Theerawit Hongnaparak and Boonsin Tangtrakulwanich
Department of Orthopedics, Faculty of Medicine, Prince of Songkla University, Songkhla 90110, Thailand

Ziyad M. Mohaidat and Ali A. Al-omari
Orthopedic & Spine Surgeon, King Abdullah University Hospital, Irbid 22110, Jordan
Orthopedic Surgery Division, Special Surgery Department, Faculty of Medicine, Jordan University of Science and Technology, Irbid 22110, Jordan

Salah R. Al-gharaibeh, Osama N. Aljararhih and Murad T. Nusairat
Orthopedic Surgery Resident, King Abdullah University Hospital, Jordan University of Science and Technology, Irbid 22110, Jordan

Sharan Mallya, Surendra U. Kamath and Rajendra Annappa
Department of Orthopaedics, Kasturba Medical College, Mangalore, Manipal Academy of Higher Education, Manipal, India

Nithin Elliot Nazareth
Department of Orthopaedics, Father Muller Medical College Hospital, Mangalore, India

Krithika Kamath and Pragya Tyagi
Kasturba Medical College, Mangalore, Manipal Academy of Higher Education, Manipal, India

Yunus Oc
Medilife Health Group, Bagcilar Hospital, Department of Orthopaedics and Traumatology, Istanbul, Turkey

Bekir Eray Kilinc
Health Science University Istanbul Fatih Sultan Mehmet Training and Research Hospital, Department of Orthopaedics and Traumatology, Istanbul, Turkey

Ali Varol
Health Ministry, Silopi State Hospital, Department of Orthopaedics and Traumatology, Sirnak, Turkey

Adnan Kara
Medipol University Istanbul, Department of Orthopaedics and Traumatology, Istanbul, Turkey

Chengxin Li, Zhizhuo Li and Qiwei Wang
Department of Orthopedics, Peking University China-Japan Friendship School of Clinical Medicine, 2 Yinghuadong Road, Chaoyang District, Beijing 100029, China

Lijun Shi
Department of Orthopedics, Graduate School of Peking Union Medical College, China-Japan Friendship Institute of Clinical Medicine, 2 Yinghuadong Road, Chaoyang District, Beijing 100029, China

Fuqiang Gao and Wei Sun
Beijing Key Laboratory of Immune Inflammatory Disease, China-Japan Friendship Hospital, 2 Yinghuadong Road, Chaoyang District, Beijing 100029, China

Antimo Moretti, Annalisa De Cicco, Giovanni Landi, Nicola Tammaro, Antonio Benedetto Cecere, Adriano Braile, Alfredo Schiavone Panni and Giovanni Iolascon
Department of Medical and Surgical Specialties and Dentistry, University of Campania "Luigi Vanvitelli", Naples, Italy

Giuseppe Toro
Department of Medical and Surgical Specialties and Dentistry, University of Campania "Luigi Vanvitelli", Naples, Italy
Department of Clinical Sciences and Translational Medicine, University of Rome Tor Vergata, Rome, Italy

Umberto Tarantino
Department of Clinical Sciences and Translational Medicine, University of Rome Tor Vergata, Rome, Italy

Daniele Ambrosio, Pasquale Florio and Giacomo Negri
Unit of Orthopaedics and Traumatology, Evangelical Hospital Betania, Naples, Italy

Raffaele Pezzella
Department of Life Health & Environmental Sciences, University of L'Aquila, Unit of Orthopaedics and Traumatology, L'Aquila, Italy

Antonio Medici
Unit of Orthopaedics and Traumatology, AORN S. Giuseppe Moscati, Avellino, Italy

Antonio Siano
Unit of Orthopaedics and Traumatology, Santa Maria Della Speranza Hospital, Battipaglia, Italy

Bruno Di Maggio
Unit of Orthopaedics and Traumatology, "Ave Gratia Plena" Civil Hospital, Piedimonte Matese, Italy

Giampiero Calabrò
Unit of Orthopaedics and Traumatology, San Francesco D'Assisi Hospital, Oliveto Citra, Italy

Nicola Gagliardo
Unit of Orthopaedics and Traumatology, San Giuliano Hospital, Giugliano, Italy

Ciro Di Fino
Unit of Orthopaedics and Traumatology, AOR San Carlo, Potenza, Italy

Gaetano Bruno
Unit of Orthopaedics and Traumatology, AORN Sant'Anna e San Sebastiano, Caserta, Italy

Achille Pellegrino
Unit of Orthopaedics and Traumatology, San Giuseppe Moscati Hospital, Aversa, Italy

Vincenzo Monaco
Unit of Orthopaedics and Traumatology, Santa Maria Incoronata Dell'Olmo Hospital, Cava de' Tirreni, Italy

Michele Gison and Antonio Toro
Unit of Orthopaedics and Traumatology, Villa Malta Hospital, Sarno, Italy

Syed Imran Ghouri, Abduljabbar Alhammoud and Mohammed Mubarak Alkhayarin
Hamad Medical Corporation, Doha, Qatar

Shannon M. Kaupp, Kenneth A. Mann, Mark A. Miller and Timothy A. Damron
SUNY Upstate Medical University, Department of Orthopedic Surgery, 750 East Adams Street, Syracuse, NY 13210, USA

Dana El-Mughayyar, Erin Bigney and Eden Richardson
Canada East Spine Centre, Saint John Regional Hospital, 400 University Ave, Saint John, New Brunswick E2L 4L4, Canada

Neil Manson and Edward Abraham
Canada East Spine Centre, Saint John Regional Hospital, 400 University Ave, PO Box 2100, Saint John, New Brunswick E2L 4L4, Canada
Saint John Regional Hospital, Horizon Health Network, 400 University Ave, Saint John, New Brunswick E2L 4L4, Canada
Department of Surgery, Dalhousie University, 100 Tucker Park Rd, Saint John, New Brunswick E2K 5E2, Canada

Thomas Gatt, Daniel Cutajar, Lara Borg and Ryan Giordmaina
Department of Orthopaedics and Trauma, Mater Dei Hospital, Msida MSD2090, Malta

Michael Serra-Torres
DHR Health Orthopedic Institute, Edinburg, TX 78539, USA
DHR Health Institute for Research and Development, Edinburg, TX 78539, USA

David Weaver and Annelyn Torres-Reveron
DHR Health Institute for Research and Development, Edinburg, TX 78539, USA

Raul Barreda
DHR Health Institute for Research and Development, Edinburg, TX 78539, USA
DHR Health Surgery Institute, McAllen, TX 78504, USA

Ivan Micic
Clinic for Orthopaedic Surgery and Traumatology, Clinical Center Nis, Nis, Serbia

Erica Kholinne
Department of Orthopedic Surgery, St. Carolus Hospital, Jakarta, Indonesia
Department of Orthopedic Surgery, Asan Medical Center, University of Ulsan College of Medicine, Seoul, Republic of Korea

Jae-Man Kwak and In-Ho Jeon
Department of Orthopedic Surgery, Asan Medical Center, University of Ulsan College of Medicine, Seoul, Republic of Korea

Yucheng Sun
Department of Orthopedic Surgery, Asan Medical Center, University of Ulsan College of Medicine, Seoul, Republic of Korea
Department of Hand Surgery, Affiliated Hospital of Nantong University, Nantong, Nantong University, Jiangsu, China

Afif Harb, Emmanouil Liodakis, Sam Razaeian, Christian Krettek and Nael Hawi
Trauma Department, Hannover Medical School (MHH), Carl-Neuberg-Str. 1, Hannover 30625, Germany

Bastian Welke and Christof Hurschler
Laboratory for Biomechanics and Biomaterials, Department of Orthopaedic Surgery, Hannover Medical School, Hannover, Germany

Dafang Zhang
Department of Orthopaedic Surgery, Brigham and Women's Hospital, 75 Francis St, Boston, MA 02115, USA

Elias Saidy
Department of Orthopedic Surgery and Traumatology, Saint George Hospital University Medical Center, Balamand University, Achrafieh, Beirut 1100 2807, Lebanon

Antonios Tawk, Georges Katoul Al Rahbani and Aida Metri
Faculty of Medicine and Medical Sciences, University of Balamand, Aschrafieh, Beirut, Lebanon

Gerard El-Hajj
Department of Medical Imaging and Radiology, Saint George Hospital University Medical Center, Balamand University, Achrafieh, Beirut 1100 2807, Lebanon

Ryogo Furuhata, Yusaku Kamata, Aki Kono, Yasuhiro Kiyota and Hideo Morioka
Department of Orthopedic Surgery, National Hospital Organization Tokyo Medical Center, 2-5-1, Higashigaoka, Meguro-ku, Tokyo 152-8902, Japan

Takayuki Tani, Natsuo Konishi, Hitoshi Kubota, Shin Yamada, Hiroshi Tazawa, Norio Suzuki, Keiji Kamo, Yoshihiko Okudera, Ken Sasaki and Tetsuya Kawano
Akita Hip Research Group, Akita 010-8543, Japan

Hiroaki Kijima, Masashi Fujii, Yosuke Iwamoto, Itsuki Nagahata and Yoichi Shimada
Akita Hip Research Group, Akita 010-8543, Japan
Department of Orthopedic Surgery, Akita University Graduate School of Medicine, Hondo, Akita 010 8543, Japan

Naohisa Miyakoshi
Department of Orthopedic Surgery, Akita University Graduate School of Medicine, Hondo, Akita 010 8543, Japan

Mohamed I. Abulsoud, Mohammed Elmarghany, Tharwat Abdelghany, Mohamed Abdelaal and Mohamed F. Elhalawany
Department of Orthopedic Surgery, Faculty of Medicine, Al-Azhar University, Cairo, Egypt

Ahmed R. Zakaria
Department of Orthopedic Surgery, Helwan University, Helwan, Egypt

Giuseppe Maccagnano, Giovanni Noia, Antonio Luciano Sarni, Raffaele Quitadamo, Costantino Stigliani and Vito Pesce
Orthopaedics Unit, Department of Clinical and Experimental Medicine, Faculty of Medicine and Surgery, University of Foggia, Policlinico Riuniti di Foggia, Foggia, Italy

Giuseppe Danilo Cassano
Orthopaedics Unit, Department of Basic Medical Science, Neuroscience and Sensory Organs, Faculty of Medicine and Surgery, University of Bari, Policlinico di Bari, Bari, Italy

Francesco Liuzza and Raffaele Vitiello
Fondazione Policlinico Universitario A. Gemelli IRCCS, Rome, Italy

Aditya Prinja, Antony Raymond and Mahesh Pimple
Whipps Cross University Hospital, London, UK

Hossam Fathi Mahmoud, Ahmed Hatem Farhan and Fahmy Samir Fahmy
Orthopedic Surgery Department, Faculty of Medicine, Zagazig University, Zagazig, Egypt

Ahmed Elabd
Department of Orthopaedic Surgery, Medstar Washington Hospital Center, Washington, DC, USA

Ramy Khalifa, Zainab Alam and Ahmed M Thabet
Department of Orthopaedic Surgery and Rehabilitation, TTUHSC-El Paso, Paul L. Foster SOM, Elpaso, TX, USA

Ehab S. Saleh
Department of Orthopaedic Surgery, Oakland University William Beaumont School of Medicine, Rochester, MI, USA

Amr Abdelgawad
Department of Orthopaedic Surgery, Maimonides Medical Center, Brooklyn, NY11204, USA

Takamitsu Mondori and Yoshiyuki Nakagawa
Department of Orthopaedics, Uda City Hospital, Nara Shoulder & Elbow Center, 815 Hagiwara, Haibara, Uda, Nara 633-0298, Japan

Shimpei Kurata, Kazuya Inoue and Yasuhito Tanaka
Department of Orthopaedics, Nara Medical University, 840 Shijyo, Kashihara, Nara 634-8521, Japan

Shuhei Fujii
Department of Orthopaedics, Nara Prefecture Seiwa Medical Center, 1-14-16 Mimuro, Sangou-cho, Ikoma-gun, Nara 636-0802, Japan

Takuya Egawa
Department of Orthopaedics, Okanami General Hospital, 1734 Ueno Kuwamachi, Iga, Mie 518-0842, Japan

Vineet Kumar, Sachin Avasthi and Swagat Mahapatra
Department of Orthopaedics, Dr RMLIMS, Lucknow, India

Shah Waliullah
Department of Orthopaedics, KGMU, Lucknow, India

Ajai Singh and Sabir Ali
Department of Paediatric Orthopaedics, KGMU, Lucknow, India

Mohamed Mosa Mohamed Mahmoud, Bahaaeldin Ibrahim, Amr Abdelhalem Amr and Maysara Abdelhalem Bayoumy
Orthopaedic and Traumatology Department, Faculty of Medicine in Assiut, Al-Azhar University, Assiut 71524, Egypt

Ferdinand Wagner
Institute of Health and Biomedical Innovation, Queensland University of Technology, 60 Musk Ave, QLD 4059, Brisbane, Australia

Department of Orthopaedic Surgery, Ludwig-Maximilians-University, Marchioninistrasse 15, 81337 Munich, Germany
Dr. von Hauner Children's Hospital, Ludwig-Maximilians University of Munich, Lindwurmstrasse 4, 80337 Munich, Germany

Jochen Hubertus
Dr. von Hauner Children's Hospital, Ludwig-Maximilians University of Munich, Lindwurmstrasse 4, 80337 Munich, Germany

Günther Maderbacher, Jan Matussek, Sven Anders, Sebastian Winkler, Joachim Grifka and Armin Keshmiri
Department of Orthopaedic Surgery for the University of Regensburg at the Asklepios Clinic Bad Abbach, Kaiser-Karl-V. Allee 3, 93077 Bad Abbach, Germany

Boris M. Holzapfel
Institute of Health and Biomedical Innovation, Queensland University of Technology, 60 Musk Ave, QLD 4059, Brisbane, Australia
Orthopedic Center for Musculoskeletal Research, University of Wuerzburg, Koenig-Ludwig-Haus, Brettreichstr. 11, 97074 Wuerzburg, Germany

Birgit Kammer
Pediatric Radiology, Department of Radiology, Dr. von Hauner Children's Hospital, Ludwig-Maximilians University, Lindwurmstrasse 4, 80337 Munich, Germany

Abdul R. Arain, Curtis T. Adams, Stefanos F. Haddad, Muhammad Moral, Joseph Young, Khusboo Desai and Andrew J. Rosenbaum
Albany Medical Center, Albany, NY, USA

Gerard El-Hajj and Raja Ashou
Department of Radiology, Saint George Hospital University Medical Center, University of Balamand, Achrafieh, Beirut 1100 2807, Lebanon

Hicham Abdel-Nour, Rami Ayoubi, Joseph Maalouly, Fouad Jabbour and Alexandre Nehme
Department of Orthopedic Surgery and Traumatology, Saint George Hospital University Medical Center, University of Balamand, Achrafieh, Beirut 1100 2807, Lebanon

Index

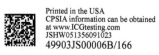

Printed in the USA
CPSIA information can be obtained
at www.ICGtesting.com
JSHW051356091023
49903JS00006B/166